*Methods in Community-Based Participatory
Research for Health*

Methods in Community-Based Participatory Research for Health

Barbara A. Israel, Eugenia Eng,
Amy J. Schulz, and Edith A. Parker

Editors

Foreword by David Satcher

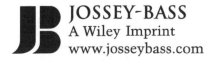

JOSSEY-BASS
A Wiley Imprint
www.josseybass.com

Published by Jossey-Bass
A Wiley Imprint
989 Market Street, San Francisco, CA 94103-1741   www.josseybass.com

Jossey-Bass books and products are available through most bookstores. To contact Jossey-Bass directly call our Customer Care Department within the U.S. at 800-956-7739, outside the U.S. at 317-572-3986, or fax 317-572-4002.

Jossey-Bass also publishes its books in a variety of electronic formats. Some content that appears in print may not be available in electronic books.

Portions of Chapter Eight have appeared in Zenk, S. N., Schulz, A. J., Israel, B. A., House, J. S., Benjamin, A., & Kannan, S. (2005). Use of community-based participatory research to assess environmental determinants of health: Challenges, facilitators, and implications for universities. *Metropolitan Universities Journal, 16*(1), 107–125. Included with the permission of the publisher. Reprinted with permission from Indiana University Purdue University Indianapolis (IUPUI), University College.

Library of Congress Cataloging-in-Publication Data
Methods in community-based participatory research for health/Barbara A. Israel . . . [et al.]; foreword by David Satcher.—1st ed.
p.; cm.
Includes bibliographical references and index.
ISBN-13 978-0-7879-7562-3
ISBN-10 0-7879-7562-1 (alk. paper)
1. Public health—Research—Citizen participation—Case studies. 2. Public health—Research—Methodology—Case studies. 3. Community health services—Case studies.
[DNLM: 1. Public Health—methods—Case Reports. 2. Research—methods—Case Reports. 3. Consumer Participation—methods—Case Reports. 4. Cultural Diversity—Case Reports. WA 20.5 M592 2005]. I. Israel, Barbara A.
RA440.85.M475 2005
362.1'072—dc22
2005012788

Printed in the United States of America
FIRST EDITION

HB Printing   10 9 8 7 6 5 4 3 2 1

CONTENTS

FIGURES AND TABLES

FIGURES

TABLES

FOREWORD

David Satcher, M.D., Ph.D.

As director of the Centers for Disease Control and Prevention (CDC) in the mid-1990s, I had the opportunity to initiate the Urban Research Centers Program. At that time, we were able to fund three inaugural programs representing partnerships between communities and academic institutions. The original programs were in Detroit, Michigan, Seattle, Washington, and New York, New York. Although we were not able to expand the programs as we had hoped, we learned and continue to learn valuable lessons from them. Many of these lessons were included in the first comprehensive federal programs geared toward the reduction and ultimate elimination of disparities in health: The CDC's Racial and Ethnic Approaches to Community Health (REACH). Currently, more than forty communities have been funded through REACH. These communities are funded and empowered to contract with academic health centers to conduct community-based participatory research.

Community-based participatory research brings the best and latest technology for design and measurement to the major issues impacting community health. In communicating the goals, objectives, and strategies of *Healthy People 2010,* we settled on a design that showed the interaction among determinants of health. The major components included the individual and his or her behavior (downstream), the physical and social environment including healthcare (midstream), and the various policies that impact this interaction (upstream). We tried to show that the components do not exist in isolation; that there is intense interaction among them. It is increasingly clear that in order to reach the goals of improving quality as well as increasing years of healthy life and eliminating disparities in health among different racial, ethnic, and socioeconomic groups, we must target all of the determinants of health where disparities have their roots. We must close the gaps that exist in access to quality health care, practice of healthy lifestyles, quality of physical and social environments, and policies that impact these areas. For research aimed at understanding and closing these gaps, community-based participatory research is a viable approach.

As more and more programs in community-based participatory research are funded and initiated, it is important that the lessons learned and problems solved in this area over the last thirty or more years are captured and shared. This book, *Methods in Community-Based Participatory Research for Health,* is a major contribution to this field. The editors are some of our most outstanding leaders in community-based participatory research. The writing of this book represents an unusual partnership among diverse participants whose involvements with communities make them experts in their own right. They bring a broad range of perspectives to this research approach, grounded in extensive community involvement and experience. What brings them together in this book is their respect for the dignity of community and the tremendous challenges and opportunities found in communities for enhancing health. Because they have found each other, and have come together around this common theme from their diverse backgrounds of race, ethnicity, and perspective, we are the beneficiaries of this outstanding text.

Critical to each case example of community-based participatory research discussed in this book is the development of meaningful partnerships. These partnerships must exist in order that when the question is asked, "Who is the community?," the answer can reliably be, "We are the community," who have engaged in meaningful partnerships, made the investments, developed the relationships, suffered the pains, and reaped the benefits of the community. These partnerships are entrenched in the community, they are as diverse as the community, and they are devoted to meaningful change and progress in the community. They share knowledge, resources, and control at every level of the community. They are trusted, not because of what they say, but because of who and where they are, and with whom they share information, methodology, and control of the research agenda. They are interested in bringing the best technology and methodology to bear on problems and opportunities within the community. Community-based participatory research deals with all the determinants of health and the dynamic nature of the interactions within the community. This research approach holds the promise of getting to the root cause of disability and of strategies for enhancing health as well as the involvement of persons at every level of community. In her book *Night Falls Fast,* which deals with teenage suicide,

Kay Redfield Jamison says, "The gap between what we know and what we do is lethal." Community-based participatory research holds the promise of removing these tremendous gaps and adding significantly to what we know.

To move our field forward in accomplishing these aims, this volume provides an excellent compendium of chapters on the methods and processes of community-based participatory research.

ACKNOWLEDGMENTS

This book would not have been possible without the insightful contributions from the numerous authors who so graciously shared their time and experiences in writing these chapters. It was important to us that each chapter reflected the principles of community-based participatory research (CBPR), involving community partners as well as academics and health practitioners as coauthors. We extend to each writing team, therefore, our deepest appreciation for the privilege of witnessing, and temporarily joining, their collaboration throughout the writing process.

And to those with whom we have collaborated through our CBPR partnerships over the years we are tremendously indebted. We consider ourselves most fortunate to have worked with, learned from, and been inspired by many partners. To our community and health practitioner partners and staff we are especially grateful for their wisdom and tireless efforts to effect meaningful change in their communities, and in us. We have also been most fortunate to count among our academic partners faculty colleagues, students, and postdoctoral fellows whose hard work and enthusiastic engagement continue to renew our energy and our perspectives on the value of CBPR. Specifically, although too numerous to mention by name, we would like to acknowledge and thank the many community and academic partners who have been involved with us through the following CBPR partnerships: Bi-Cultural Bi-Lingual Medicaid Managed Care Project, Broome Team in Flint, Carolina-Shaw Partnership to Eliminate Health Disparities, Chatham Communities in Action, Chatham Social Health Council,

Community Action Against Asthma, Detroit Community-Academic Urban Research Center, Detroit-Genesee County Community-Based Public Health Consortium, East Side Village Health Worker Partnership, Healthy Environments Partnership, Men As Navigators for Health, North Carolina Community-Based Public Health Initiative, Partners for Improved Nutrition and Health, Promoting Healthy Eating in Detroit, REACH Detroit, Save Our Sisters, Strengthening the Black Family, Inc., Stress and Wellness Project, Partnership Project of Greensboro, and United Voices of Efland-Cheeks, Inc.

We are also indebted to friends and colleagues who were not involved with these partnerships but who have had an impact on our thinking and commitment to CBPR. Current and former colleagues and mentors at the University of Michigan include Cleo Caldwell, Barry Checkoway, Mark Chesler, Noreen Clark, Jim Crowfoot, Libby Douvan, Larry Fine, Cathy Heaney, Maggie Hugentobler, Hy Kornbluh, Joyce Kornbluh, and Sue Schurman. Similarly, at the University of North Carolina at Chapel Hill, we are indebted to Marci Campbell, Tim Carey, Leonard Dawson, John Hatch, Michel Ibrahim, Ethel Jean Jackson, Laura Linnan, Betsy Randall-David, Allan Steckler, Guy Steuart, Jim Thomas, Rosalind Thomas, and Steve Wing.

We also thank the many other academic and practitioner colleagues who have influenced and supported our CBPR endeavors, including Clive Aspin, Heather Danton, Nancy Epstein, Jean Forster, Mark Freedman, Jack Geiger, Myles Horton, Ron Labonte, Mubiana Macwangi, Kathleen Parker, Baba Phillip-Ouattara, Ted Parrish, Jesus Ramirez-Valles, Sarena Seifer, Jackie Smith, Meera Viswanathan, and Tony Whitehead. Barbara owes a special debt to her colleagues in New Zealand at the Department of Public Health and the Eru Pōmare Center, Wellington School of Medicine, University of Otago, for hosting and supporting her during the sabbatical year in which much of the work on this book occurred. They include Peter Crampton, Philippa Howden-Chapman, Anna Matheson, Clare Salmond, and Alistair Woodward.

We have been most fortunate in and appreciative of the funding we have received from a number of federal and foundation sources, which has enabled us to engage in CBPR endeavors. We are especially indebted to the following institutions and individuals for the leadership they have provided in supporting CBPR for us and countless others: the W. K. Kellogg Foundation and Tom Bruce, Barbara Sabol, Steven Uranga-McKane, and Terri Wright; the National Institute of Environmental Health Sciences and Gwen Coleman, Allen Dearry, Liam O'Fallon, Ken Olden, Shobha Srinivasan, and Fred Tyson; the Centers for Disease Control and Prevention and Lynda Anderson, Larry Green, Donna Higgins, and David Satcher; the National Cancer Institute and Jon Kerner; and the Agency for Healthcare Research and Quality and Kaytura Felix-Allen.

An edited book such as this requires considerable organizational skill and attention to detail. We owe tremendous thanks to Sue Andersen, whose continuous assistance and ability to anticipate what needed to be done were invaluable to the completion of this volume.

We have been most fortunate to have worked with Andy Pasternak, a senior editor at Jossey-Bass. His knowledge of the publishing process, flexibility, and sense of humor were instrumental in guiding our efforts. We thank Seth Schwartz, assistant editor at Jossey-Bass, and production editor Rachel Anderson and copyeditor Elspeth MacHattie, for their assistance. We also appreciate the thoughtful comments of the anonymous reviewers of our book proposal.

We recognize the importance of social justice as both a core value and guiding principle for this book and hence are grateful to have had parents and grandparents who instilled this commitment in us and encouraged our work. We would like to specifically acknowledge our parents, Archie and Adelaide Israel, Wah and Alice Eng, Robert and Gail Stegmier, and Jim and Hallie Parker.

To our partners and children, Richard Pipan, Ilana Israel, Daniel Goetz, Mira Eng-Goetz, Gabriel Eng-Goetz, David Schulz, and David Cohen, whose support and love are always given so unconditionally, we owe particular thanks, for we could not have completed this book without you.

To Guy W. Steuart
Whose life's work on the wisdom of communities and the power
of partnerships is our touchstone. Thank you, Guy.

To Archie Israel and Adelaide Love Israel
Your passion for creating a sense of community lives
on through the spirit and work of all the persons
and organizations you touched.
You are missed.

THE EDITORS

Barbara A. Israel is professor of health behavior and health education at the School of Public Health, University of Michigan, where she joined the faculty in 1982. She received her MPH and DrPH degrees from the University of North Carolina at Chapel Hill. She was deputy editor of *Health Education & Behavior* from 1989 to 2003 and is the author or coauthor of more than eighty journal articles and book chapters in the areas of community-based participatory research (CBPR), social support and stress, social determinants of health, evaluation, and community health education. She has over twenty-five years of experience in conducting CBPR in collaboration with partners in diverse ethnic communities and is presently involved in several CBPR projects addressing topics such as environmental triggers of childhood asthma, diabetes management and prevention, social determinants of health, and social and physical environmental factors and cardiovascular disease. She is the principal investigator for two centers engaged in CBPR efforts: the Detroit Community-Academic Urban Research Center, funded initially through the Centers for Disease Control and Prevention, and the Michigan Center for the Environment and Children's Health, funded through the National Institute of Environmental Health Sciences and the U.S. Environmental Protection Agency.

Eugenia Eng is professor of health behavior and health education at the School of Public Health, University of North Carolina at Chapel Hill, where she joined the faculty in 1984 and where she is director of the MPH degree program and the Community Health Scholars postdoctoral program. She received her MPH and DrPH degrees from the University of North Carolina at Chapel Hill. She has authored or coauthored over seventy-five journal articles, book chapters, and monographs on the lay health adviser intervention model, the concepts of community competence and natural helping, and Action-Oriented Community Diagnosis, a community assessment procedure. She has over twenty-five years of CBPR experience, including field studies conducted with rural communities in the U.S. South, West Africa, and Southeast Asia to address socially stigmatizing health problems such as pesticide poisoning, breast cancer, and STDs. Her research has been funded by the National Institutes of Health, Centers for Disease Control and Prevention (CDC), U.S. Agency for International Development, and private foundations. She was the co-scientific director for an evidence-based review of CBPR quality, funded by the Agency for Healthcare Research and Quality, and is the principal investigator for the CDC-funded Men As Navigators for Health project.

Amy J. Schulz is research associate professor of health behavior and health education at the School of Public Health, University of Michigan, where she joined the faculty in 1997, research associate professor at the Institute for Research on Women and Gender, and associate director for the Center for Research on Ethnicity, Culture and Health. She received her PhD degree in sociology and MPH degree in health behavior and health education from the University of Michigan. Her research focuses on social determinants of health in urban communities, with a particular focus on the social and physical environments as they mediate relationships between race, socioeconomic position, and health outcomes. She has over fifteen years' experience in this field and has authored or coauthored more than fifty journal articles and book chapters on the development, implementation, and evaluation of community-based partnerships, social determinants of health, and related issues. She serves as principal investigator for the National Institute of Environmental Health Sciences–funded Healthy Environments Partnership. She also serves as a board member for the Detroit Community-Academic Urban Research Center and is actively involved with the East Side Village Health Worker Partnership and with Promoting Healthy Eating in Detroit, two other community-based participatory research efforts in Detroit.

Edith A. Parker is associate professor of health behavior and health education at the University of Michigan School of Public Health, where she joined the faculty in 1995. She received her MPH and DrPH degrees from the University of North Carolina at Chapel Hill. She has authored or coauthored more than forty journal articles and book chapters about lay health advisers, community-based participatory research, community capacity, and related areas. She has over fifteen years' research experience in the development, implementation, and evaluation of community-based participatory interventions to improve health status. Currently, she serves as the principal investigator of the CBPR household intervention component of the National Institute of Environmental Health Sciences (NIEHS) and Environmental Protection Agency (EPA)–funded Michigan Center for the Environment and Children's Health (MCECH) and the NIEHS-funded Community Organizing Network for Environmental Health project, which involves a neighborhood- and policy-level CBPR intervention affiliated with MCECH.

THE CONTRIBUTORS

Alex J. Allen III is vice president of community planning and research at Isles, Inc., a community development and environmental organization that works to improve social, economic, and environmental health in distressed areas in New Jersey. He has seventeen years of experience in community development and is an experienced facilitator of diverse groups that collaborate to address a broad range of community issues, including the Detroit Community-Academic Urban Research Center. He has expertise in community-based participatory research and participatory neighborhood planning. He holds an MSA degree from Central Michigan University.

Carol A. Allen is outreach coordinator for both the Seattle Healthy Homes-II Asthma Project and Better Homes for Asthma project. Formerly, she was the director of a community-based agency serving the senior population through health-related programs and social activities. During her eleven years in this role, she managed six community-based research projects, including the Senior Immunization Study, which increased influenza immunizations among its 500 senior participants. She has worked as an asthma community health worker and was the project coordinator of the Seattle–King County Healthy Homes Project.

Leo L. Allison is past president of United Voices of Efland-Cheeks, Inc., and currently serves on its board. He has a BS degree in mathematics from North Carolina Central University and an MS degree in engineering administration from Syracuse University. Upon retiring from his position as an advisory engineer with IBM in Manassas, Virginia, he returned to Efland, North Carolina, to work with a broad range of community organizations. His experience in community development currently includes serving on the board of Friends of the Senior Center for Central Orange, chairing the board of Legal Aid for North Carolina, and serving as president of the board of Orange Congregations in Mission. He also serves on the community advisory group for the Centers for Disease Control and Prevention–funded Men As Navigators for Health Project.

Guadalupe X. Ayala is assistant professor in the Department of Health Behavior and Health Education in the School of Public Health, University of North Carolina at Chapel Hill. She completed her PhD degree in clinical health psychology at San Diego State University-University of California San Diego and an MPH in Health Promotion from San Diego State University. Her primary area of research is U.S. Latino health promotion, with a specific focus on developing family and community-based interventions to prevent obesity and improve management of chronic illnesses, and she teaches a course in U.S. Latino health promotion for graduate students.

Kelly E. Baber was the community liaison for the Eastside Access Partnership, an innovative CBPR partnership that identified uninsured children and helped their families apply for health insurance in Detroit, Michigan. She is a former executive director of the Kettering/Butzel Health Initiative, a community-based organization whose mission was to improve health status by addressing unmet health needs (especially maternal and child health) of residents of lower eastside Detroit. She is a native Detroiter, with an MSA degree in public administration from Central Michigan University and a BS degree in criminal justice from Ferris State University. Her interests include planning and implementing community health projects in Detroit and assisting city residents in seeking quality health care services for their families.

Elizabeth A. Baker is associate professor at the Saint Louis University School of Public Health. Her main areas of interest are social networks and social support, control, and other social determinants of health (such as race and income) and the ways in which they influence community and individual capacity to create desired changes. She has extensive experience in community-based participatory research in both urban and rural communities and teaches courses in behavioral science and health education. She received her MPH and PhD degrees from the University of Michigan School of Public Health.

Adam B. Becker is assistant professor in the Department of Community Health Sciences at the Tulane University School of Public Health and Tropical Medicine. He teaches courses in CBPR, group dynamics, community organizing, and monitoring and evaluation. His current CBPR projects include investigating and addressing the social determinants of violence with high school students and community residents and examining and addressing social determinants of obesity in an economically marginalized neighborhood in New Orleans. He facilitates the community advisory board of Tulane's Prevention Research Center and consults with community-based coalitions on effective collaboration and group process. He received his MPH and PhD degrees from the Department of Health Behavior and Health Education at the University of Michigan School of Public Health.

Alison Benjamin is program manager for contaminated sites for Southwest Detroit Environmental Vision. She has worked in southwest Detroit on issues related to land use and community development. She has been a member of the Healthy Environments Partnership (HEP) Steering Committee since 2001 and has represented HEP at the annual grantee meeting, contributed to the design of the HEP survey and neighborhood observational checklist, and assisted with the development of the data feedback forms. She holds a BA degree in urban planning from Washington University.

Wilma Brakefield-Caldwell received her BS degree in nursing from Wayne State University and worked for twenty-eight years with the Detroit Health Department (DHD). During her time with the DHD, she worked as a public health nurse and supervisor, a project coordinator, a public health nursing administrator, and most recently, a health care administrator. In that capacity, she served as the DHD representative to the Detroit Community-Academic Urban Research Center. She retired in 1998 but continues to serve as a community representative on the Community Action Against Asthma Steering Committee. She frequently presents at local and national conferences and has coauthored several articles on this CBPR project.

Linda Burhansstipanov (Cherokee Nation of Oklahoma) is executive director of Native American Cancer Research, a nonprofit community-based corporation. She has taught full-time at universities (California State University-Long Beach and University of California-Los Angeles) for eighteen years and has implemented public health projects from 1971 to the present. Her areas of expertise include Native American cancer issues (prevention, early detection, survivorship, quality of life, and palliative care), medically underserved communities and cancer, cultural aspects of Native American health, women's health issues, HIV/AIDS prevention and control in Indian country, genetic education, and disparity issues. She earned a master's degree and a doctorate from the University of California, Los Angeles, School of Public Health.

Alejandro M. Bustillo Martinez, one of eleven siblings, was born in the town of Tolima in the Andean region of Colombia, home to the most aromatic coffee produced in Colombia. He received a degree in agronomic engineering from the

Universidad Nacional de Colombia and traveled extensively through Latin America and Southeast Asia, working as a project leader on various agricultural production products. He currently works as a community outreach worker at El Centro Hispano in Durham, North Carolina, and has been active in the Latino community in Durham for four years. He has been a member of Horizonte Latino since 2002, a community-based participatory research group that uses ethnography.

Suzanne Christopher is associate professor in the Department of Health and Human Development at Montana State University. She received her PhD degree from the University of North Carolina at Chapel Hill School of Public Health. Her interests are women's health, social indicators of health, and community-based participatory research. She has been fortunate to work on community-based projects with members of the Apsáalooke Nation since 1996.

Altha J. Cravey is associate professor in the Department of Geography at the University of North Carolina at Chapel Hill, where she teaches courses on Latin American geography, social geography, feminist geography, and migration geographies. She earned her PhD degree from the University of Iowa, where her dissertation, later published as *Women and Work in Mexico's Maquiladoras* (1998), was supported by the four-year Iowa Fellowship. She is interested in understanding the connections between daily life, globalization, and transnationality.

Bonnie Duran is associate professor in the Masters in Public Health Program at the University of New Mexico School of Medicine. Her research areas include mental health epidemiology and interventions, health services, and health promotion and disease prevention for Native American and other communities of color. With National Institute of Mental Health and Health Resources and Services Administration funding, she currently is conducting health services research for tribes in the Southwest and plains to determine the most effective and efficient way to structure services for people with mental disorders and HIV/AIDS. She is codirector of the Center for Native American Health and the Southwest Alcohol Research Group. She holds a DrPH degree from the University of California, Berkeley.

Katherine K. Edgren is project manager of Community Action Against Asthma and works at the University of Michigan School of Public Health. Her interests include community-based participatory research, citizen participation in the political process, and psychosocial rehabilitation. She has held leadership positions in a variety of settings for over twenty-five years, including serving as executive director of two nonprofit organizations working with adults with serious mental illnesses and serving six years as a City Council member in Ann Arbor,

Michigan. She holds an MSW degree from the University of Michigan and is a certified social worker (CSW).

Kevin Foley is a clinical psychologist and director of clinical services at Na'Nizhoozhi Center, Inc. (NCI), a large substance abuse detoxification center in Gallup, New Mexico. He is the principal investigator for a Health Resources and Services Administration American Indian/Alaska Native Special Projects of National Significance HIV Integration of Services grant in the Four Corners area. He writes about cultural competency and clinical issues related to American Indians. He received his PhD degree from Sierra University.

Nicholas Freudenberg is Distinguished Professor of Urban Public Health at Hunter College, City University of New York, and has worked with community organizations and health agencies in New York City for more than thirty years. He currently directs a program in New York City for male adolescents returning from incarceration. He is an investigator for the Harlem Urban Research Center, a member of its Community Action Board and its Policy Work Group and has served as an adviser to the New York City Departments of Health and Correction on the health needs of people returning from incarceration. He received his DrPH degree from Columbia University.

Derek M. Griffith is assistant research scientist of health behavior and health education at the School of Public Health and associate director of evaluation for the Prevention Research Center of the University of Michigan. He holds MA and PhD degrees in clinical-community psychology from DePaul University. He completed a two-year fellowship as a W. K. Kellogg Foundation–funded community health scholar at the University of North Carolina at Chapel Hill School of Public Health, gaining invaluable experience collaborating with three CBPR partnerships on initiatives to examine organizational and community-level dimensions of racism and African American men's health. He is currently conducting CBPR on organizational capacity, African American men's health, social determinants of health, and institutional racism.

J. Ricardo Guzman is the chief executive officer of Community Health and Social Services Center, Inc. (CHASS), a Section 330 federally qualified health center (FQHC) with three locations in the city of Detroit. He is a long-standing community leader and activist in southwest Detroit. He has played a leadership role in increasing access to culturally appropriate, high-quality, affordable, comprehensive health services to community members who historically have not had access to such services. He is also an influential member of the National Association of Community Health Centers, and in 1994 received the National Hispanic Health Leadership Award. He holds an MSW degree from Wayne State University and an MPH degree from the University of Michigan.

James S. House is research professor and former director of the Survey Research Center in the Institute for Social Research and professor and former chair of the Department of Sociology at the University of Michigan. Throughout his career his research has focused on the role of social and psychological factors in the etiology and course of health and illness, initially on occupational stress and health, later on social relationships and support in relation to health, and currently on the role of psychosocial factors in understanding and explaining social inequalities in health and the way health changes with age. He is an elected member of the American Academy of Arts and Sciences and the Institute of Medicine of the National Academies of Science. He received his PhD degree from the University of Michigan.

Srimathi Kannan is assistant professor of environmental health sciences, University of Michigan School of Public Health. She serves as co-principal investigator for the National Institute of Environmental Health Sciences–funded Healthy Environments Partnership CBPR project. Her research interests are biological risk and protective micronutrient markers of acute and chronic exposure in humans to ambient airborne particle matter, and micronutrients and cultural food choices of relevance to infant nutrition and health. She received her PhD degree from the University of Tennessee.

Diana L. Kerr is deputy director of the Center for Health Promotion and Disease Prevention, Henry Ford Health System, Detroit, Michigan. She has thirty-five years of experience in health care, including positions in clinical practice, education, and management. She has held provider and management positions in urban primary care, older adult services, and community health in the Trinity Health System, Greater Detroit Area Health Council, Inc., and Henry Ford Health System. She has further served as clinical faculty in the School of Nursing, Continuing Education Services, University of Michigan. She is a member of the board of the Detroit Community-Academic Urban Research Center. She holds a BSN degree from Wayne State University and an MS degree from the University of Michigan.

Edith C. Kieffer is a research associate professor in the School of Social Work, University of Michigan. She received her PhD degree in medical geography and her MPH degree in maternal and child health and health services administration and planning from the University of Hawaii. Her research interests include understanding and addressing ethnic and geographical disparities in health, especially in the areas of diabetes, obesity, and pregnancy outcomes. In collaboration with Detroit community members and organizations, she is developing and implementing multilevel interventions designed to promote healthy eating and regular exercise among Latino and African American residents of southwest and eastside Detroit, including pregnant and postpartum women.

Mary A. Koch served as director of the Brightmoor Community Center in northwest Detroit for twenty-five years. She has served as the Brightmoor Community Center representative to the Healthy Environments Partnership (HEP) Steering Committee, a CBPR project in Detroit, since 2000. She has represented HEP at the annual grantee meeting, served as a member of the staff selection interview team, and contributed to the design of the survey questionnaire, interviewer training curriculum, and speaker training efforts. As a long-time resident of northwest Detroit, with a history of social service, advocacy, and political activism, she contributes an essential understanding of both historical and contemporary community dynamics and resources to the work of HEP. She holds a BA degree from Wayne State University.

James Krieger is chief of the Epidemiology, Planning and Evaluation Unit at Public Health—Seattle & King County and clinical associate professor of medicine and health services at the University of Washington. He serves as principal investigator of the Healthy Homes Project, which seeks to control asthma through community health worker home visits, and Healthy Homes/Healthy Community at High Point, which engages public housing residents in environmental justice and community-building actions. He directed Seattle Partners for Healthy Communities, a collaboration between the community, Public Health—Seattle & King County, and the University of Washington to conduct community-based participatory research, for eight years. He received his undergraduate degree at Harvard, his MD degree at the University of California-San Francisco, and his MPH degree at the University of Washington.

Paula M. Lantz is associate professor in the Department of Health Management and Policy of the University of Michigan School of Public Health, where she teaches courses on program evaluation methods and public health policy. Her PhD degree, from the University of Wisconsin, is in social demography, and she also has an MS degree in epidemiology from the University of Wisconsin and an MA degree in sociology from Washington University. She has over twenty years of experience in conducting program and policy evaluations in health and human services. She also conducts research into socioeconomic inequalities in health and cancer prevention and control.

Ellen D. S. López is assistant professor at the University of Florida College of Public Health and Health Professions. She completed her MPH degree at the University of Washington at Seattle School of Public Health and Community Medicine and her PhD degree at the University of North Carolina at Chapel Hill School of Public Health, where her dissertation research involved a CBPR approach and blended the methods of photovoice and grounded theory as a means to explore quality of life with African American breast cancer survivors from rural eastern North Carolina. Prior to joining the University of Florida faculty, she completed a two-year fellowship as a W. K. Kellogg Foundation–funded community health scholar at the University of Michigan School of Public Health where she further enhanced her expertise, working on several initiatives that applied a CBPR approach.

Siobhan C. Maty is assistant professor of Community Health at Portland State University, where she teaches graduate and undergraduate courses in epidemiology, women's health, and gender, race, class, and health. She completed her MPH degree at John Hopkins University and her PhD degree in epidemiology, with an emphasis in social epidemiology, at the University of Michigan School of Public Health. Her research interests include the social determinants of health and disease, health disparities, the epidemiology of diabetes and obesity, and the translation of research into action to achieve social change.

Alma Knows His Gun-McCormick (Crow) is project coordinator for Messengers for Health, a CBPR project on the Apsáalooke Reservation in Montana that uses a lay health adviser approach to increase women's participation in cervical cancer screening. She has been involved in community-based health programs with children, youths, parents, women, and elders. She is interested in helping to enhance the health of the Crow Indian people.

Robert J. McGranaghan is project manager for the Detroit Community-Academic Urban Research Center (URC), based at the University of Michigan School of Public Health, and has been involved with the Detroit URC since its inception in 1995. His current interests include working to disseminate lessons learned and recommendations for conducting community-based participatory research (CBPR), helping new and emerging community-institutional partnerships to understand and use the CBPR model, and advocating for community-based interests in public health. He received his MPH degree from Temple University.

Chris McQuiston is associate professor at the University of North Carolina at Chapel Hill School of Nursing. She is a member of El Centro Hispano, a Latino community-based organization located in Durham, North Carolina, and has had an active presence in that Latino community for the past eight years. She worked collaboratively with the community to develop and deliver culture-specific HIV interventions, to identify measurement concerns with recently arrived Mexicans, and to identify a Latino model for sexual prevention of HIV. Presently, she is the co-principal investigator of a binational study (Migration, Gender and HIV Among Mexicans) funded by the National Institute of Nursing Research (NINR), and director of the NINR-funded Center for Innovations in

Health Disparities Research. She received her BSN degree from the University of Cincinnati and her PhD degree from Wayne State University.

Elvira M. Mebane is president and a founding member of United Voices of Efland-Cheeks, Inc. With the Orange County Health Department, Central Administrative Services, she is the deputy vital records clerk, and she serves on the United Village of Orange Committee to guide the health department's dismantling racism process. She plays leadership roles in the local chapter of the NAACP and McCoy Temple. She serves on the community advisory group for the Centers for Disease Control and Prevention–funded Men As Navigators for Health Project.

Meredith Minkler is professor of health and social behavior and director of the DrPH Leadership Program at the School of Public Health, University of California, Berkeley. She has close to thirty years experience in community organizing and community-based participatory research with diverse underserved populations and has published several books, including the coedited volume, *Community-Based Participatory Research for Health* (with Nina Wallerstein, 2003) and *Community Organizing and Community Building for Health* (with Nina Wallerstein, 2004). She earned her DrPH degree from the University of California, Berkeley.

Karen Strazza Moore is project director with the North Carolina Center for Children's Healthcare Improvement. In the recent past she served as clinical instructor for the Department of Health Behavior and Health Education and as field training coordinator with the Department of Maternal and Child Health at the University of North Carolina at Chapel Hill. She has also served as lead health educator with the North Carolina Breast and Cervical Cancer Control Program and project director for the North Carolina Community-Based Public Health Initiative. She has been involved in refugee assistance and community development in Southeast Asia with UNICEF, CARE, and Save the Children. Throughout her career, she has worked collaboratively with diverse communities to address health issues in a manner that emphasizes community participation and control. She holds a BA degree from Lewis and Clark University and an MPH degree from the University of North Carolina at Chapel Hill.

Rachel Morello-Frosch is assistant professor in the Center for Environmental Studies and the Department of Community Health, School of Medicine, at Brown University. Her research examines race and class determinants of the distribution of health risks associated with air pollution among diverse U.S. communities. Her current research and publications focus on comparative risk assessment and environmental justice, developing models for community-based environmental health research, science and environmental health policymaking, children's environmental health, and the intersection between economic restructuring and environmental health. Her collaborative projects include work with Communities for a Better Environment in California and the Silent Spring Institute in Massachusetts. She earned her PhD degree in environmental health sciences from the University of California, Berkeley, School of Public Health.

Freda L. Motton is field coordinator of the Bootheel Heart Health Project in southeast Missouri, which involves programs aimed at reducing risky health behaviors associated with cardiovascular disease. She also serves as regional director in the midwest region for the National Community Committee for the Prevention Research Centers funded by the Centers for Disease Control and Prevention. Her areas of interest include building community capacity to improve health and education. She earned her BS degree from Southeast Missouri State University.

Sister Mary Nerney is executive director of STEPS to End Family Violence, a multiservice organization working to improve the lives of women in East Harlem. She is active in numerous local and citywide advocacy organizations and is a long-time activist in the movement to end violence against women. She testifies frequently before legislative bodies and is a member of the Harlem Urban Research Center Community Action Board and its Policy Work Group. She has been honored for her work by numerous local, statewide, and national organizations.

Angela M. Odoms-Young is assistant professor in public and community health in the School of Allied Health Professions at Northern Illinois University. She earned a BS degree in foods and nutrition from the University of Illinois-Urbana/Champaign and MS and PhD degrees from Cornell University in human nutrition and community nutrition, respectively. She completed a W. K. Kellogg Foundation–funded Community Health Scholars postdoctoral fellowship at the University of Michigan School of Public Health in 2000, and a Family Research Consortium postdoctoral fellowship in 2003. Her research and teaching interests focus on race, poverty, nutrition, and health; community-based participatory research; obesity prevention and management; and religion and health.

Julio César Olmos-Muñiz is a computer systems engineer from Tamaulipas, Mexico. He came to the United States five years ago with his wife and two children. He worked as a volunteer for the National AIDS Prevention Program (CONASIDA) in his home country, and after his arrival in the United States, he worked as a lay health adviser for HIV prevention and as an outreach worker for the Syphilis Elimination Project. He has been a guest lecturer at workshops on community-based participatory research and teenage pregnancy prevention. He is currently outreach coordinator for Project LIFE, an HIV education and prevention program at El Centro

Hispano in Durham, North Carolina. His computer system technician degree is from Centro de Estudios Tecnologicos de Monterrey.

Emilio A. Parrado is assistant professor of sociology at Duke University. His research focuses on issues of health, migration dynamics, and adaptation among Latinos. Recently, he has concentrated on Latino migration to new areas of destination in the Southwestern United States, including the issues of occupational representation, social demands, and HIV risks. In addition, he has worked collaboratively with the Durham, North Carolina, Latino community to better understand the social and cultural forces shaping migrants' lives. He is currently co-principal investigator of a binational study funded by the National Institute of Nursing Research and titled Migration, Gender and HIV Among Mexicans. He earned his BA from the University of Buenos Aires and his PhD degree from the University of Chicago.

Manuel Pastor Jr. is professor of Latin American and Latino studies and director of the Center for Justice, Tolerance, and Community at the University of California, Santa Cruz. His most recent books are *Searching for the Uncommon Common Ground: New Dimensions on Race in America* (with Angela Glover Blackwell and Stewart Kwoh, 2002) and *Regions That Work: How Cities and Suburbs Can Grow Together* (with Peter Dreier, Eugene Grigsby, and Marta Lopez-Garza, 2000). He is currently working on issues of environmental justice with support from both The California Endowment and the California Wellness Foundation and in collaboration with Communities for a Better Environment, an environmental justice organization. He earned his PhD in economics from the University of Massachusetts, Amherst.

Carlos Porras is a former executive director of Communities for a Better Environment (from 1999 to 2004), an environmental justice organization in Southern California. He has more than thirty years of experience as a labor, community, and environmental leader and organizer through his work in the Chicano and prisoners' rights movements in Texas. He is a graduate of the Community Scholars Program in Urban Planning at the University of California-Los Angeles (UCLA) and received the Lucy and Harry Lang Fellowship from the UCLA Center for Labor Research and Education. He is a former member of the National Environmental Justice Advisory Council, the Environmental Justice Advisory Committee to the California Environmental Protection Agency, and a recipient of the Environment Now Wells Family Award for Urban Renewal from Vice President Al Gore.

Michele Prichard, director of special projects at the Liberty Hill Foundation in Los Angeles, began her involvement with philanthropy in 1982 as a community activist. As Liberty Hill's executive director from 1989 to 1997, she helped create new grant programs addressing poverty, race relations, and environmental health. Liberty Hill now awards over $3 million annually and is one of the most innovative public foundations in the country. She has served on the boards of several philanthropic organizations, including the Southern California Association for Philanthropy, the L.A. Urban Funders, and the Funding Exchange. She also serves on the board of the Human Services Alliance and on the advisory board to the Los Angeles Coalition to End Hunger and Homelessness. She received her MA degree from the University of California-Los Angeles School of Urban Planning.

Scott D. Rhodes is assistant professor in the Wake Forest University School of Medicine, Department of Public Health Sciences. He has an MPH degree from the University of South Carolina and a PhD degree from the University of Alabama at Birmingham. He completed a two-year postdoctoral fellowship with the W. K. Kellogg Foundation–funded Community Health Scholars Program at the University of North Carolina at Chapel Hill, gaining valuable skills in establishing a CBPR partnership with a Latino community. He is currently principal investigator for the Centers for Disease Control and Prevention-funded project HoMBReS: Hombres Manteniendo Bienestar y Relaciones Saludables (Men Maintaining Wellness and Healthy Relationships), designed to reduce the risk of sexually transmitted disease infection among Latino migrant and seasonal farmworkers.

Cassandra Ritas worked for three years (2000 to 2003) with the Harlem Urban Research Center Community Action Board to advance community-based recommendations for criminal justice policy. In 2002, she received a fellowship from Community-Campus Partnerships for Health to develop a guide to policy work for CBPR practitioners, entitled, "Speaking Truth, Creating Power" (now available on the Web). She earned her MPP degree from the Kennedy School at Harvard. Presently, she works for a progressive New York state senator. In this role and others she seeks to facilitate the creation of community-based public policy.

John W. Roberts is a consulting engineer and president of Engineering Plus, Inc., where he specializes in assessing and managing exposures and risks from pollutants in house dust. He is the codeveloper of the High Volume Small Surface Sampler (HVS3) for measuring pollutants in house dust in carpets and on bare floors, and he also developed the High Volume Furniture Sampler for measuring pollutants in dust on furniture, floors, and bare surfaces. He has served as a consultant to Public Health—Seattle & King County on the projects Healthy Homes-I and Healthy Homes-II and also to the Master Home Environmentalist Program (MHEP) of the American Lung Association of Washington. He has authored or coauthored twenty-seven publications on air pollution, indoor air, fugitive dust, house dust, and total exposure of children. He holds an MS degree and an MEd degree from the University of Washington and is a licensed professional engineer (PE).

Thomas G. Robins is a professor in the Department of Environmental Health Sciences at the University of Michigan School of Public Health. He is director of the University of Michigan Education and Research Center, funded by the National Institute for Occupational Health and Safety, and of the University of Michigan Southern Africa Program in Environmental and Occupational Health, funded by NIH. He is an occupational and environmental physician and epidemiologist. He has served as the principal investigator on a number of large-scale epidemiological studies of environmental exposures and health outcomes, both in United States and internationally. He is the principal investigator for the Exposure and Health Effects Research Project, which is a component of Community Action Against Asthma. He received his MD degree from Tufts University and his MPH degree from the University of Michigan.

Naomi Robinson is project coordinator of the Surviving Angels—Eastern North Carolina Witness for Life Program. In this capacity, she coordinates a three-county breast and cervical cancer program for African American women. She is also involved in a number of community-based programs, including those targeting cancer survivorship and obesity prevention. She received her BA degree in business administration from North Carolina Central University and her MAT degree from Trinity College.

Marc A. Rogers was director of the New York City Community Reintegration Project at the Hunter College Center on AIDS, Drugs, and Community Health from 2002 to 2004. During this time he was also a member of the Harlem Urban Research Center Community Action Board and the East Harlem HIV Care Network Steering Committee; he has served as coordinator for the New York City Community Reintegration Network as well. He earned his PhD degree in political science from American University in Washington, DC, specializing in public policy analysis, public opinion, survey research, and health policy. He is adjunct assistant professor in political science at Hunter College and currently works as research director with the Roper Global Diabetes Program at NOP World Health in New York City.

Lisa Carol Ross has worked in public health for over ten years. She has participated in community-based education and research projects, including dental disease prevention, tobacco prevention and control, cancer prevention, and for the last four years, asthma in children. She is currently research manager for two asthma-related, community-based research studies: Healthy Homes-II (funded by the National Institute of Environmental Health Sciences), and Better

Homes for Asthma (funded by the Department of Housing and Urban Development). She holds an MPH degree from the University of Washington.

James L. Sadd is associate professor of environmental science and chair of the Geology Department at Occidental College in Los Angeles. His research includes spatial analysis using geographical information systems and remote sensing tools, particularly to evaluate environmental justice questions. He is also conducting active research programs in the reconstruction of sedimentation and pollution histories in coastal and marine environments. His current research is supported by grants from the Andrew W. Mellon Foundation, U.S. Army Corps of Engineers, U.S. Navy Office of Naval Research, California Wellness Foundation, and The California Endowment. He earned his PhD degree from the University of South Carolina.

Yamir Salabarría-Peña is a health scientist in the Division of STD Prevention, Centers for Disease Control and Prevention. She received her BS and MPH degrees in health education from the University of Puerto Rico and her DrPH degree in health education from Loma Linda University, and she completed the W. K. Kellogg Foundation–funded Community Health Scholars Program at the University of Michigan School of Public Health in 2002. Her research addresses social and cultural factors that influence individuals' decisions regarding health-related issues such as HIV and STD prevention, diabetes control and prevention, and chronic disease risk in Latino populations, as well as health disparities among racial and ethnic minorities and racism and discrimination issues in health.

Kate Shirah is clinical instructor and field training coordinator in the Department of Health Behavior and Health Education at the University of North Carolina at Chapel Hill (UNC-CH) School of Public Health. She also serves as project manager for the Centers for Disease Control and Prevention–funded Men As Navigators for Health Project. Her BSPH degree in health policy and administration and MPH degree in health behavior and health education are from UNC-CH. Prior positions she has held include coordinator for the North Carolina Division of Public Health statewide Winner's Circle Program to increase healthy eating and project manager for the CDC-funded Families for Safe Dates Project to prevent adolescent dating violence.

Carmen A. Stokes is a member of the teaching faculty at the University of Detroit-Mercy McAuley School of Nursing. She is the course director for Fundamentals of Nursing, Pharmacology, and an introductory course on the profession of nursing, and assists in instruction in the graduate nursing program. A past resident of northwest Detroit, she has been a member of the Healthy Environments Partnership (HEP) Steering Committee, a CBPR project in Detroit, since 2001.

She has served as a member of the HEP Survey Subcommittee, has assisted in conducting focus groups with community residents, and has represented HEP at the annual meeting of the American Public Health Association. She received her MSN degree from the University of Detroit-Mercy and her BSN degree from Wayne State University, and she is a certified family nurse practitioner (FNP).

Tim K. Takaro is a member of the faculty of the University of Washington Occupational and Environmental Medicine Program and Fred Hutchinson Cancer Research Center. His primary work is directed toward determining whether linkages exist between occupational or environmental exposures and disease and finding public health–based preventive solutions where such hazards exist. His primary research interests are in exposure, surveillance, and genetic factors in immunologic lung disease, and he is conducting ongoing research in the use of biomarkers for medical surveillance and risk assessment. As part of this program he is actively studying hazardous exposures, including mold, in homes of low-income children with asthma and testing the efficacy of home environmental interventions for these exposures. He received his MS degree from the University of Washington and his MPH and MD degrees from the University of North Carolina.

Nina Wallerstein is professor and director of the Masters in Public Health Program in the School of Medicine, University of New Mexico. She has been developing participatory research methodologies and empowerment intervention research for twenty-five years, and her latest coedited volume, *Community-Based Participatory Research for Health* (with Meredith Minkler, 2003), covers these fields. She has worked in North American and Latin American contexts in participatory evaluation of healthy city initiatives, in adolescent and women's health intervention research, and in community health development. For the past five years she has conducted participatory research with tribes to develop better understanding of tribal community capacities, public health infrastructure, and measures of social capital, and she is codeveloping a minority Southwest alcohol research center. She received her DrPH degree from the University of California, Berkeley.

Caroline C. Wang is assistant professor in the Department of Health Behavior and Health Education at the University of Michigan School of Public Health. With Mary Ann Burris, she originated the photovoice methodology, an innovative participatory action research approach based on the principles that images teach, pictures can influence policy, and community people ought to help create and define the images that make healthful public policy and programs. She is coeditor of the book *Visual Voices: 100 Photographs of Village China by the Women of Yunnan Province,* and editor of *Strength to Be: Community Visions and Voices,* a project based in Flint, Michigan. Additional information can be found at http://www.photovoice.com. She received her MPH degree and her DrPH degree from the University of California, Berkeley.

Lucille H. Webb is a long-time resident of Wake County, North Carolina. She is a former teacher and current president of the board of directors of Strengthening the Black Family, Inc. in Raleigh, North Carolina, a coalition of more than forty organizations dedicated to improving the life of black families in Wake County. She has served as an exemplary community mentor for numerous postdoctoral community health scholars (CHSs) involved in the W. K. Kellogg Foundation–funded CHS program.

Donele J. Wilkins has over two decades of experience in occupational and environmental health as an educator, consultant, trainer, administrator, and advocate. In 1994, she cofounded and currently serves as the executive director of Detroiters Working for Environmental Justice, a nonprofit organization addressing urban environmental issues in the City of Detroit. She is sought after as a public speaker, addressing local and national audiences, and as a consultant on topics addressing community-driven sustainable development, environmental justice, and occupational and environmental health advocacy. She has coordinated and organized several conferences and gatherings to highlight the plight of her community. She is a mom of two—which motivates her to change conditions in her community so that they can have a brighter future.

Sharla K. Willis is adjunct assistant professor in the Division of Health Behavior and Health Promotion, School of Public Health, Ohio State University. She received an MPH degree in international population and family health, an MA degree in Latin American studies from the University of California-Los Angeles, and a DrPH degree at the University of Illinois at Chicago, and she completed the W. K. Kellogg Foundation–funded Community Health Scholars postdoctoral program at the University of Michigan School of Public Health in 2000. Her research focuses on the use of qualitative research methods in collaboration with Latino and African American women to identify community-based health needs and strategies to address those needs.

Shannon N. Zenk is postdoctoral research associate in cancer control and population sciences at the University of Illinois at Chicago. Her research interests focus on how places contribute to racial and socioeconomic disparities in health. While earning her PhD degree at the University of Michigan School of Public Health, she was actively involved in a number of community-based participatory research efforts: the Healthy Environments Partnership (HEP), the East Side Village Health Worker Partnership, and the Healthy Eating and Exercising to Reduce Diabetes program. She has worked with HEP since its inception.

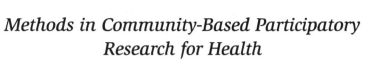

Methods in Community-Based Participatory
Research for Health

INTRODUCTION TO METHODS IN COMMUNITY-BASED PARTICIPATORY RESEARCH FOR HEALTH

Introduction to Methods in Community-Based Participatory Research for Health

Barbara A. Israel, Eugenia Eng,
Amy J. Schulz, and Edith A. Parker

Public health problems are complex, and their solutions involve political and social, as well as biomedical, dimensions. Researchers, practitioners, community members, and funders have increasingly recognized the importance of comprehensive and participatory approaches to research and intervention, and opportunities for such partnership approaches to research and intervention continue to emerge. As they do, so does the demand for concrete skills and knowledge about how to conduct community-based or other participatory approaches to research. Both new and established partnerships continue to search for information about strategies, skills, methods, and approaches that support the equitable participation and influence of diverse partners, toward the end of developing a clearer understanding of public health problems and working collectively to address them. This book is intended to be a resource for students, practitioners, researchers, and community members seeking to use community-based participatory research (CBPR) approaches to improve the health and well-being of communities in general and to eliminate health disparities in particular. In the introduction to this volume, we discuss the background to and growing support for CBPR, the principles of CBPR, the broad cultural and socioeconomic environmental context in which CBPR is conducted, and the purposes and goals of this book, and we present the organization and brief descriptions of the chapters.

BACKGROUND

There is increasing recognition that more comprehensive and participatory approaches to research and interventions are needed in order to address the complex set of determinants associated with public health problems that affect populations generally and those factors associated more specifically with racial and ethnic disparities in health (Butterfoss, Goodman, & Wandersman, 1993; Green & Mercer, 2001; Israel, Schulz, Parker, & Becker, 1998; Minkler & Wallerstein 2003; Schulz, Williams, Israel, & Lempert, 2002; Williams & Collins, 1995). Concomitantly, the number of funding opportunities that support partnership approaches to research that addresses these problems has grown. These include, for example, the Centers for Disease Control and Prevention's (CDC's) Urban Research Centers program, initiated by then CDC Director David Satcher (Higgins, Maciak, & Metzler, 2001; CDC, 1994), Racial and Ethnic Approaches to Health initiative—REACH 2010 (CDC, 1999), and community-based participatory prevention research projects from the Prevention Research Initiative (Green, 2003); the National Institute of Environmental Health Sciences' Environmental Justice Initiative and Children's Health Initiative (NIEHS, 1997; O'Fallon & Dearry, 2002); and the W. K. Kellogg Foundation's Community-Based Public Health Initiative (Bruce & Uranga-McKane, 2000), Turning Point Initiative (Sabol, 2002), and Community Health Scholars Program (2004). In addition, the emergence of the National Institutes of Health Interagency Workgroup on Community-Based Participatory Research, which aims to further advance the use of partnership approaches for examining and addressing these complex health problems, illustrates the growth of interest in and support for the CBPR approach.

Partnership approaches to research exist in many different academic disciplines and fields. In the field of public health, partnership approaches to research have been called, variously, "community-based participatory," "involved," "collaborative," and "centered-research" (see Israel et al., 1998, for a review of this literature). In addition, a large social science literature has examined research approaches in which participants are actively involved in the process. Examples include discussions of "participatory research" (deKonig & Martin, 1996; Green et al., 1995; Hall, 1992; Kemmis & McTaggart, 2000; Park, 1993; Tandon, 1996), "participatory action research" (Whyte, 1991), "action research" (Peters & Robinson, 1984; Reason & Bradbury, 2001; Stringer, 1996), "participatory feminist research" (Maguire, 1987), "action science/inquiry" (Argyris, Putnam, & Smith, 1985; Torbert, 2001), "cooperative inquiry" (Heron & Reason, 2001; Reason, 1994), "critical action research" (Kemmis & McTaggart, 2000), "empowerment evaluation" (Fetterman, Kaftarian, & Wandersman, 1996), and "participatory community research" (Jason, Keys, Suarez-Balcazar, Taylor, & Davis, 2004). Although there are differences among these approaches, they all involve a commitment to conducting research that shares power with and engages community partners in the research process and that benefits the communities involved, either through direct intervention or by translating research findings into interventions and policy change.

In public health, nursing, social work, and related fields, the term *community-based participatory research* (CBPR) is increasingly used to represent such collaborative approaches (Israel et al., 2001; Minkler & Wallerstein, 2003), while recognizing that there are other approaches with different labels that share similar values and methods. Community-based participatory research in public health is a partnership approach to research that equitably involves, for example, community members, organizational representatives, and researchers in all aspects of the research process and in which all partners contribute expertise and share decision making and ownership (Israel et al., 1998, 2003). The aim of CBPR is to increase knowledge and understanding of a given phenomenon and integrate the knowledge gained with interventions and policy and social change to improve the health and quality of life of community members (Israel et al., 1998, 2003).

Associated with the developments just described, the recent Institute of Medicine Report *Who Will Keep the Public Healthy? Educating the Public Health Professionals for the 21st Century* (Gebbie, Rosenstock, & Hernandez, 2003) identifies community-based participatory research as one of the eight areas in which all public health professionals need to be trained. As stated in the report, "the committee believes that public health professionals will be better prepared to address the major health problems and challenges facing society if they achieve competency in the following eight content areas," and the text goes on to list and discuss CBPR as one of "these eight areas of critical importance to public health education in the 21st century" (p. 62).

Further recognition of the relevance of CBPR for professionals can be found in the increasing number of participatory research courses being taught in schools and departments of public health, nursing, sociology, social work, psychology, and the like. In addition the number of CBPR workshops and conference sessions offered in local communities as well as at regional and national meetings has expanded over the past decade as participants strive to enhance their knowledge and skills related to partnership approaches to research. There are now a number of excellent books that examine the theoretical underpinnings of participatory approaches and provide case studies that illustrate implementation issues (see, for example, deKoning & Martin, 1996; Jason et al., 2004; Minkler & Wallerstein, 2003; Reason & Bradbury, 2001; Stringer, 1996). Several journals, such as the *Journal of General Internal Medicine* ("Community-Based Participatory Research," 2003) and *Health Education & Behavior* ("Community-Based Participatory Research—Addressing Social Determinants of Health: Lessons from the Urban Research Center," 2002), have recently published entire issues devoted to CBPR. Special sections on CBPR have appeared in such journals as the *American Journal of Public Health* ("Community-Based Participatory Research," 2001) and *Environmental Health Perspectives* ("Community-Based Participatory Research," in press). Finally, the Agency for Healthcare Research and Quality commissioned a systematic, evidence-based review that consolidates and analyzes the body of literature produced to date on (1) what defines CBPR, (2) how CBPR has been implemented with regard to the quality of research methodology and community involvement, (3) the evidence that CBPR efforts have resulted in the intended outcomes, and (4) criteria and processes that should be used for review of CBPR in grant proposals (Viswanathan et al., 2004).

As opportunities for conducting and learning about CBPR expand, so does the demand for knowledge and skills in this area. Practitioners and scholars ask for information about specific participation structures and procedures needed to establish and maintain equitable partnerships among individuals and groups from diverse cultures. They ask how specific data collection methods, such as survey questionnaires, in-depth interviews, and focus groups, can be designed and implemented to follow participatory principles, and how to engage all CBPR partners in disseminating research findings and translating results into action and policy change. This book is designed as a resource for students, practitioners, community members, and researchers in public health and related disciplines, with the aim of expanding their repertoire of skills and methods for supporting partnership approaches to research intended to improve the health and well-being of communities in general and eliminate health disparities in particular.

PRINCIPLES OF CBPR

Based on an extensive review of the literature, the following discussion briefly presents nine guiding principles of CBPR (see Israel et al., 2003, for a more detailed examination). These principles are offered with the caution that no one set of principles is applicable to all partnerships. Rather, the members of each research partnership need jointly to decide on the core values and guiding principles that reflect their collective vision and basis for decision making. However, as partnerships go about the process of making these decisions, they may be informed by the considerable experience and many lessons learned over the past several decades of participatory forms of research as well as by the literature on partnerships and group functioning. Developing or existing partnerships may choose to draw on the principles presented here, as appropriate, as well as to develop additional or alternative principles that facilitate equitable participation and influence in each partnership's particular context. We suggest that partnerships consider the principles they adopt as ideals or goals to strive for, and evaluate the extent to which they are able to do so as one aspect of partnership capacity building (Cornwall, 1996; Green et al., 1995; Israel et al., 2003). As will be evident throughout this volume, these and similar principles have been applied in numerous ways by the authors of these chapters, reflecting multiple approaches to CBPR.

1. *CBPR acknowledges community as a unit of identity.* Units of identity refer to entities in which people have membership, for example, a family, social network, or geographical neighborhood; they are socially created dimensions of identity, created and re-created through social interactions (Hatch, Moss, Saran, Presley-Cantrell, & Mallory, 1993; Steuart, 1993). Community as a unit of identity is defined by a sense of identification with and emotional connection to others through common symbol systems, values, and norms; shared interests; and commitments to meeting mutual needs. Communities of identity may be geographically bounded (people in a particular physical neighborhood may form such a community, for example) or geographically dispersed but sharing a common identity or sense of common interests (as members of an ethnic group or gay men may do, for example). A city, town, or geographical area may represent a community of identity, or then again it may be an aggregate of individuals who do not have a common identity or it may comprise multiple overlapping communities of identity. CBPR partnerships seek to identify and work with existing communities of identity, extending beyond them as necessary, to improve public health (Israel et al., 1998, 2003).

2. *CBPR builds on strengths and resources within the community.* CBPR recognizes and builds on the strengths, resources, and assets that exist within communities of identity, such as individual skills, social networks, and organizations, in order to address identified concerns (Balcazar et al., 2004; Israel et al., 1998, 2003; McKnight, 1994; Steuart, 1993).

3. *CBPR facilitates a collaborative, equitable partnership in all phases of research, involving an empowering and power-sharing process that attends to social inequalities.* To the extent possible, all partners participate in and share decision making and control over all stages of the research process, such as defining the problem, collecting and interpreting data, disseminating findings, and applying the results to address community issues (Balcazar et al., 2004; deKoning & Martin, 1996; Green et al., 1995; Israel et al., 1998, 2003; Park, Brydon-Miller, Hall, & Jackson, 1993; Stringer, 1996). Researchers involved in CBPR recognize the inequalities that exist between themselves and community partners

and attempt to address these inequalities through developing relationships based on trust and mutual respect and by creating an empowering process that involves open communication and sharing information, decision-making power, and resources (Blankenship & Schulz, 1996; Israel et al., 1998, 2003: Labonte, 1994; Suarez-Balcazar et al., 2004).

4. *CBPR fosters co-learning and capacity building among all partners.* CBPR is a co-learning process that fosters the reciprocal exchange of skills, knowledge, and capacity among all partners involved, recognizing that all parties bring diverse skills and expertise and different perspectives and experiences to the partnership process (deKoning & Martin, 1996; Freire, 1973; Israel et al., 1998, 2003; Stringer, 1996; Suarez-Balcazar et al., 2004).

5. *CBPR integrates and achieves a balance between knowledge generation and intervention for the mutual benefit of all partners.* CBPR aims to contribute to science while also integrating and balancing the knowledge gained with interventions and policies that address the concerns of the communities involved (Green et al., 1995; Park, Brydon-Miller, Hall, & Jackson, 1993; Israel et al., 1998, 2003). Although a given CBPR project may not include a direct intervention component, it will have a commitment to the translation of research findings into action strategies that will benefit the community (deKoning & Martin, 1996; Green et al., 1995; Israel et al., 2003; Schulz, Israel, Selig, Bayer, & Griffin, 1998).

6. *CBPR focuses on the local relevance of public health problems and on ecological perspectives that attend to the multiple determinants of health.* CBPR addresses public health concerns that are of local relevance to the communities involved, and it emphasizes an ecological approach to health that pays attention to individuals, their immediate context (for example, the family or social network), and the larger contexts in which these families and networks exist (for example, the community and society) (Bronfenbrenner, 1990; Israel et al., 1998, 2003; Stokols, 1996). Thus CBPR efforts consider the multiple determinants of health and disease, including biomedical, social, economic, cultural, and physical environmental factors, and necessitate an interdisciplinary team of researchers and community partners (Israel et al. 1998, 2003; Suarez-Balcazar et al., 2004).

7. *CBPR involves systems development using a cyclical and iterative process.* CBPR addresses systems development, in which a system, for example, a partnership, draws on the competencies of each partner to engage in a cyclical, iterative process that includes all the stages of the research process, such as community assessment, problem definition,

research design, data collection and analysis, data interpretation, dissemination, determination of intervention and policy strategies, and action taking, as appropriate (Altman, 1995; Israel et al., 1998, 2003; Stringer, 1996).

8. *CBPR disseminates results to all partners and involves them in the wider dissemination of results.* CBPR emphasizes the dissemination of research findings to all partners and communities involved and in ways that are understandable, respectful, and useful (Israel et al., 1998, 2003; Schulz et al., 1998). This dissemination principle also emphasizes that all partners engage in the broader dissemination of results, for example as coauthors of publications and copresenters at meetings and conferences (Israel et al., 2003).

9. *CBPR involves a long-term process and commitment to sustainability.* CBPR involves a long-term process and commitment to sustainability in order to establish and maintain the trust necessary to successfully carry out CBPR endeavors, and to achieve the aims of addressing multiple determinants of health (Hatch et al., 1993; Israel et al., 2003; Mittelmark, Hunt, Heath, & Schmid, 1993). This long-term commitment frequently extends beyond a single research project or funding period, and although partners may reach a point at which they decide to no longer continue as a partnership, they retain a commitment to the relationships that exist and that can be called on in the future to the extent that partners feel is needed and desired (Israel et al., 2003).

CBPR AND HEALTH DISPARITIES: CULTURAL, SOCIAL, ECONOMIC, AND ENVIRONMENTAL CONTEXT

Although CBPR is appropriate for addressing many health problems in community contexts, in the United States such partnership efforts have been carried out primarily in predominantly low-income communities, often communities of color (Minkler, 2004). African American, Latino, Native American, and other ethnic communities have historically been economically and politically marginalized and have compelling reasons to distrust research and researchers (Gamble, 1997; Minkler, 2004; Ribisl & Humphreys, 1998; Sloane et al., 2003). Furthermore, communities of color disproportionately experience the burden of higher rates of morbidity and mortality accompanied by lower socioeconomic position (Cooper et al., 2000; House & Williams, 2000; Krieger, Rowley, Herman, Avery, & Phillips, 1993; Schulz, Williams, et al., 2002). These health disparities are associated with sociostructural and physical environmental determinants of health status, such as poverty, inadequate housing, racism, lack of access to community services and employment opportunities, air pollution, and exposure to toxic substances (Collins & Williams, 1999; Krieger et al., 1993; Schulz, Williams, et al., 2002; Schulz & Northridge, 2004). Thus it is critical that CBPR efforts strive to understand and address the social, economic, and environmental contexts that have an impact on the communities involved. In addition, as elaborated upon here, it is essential that the cultural context of communities be understood and respected and that this context inform partnership approaches to research.

CBPR is intended to bring together researchers and communities to establish trust, share power, foster co-learning, enhance strengths and resources, build capacity, and examine and address community-identified needs and health problems. Given that academically based researchers involved in CBPR are often from "outside" the community in which the research is taking place and are often different from community partners in terms of, for example, class, ethnicity, and culture, a number of power issues and tensions may arise and need to be addressed (Chávez, Duran, Baker, Avila, & Wallerstein, 2003; Minkler, 2004; Nyden & Wiewel, 1992; Wallerstein, 1999). These differences require researchers to gain the self-awareness, knowledge, and skills to work in multicultural contexts.

Two concepts are particularly germane to our focus on CBPR and to efforts to work effectively in cultures different from one's own. First, the concept of *cultural humility* has its roots in medical education in the United States (Tervalon & Murray-Garcia, 1998). Second, the concept of *cultural safety* originated in nursing education and has been applied to medical education in New Zealand (Crampton, Dowell, Parkin, & Thompson, 2003; Ramsden, 1997). Here are brief descriptions of the ways in which each concept provides a framework for considering the many methods and issues addressed in this volume.

As articulated by Tervalon and Murray-Garcia (1998), cultural humility rather than *cultural competence* is the goal for professionals to strive to achieve, because achieving a "static notion of competence" (p. 120) is not possible. That is, professionals cannot fully master another's culture. Tervalon and Murray-Garcia recommend a process that requires humility and commitment to ongoing self-reflection and self-critique, including identifying and examining one's own patterns of unintentional and intentional racism and classism, addressing existing power imbalances, and establishing and maintaining "mutually beneficial and non-paternalistic partnerships with communities" (p. 123). Achieving cultural humility is reflected in the principles of CBPR, given its emphasis on co-learning, which requires relinquishing one's role as the "expert" in order to recognize the role of community members as full partners in the learning process.

Also reflected in CBPR principles is the concept of cultural safety, which was first defined in New Zealand during the processes of examining how relationships and power imbalances affect and are affected by racism and of investigating the health disparities that exist between Māori (the colonized indigenous peoples of New Zealand) and non-Māori (Crampton et al., 2003; Ramsden, 1997). A policy of cultural safety gives the power to community members to say whether or not they feel safe, and professionals need to enable the community members to express the extent to which they feel risk or safety, resulting in changes in the behaviors of health professionals as appropriate. The concept of cultural safety purports that cultural factors, such as differences in worldview and language, have a major influence on current relationships between professionals and communities. Hence professionals need to acknowledge and understand that these cultural factors, as well as the social, economic, political, and historical determinants of health disparities, can contribute to communities' distrust of and not feeling safe about collaboration (Ramsden, 1997). To achieve cultural safety within a CBPR partnership, it is essential to establish deliberation and decision-making structures and procedures whereby all partners are required to express and critically examine their own realities and the attitudes they bring to the issue at hand, be open-minded toward others whose views are different from their own, consider the influences of social and historical processes on their present situation, and work toward becoming members of a partnership that anticipates differences and conflict by addressing them through processes that have been defined by all partners, and particularly by community partners, to be culturally safe (Crampton et al., 2003; Ramsden, 1997). The concepts of cultural humility and cultural safety are integral to the purpose and goals of this book.

PURPOSES AND GOALS OF THIS BOOK

The overall purpose of this book is to provide students, practitioners, researchers, and community members with the knowledge and skills necessary to conduct research that is guided by community-based participatory research principles. CBPR is *not* a particular research design or method. Rather, it is a collaborative approach to research that may draw on the full range of research designs (from case study, etiological, and other nonexperimental designs to randomized control trial, longitudinal, and other experimental or quasi-experimental designs). CBPR data collection and analysis methods may involve both quantitative (for example, psychometric scaling and survey questionnaire) and qualitative (for example, in-depth interview and participant observation) approaches. What distinguishes CBPR from other approaches to research is the integral link between the researcher and the researched whereby the concepts of cultural humility and cultural safety are combined with process methods and procedures (such as group facilitation) to establish and maintain the research partnership.

The chapters in this volume provide a wide range of concrete examples of CBPR study designs, specific data collection and analysis methods, and innovative partnership structures and process methods. Each chapter addresses one or more methods for data collection and analysis and presents a detailed case example of CBPR from the authors' experience to examine challenges, lessons learned, and implications that can be applied to other contexts. The purpose is not to provide detailed explanations of how to administer such data collection methods as survey questionnaires and in-depth interviews—there are numerous excellent books that do that (for example, Nardi, 2002; Patton, 2002), and they are referred to throughout this volume. Rather, the focus is on how to conduct these methods in ways that involve all partners and that attend to issues of equity, power sharing, cultural differences, and research dissemination and benefits. The chapters that discuss different process methods also provide numerous examples from the authors' experiences in multiple settings. In keeping with the principles of CBPR, all chapters have community partners as coauthors, ensuring that community partners' voices are reflected in the descriptions and recommendations provided.

Our work has been greatly enhanced by Minkler and Wallerstein's excellent volume *Community-Based Participatory Research for Health* (2003), which provides an in-depth discussion of what CBPR is, its history, and its theoretical roots (Wallerstein & Duran, 2003); issues related to power and trust (Chávez et al., 2003); and case examples of CBPR efforts that examine topics such as ethical considerations (Farquhar & Wing, 2003) and conducting CBPR with and by diverse populations (Cheatham & Shen, 2003). *Community-Based Participatory Research for Health* is an outstanding precursor to and companion volume for this one.

We also acknowledge the international body of work in participatory research that has laid the foundation for CBPR (for examples of work in Australia and Canada and in Asia, Latin America, and Africa, see deKoning & Martin, 1996; Fals-Borda & Rahman, 1991; Park, Brydon-Miller, Hall, & Jackson, 1993; Reason & Bradbury, 2001; Stringer & Genat, 2004). While recognizing and drawing upon this important work, we have chosen to focus this CBPR methods book on case examples from the United States, given the necessity to attend to the context within which CBPR is conducted (Minkler & Wallerstein, 2003). Our intent is that readers will embrace the lessons learned by the authors of the chapters in this book and gain the skills needed to apply them throughout the United States and to adapt them as appropriate to the particular context of other countries as well.

ORGANIZATION OF THIS BOOK

The chapters in this book are organized into six parts:

1. An introduction to methods in CBPR and to the five specific phases of the CBPR approach that are discussed in the subsequent parts
2. Partnership formation and maintenance
3. Community assessment and diagnosis
4. Definition of the issue
5. Documentation and evaluation of the partnership process
6. Feedback, interpretation, dissemination, and application of results

Although these phases are presented in the book as distinct entities, we understand that CBPR is an iterative process in which a partnership will cycle through earlier phases at various points in time.

Each chapter examines one or more methods organized around a case study and includes an overview of each method, background on the CBPR partnership and project to be discussed, a description of how the method was designed and implemented within a particular phase of the CBPR process, an analysis of the challenges and limitations of the method within the context of CBPR, and an examination of the lessons learned, the implications, and recommendations for using the data collection method in CBPR projects more broadly. When a method examined in relation to a particular phase of CBPR is also applicable to another phase, readers are referred to relevant chapters elsewhere in the book. In addition, a few methods are covered in more than one part of the book because their application differs depending on the phase of CBPR in which they are used.

Part Two (Chapters Two and Three) focuses on one of the most critical aspects of CBPR, partnership formation and maintenance. In any CBPR project, regardless of the specific focus of the project and the data collection methods used, a number of important questions need to be addressed regarding the creation of a partnership. Such questions include the following: How is the community defined? Who will be involved, and who decides on that involvement? Are community members involved as individuals or representatives of organizations? To what extent do members of the partnership represent the community in terms of class (income and education level), gender, race, or ethnicity, and language(s) spoken? How will partners be involved? How will trust and open communication be established and maintained? How will issues of power and conflict be addressed? And how will equitable participation and influence be achieved across all partners? To address these questions and the issue of developing and maintaining effective partnerships, Chapters Two and Three examine *process methods* that can be used. Although this phase is presented as the beginning of a CBPR effort, it is essential to give continued attention to these partnership formation methods throughout all phases of a CBPR endeavor in order to maintain the partnership.

In Chapter Two, Wallerstein, Duran, Minkler, and Foley share their experiences in building and maintaining university-community research partnerships in New Mexico and California. They describe the how-to methods and challenges of partnership development and maintenance, framed specifically for academic and other outside research partners. However, all readers, including community partners and those new to CBPR, will benefit from the self-reflection and dialogue methods provided. They examine different starting points and strategies for establishing partnerships, process methods for creating and incorporating collaborative principles to foster effective partnerships, the dilemmas and challenges of collaboration between outside researchers and communities that are built into the various contexts represented and strategies for addressing these challenges (such as ways to achieve cultural humility), and process methods for maintaining partnerships over the long haul.

In Chapter Three, Becker, Israel, and Allen describe group process methods and facilitation strategies to establish and maintain effective partnerships. Based on concepts and findings from the field of group dynamics, they present specific techniques and activities for facilitating CBPR groups, drawing from a number of CBPR efforts in Michigan and Louisiana in which they have been involved. This chapter is organized around twelve elements of group dynamics (including equitable participation and open communication, developing trust, addressing power and influence, conflict resolution, and working in culturally diverse groups) relevant to CBPR partnerships. For each element the authors provide useful strategies and techniques for improving the partnership process with the aim of achieving the ultimate outcomes of a given CBPR effort.

Part Three (Chapter Four) examines the important phase of community assessment and diagnosis. Unlike a needs assessment that focuses on identifying health needs and problems often out of context, this phase focuses on gaining a better understanding of what it is like to live in a given community. Such understanding includes, for example, the strengths and resources that exist within the community; the history and involvement of its members and organizations; community values, language, communication, and helping patterns; and community needs and concerns (Eng & Blanchard, 1991–1992; Kretzmann & McKnight, 1993; Steuart, 1993). Eng, Moore, Rhodes, Griffith, Allison, Shirah, and Mebane, the authors of Chapter Four, refer to this phase as *action-oriented community diagnosis* (AOCD). As in the phase of partnership formation (although it is necessary for AOCD to occur early in a CBPR partnership), gaining entry to a community and establishing relationships is a long-term, ongoing process for outsiders.

Eng and colleagues examine several different methods for collecting and interpreting data (participant observation, key informant in-depth interviews, key informant focus group interviews, and community forums) as part of an AOCD community assessment procedure. They provide a case example of their experience with conducting an AOCD in Efland-Cheeks, North Carolina, describing in detail the CBPR approach they have used to engage community members and outsider researchers throughout the process, including formulating the AOCD case study research design, selecting and using multiple data collection methods, analyzing data using the technique of constant comparison to identify differences and similarities, and interpreting the findings and determining next action steps to address them. They highlight the challenges and limitations and the lessons learned and implications of using this multimethod community assessment approach within the context of CBPR.

As discussed in Part Four (Chapters Five through Eleven), whether a CBPR project is examining a basic research question, an intervention evaluation question, or both, a major phase is defining the issue or health problem that will be the focus of the project. As in all phases of CBPR, a key aspect is obtaining the active involvement of all partners in the process, ideally from the very beginning. These chapters examine various data collection methods (survey questionnaires, focus group interviews, neighborhood observational checklists, social mapping, ethnography, and exposure assessments) used to identify the issue(s) that a research partnership will investigate and address. Although the methods examined in each chapter are quite different, the lessons learned with regard to their application as part of a CBPR effort are similar. For example, lessons are offered on the role of community partners in developing measurement instruments, in tailoring language and data collection procedures to the local culture of the community, and in training and involving community members as data collectors.

In Chapter Five, Schulz, Zenk, Kannan, Israel, Koch, and Stokes draw on their experience with the Healthy Environments Partnership in Detroit, Michigan. Their case example illustrates collaboration among community members and the partners in jointly developing and implementing a population-based survey administered to a stratified random sample of community residents. They give particular attention to processes through which representatives from diverse groups were actively engaged and the contributions of these various forms of engagement to such aspects of the survey as conceptualization, identification of specific topics and items, selection of language and wording, and administration. The authors discuss challenges, lessons learned, and implications for CBPR partnerships seeking to jointly develop and implement community surveys.

In Chapter Six, Christopher, Burhansstipanov, and Knows His Gun McCormick discuss the CBPR process they used to modify interviewer training protocols developed originally for use with non-Native groups, in order to increase the cultural acceptability and accuracy of the survey data gathered by and from women on the Apsáalooke Reservation in Montana. They describe a history of inequality, manifested in the community's past disrespectful interactions with researchers and the community's inability to access, influence, or make use of information generated through research to improve the health of community members. The authors discuss how this history has shaped the community's current perspectives and responses to research, and the implications for training survey interviewers. Some of the training implications they address relate to issues of recruitment and enrollment of interviewees, the manner of interviewers, beginning the interview, language use, and dissemination of findings. The authors provide a summary of the lessons learned in this process and the implications for public health research and interventions.

In Chapter Seven, Kieffer, Salabarría-Peña, Odoms-Young, Willis, Baber, and Guzman describe how they have used focus group interviews in several CBPR projects in Detroit. They provide an in-depth examination of one partnership, Promoting Healthy Lifestyles Among Women, emphasizing the role and contributions of community partners throughout the focus group interview process. The process includes developing focus group guides, recruiting and training focus group moderators and note takers, recruiting participants, collecting and analyzing data, reporting the findings to the community, and engaging community members in the interpretation of results. The authors discuss challenges and limitations, lessons learned, and the implications for using a participatory approach in conducting focus group interviews.

In Chapter Eight, Zenk, Schulz, House, Benjamin, and Kannan begin by reviewing the ways in which direct neighborhood observation has been used in research, including CBPR, and then they describe how community and academic partners of the Healthy Environments Partnership in Detroit worked together to design and conduct an assessment using an observational tool, the Neighborhood Observational Checklist (NOC). The authors highlight how they obtained input from and engaged other community residents in this process. They emphasize the role of community partners and other residents in content discussions regarding the NOC (clarifying the purpose of the NOC, probing the meaning and examining the appropriateness of items, and adding items to better reflect community strengths and assets, for example) and in discussions on pilot testing and implementing the NOC. The authors examine challenges and lessons learned in applying a CBPR approach to the design of a neighborhood observational tool, with specific attention to implications for the use of neighborhood observation in future CBPR endeavors.

In Chapter Nine, Ayala, Maty, Cravey, and Webb examine the concept of mapping social and environmental influences using a CBPR approach. They consider not only the question of why one should use mapping techniques but also the important question of how one can engage a community in a mapping activity. They describe the methods used in two CBPR projects in North Carolina, one in Raleigh, Wake County, and the other in Burlington, Alamance County. The authors specifically address the role of community and academic partners in the development of the mapping protocol, selection and recruitment of participants, data collection and analysis, and data feedback, interpretation and discussion. They present challenges and limitations of social-mapping techniques and lessons learned and implications for the use of these techniques in CBPR partnerships.

In Chapter Ten, McQuiston, Parrado, Olmos, and Bustillo demonstrate how to conduct ethnography as CBPR. Community-based ethnographic participatory research (CBEPR) focuses on culture and cultural interpretation and uses a participatory process. These authors discuss the example of a case in Durham, North Carolina, involving Latinos who have recently immigrated to the area. They examine the roles of community and academic partner organizations and community members in proposal development, ethnographic survey development and administration, training community members as ethnographers and participant observers, and analysis and interpretation of findings. The authors also reflect on the capacity building of the partners involved and discuss challenges and limitations, lessons learned, and implications for practice.

In Chapter Eleven, Krieger, Allen, Roberts, Ross, and Takaro describe how to conduct exposure assessments of harmful substances in the environment associated with adverse health effects. Drawing from their experience with the Healthy Homes Project in Seattle, Washington, they examine the role of community partners and other community members trained as community health workers in the development and implementation of exposure data collection instruments and protocols (such as dust sampling and measuring surface moisture). These authors discuss the benefits of and lessons learned from involving community partners, community staff, and participants in this process.

As discussed in Part Five (Chapter Twelve), it is essential that CBPR partnerships continually document and evaluate their progress toward achieving an effective collaborative process (Israel et al., 2003; Lasker, Weiss, & Miller, 2001; Parker et al., 2003; Schulz, Israel, & Lantz, 2003; Sofaer, 2000; Wallerstein, Polacsek, & Maltrud, 2002; Weiss, Anderson, & Lasker, 2002). Such an evaluation involves focusing on the partnership's adherence to its CBPR principles, such as those described earlier (determining, for example, whether the partnership fosters co-learning and capacity building; involves equitable participation, influence, and power sharing; and achieves balance between knowledge generation and action). The rationale is that it is essential to determine whether and how well a research partnership is achieving, as intermediate outcomes, principles that it must use to refine and improve its methods to accomplish its long-term outcomes (Lantz, Viruell-Fuentes, Israel, Softley, & Guzman, 2001; Rossi, Freeman & Lipsey, 1999; Schulz et al., 2003; Weiss et al., 2002).

In Chapter Twelve, Israel, Lantz, McGranaghan, Kerr, and Guzman describe the use of two data collection methods, in-depth, semi-structured interviews and closed-ended survey questionnaires, for assessing the process and impact of the collaborative dimensions of CBPR partnerships (for example, participatory decision making, two-way open communication, and constructive conflict resolution). They also present a conceptual framework for assessing CBPR partnerships and the use of this framework in guiding the Detroit Community-Academic Urban Research Center's application of the two data collection methods. The authors emphasize the role of academic and community partners in the participatory process used in designing, conducting, feeding back, and interpreting the results of these two data collection methods for evaluating this CBPR partnership. They examine the challenges and limitations, lessons learned, and implications for the use of these methods.

Part Six (Chapters Thirteen through Seventeen) focus on the CBPR phase of ensuring active engagement of all partners in the feedback, interpretation, dissemination, and application of results. There are process methods that can be used to foster the steps in this phase, such as the collaborative development of dissemination guidelines (as discussed in Chapter Thirteen). In addition, four of the chapters in Part Six include case examples of using group dialogue, photovoice, document review, survey questionnaire, focus group interview, and secondary data analysis methods of data collection.

In Chapter Thirteen, Parker, Robins, Israel, Brakefield-Caldwell, Edgren, and Wilkins describe how they established and implemented dissemination guidelines in a CBPR project in order to ensure widespread dissemination of results and participation of all partners in the process. The case example draws on their experience with Community Action Against Asthma, a CBPR effort of the Michigan Center for the Environment and Children's Health. The authors examine the role of community and academic partners in deciding how to address issues in the dissemination guidelines. These issues included developing a process for selecting members to participate in presentations, establishing ground rules for collaborative authorship, drafting a list of proposed core articles and presentations, and providing feedback of results to participants and the wider community. The authors discuss the challenges and the lessons learned in creating and applying dissemination guidelines.

In Chapter Fourteen, Baker and Motton focus on the data collection method of in-depth group interviews, examining the stages involved in collecting data and using data to develop action within a CBPR project. The case example concerns a partnership in rural southeast Missouri involving a series of group interviews conducted with the Bootheel Heart Health Coalitions over an eleven-month period. The authors consider the role of community and academic partners in development of the interview guide, recruitment and data collection, data analysis, data feedback and member checking, and interpretation of the results. They discuss the challenges and limitations of the method and the lessons learned and implications for its application within CBPR efforts.

In Chapter Fifteen, López, Eng, Robinson, and Wang discuss the use of photovoice in the context of a CBPR approach. Photovoice is a participatory method in which community members use cameras to take pictures that represent their experiences and communicate those experiences to others (Wang & Burris, 1994). Following a brief review of the origins, diverse applications, and theoretical underpinnings of photovoice, the authors present a case example of the Inspirational Images Project that was conducted in three counties in rural, eastern North Carolina using photovoice as the primary data collection method. They examine the role of academic and community partner organizations and individual breast cancer survivors, who were coinvestigators in this effort, in deciding on the design of the study and research protocol, the selection and recruitment of participants, photovoice training, data collection and theoretical sampling, data management and grounded theory analysis, data feedback and interpretation, and the engagement of local policymakers in discussing the findings. The authors share lessons learned, and draw from feedback provided by photovoice participants to describe implications of the method for CBPR.

In Chapter Sixteen, Freudenberg, Rogers, Ritas, and Nerney describe participatory policy research (PPR), an approach to CBPR designed to analyze the impact of policies on public health and to use these analyses to mobilize action to change harmful policies. They illustrate the multiple methods used in PPR through their experiences in a multipronged partnership process in New York City. They examine the role of different stakeholders in applying diverse methods to understand issues and change policies, methods such as review of public data, review of relevant legislation and agency regulations, surveys, focus group interviews, literature reviews, opinion polls, and meeting with legislators, staff, and executive branch officials. The authors discuss limitations and challenges, the lessons learned, and the implications of using such a multimethod approach.

In Chapter Seventeen, Morello-Frosch, Pastor, Sadd, Porras, and Prichard demonstrate how the Southern California Environmental Justice Collaborative has applied a CBPR approach to conducting research in the region using secondary data sources. They discuss the rationale for the use of secondary data analysis and focus on how the collaborative has collectively developed research projects, interpreted data, disseminated study findings, and leveraged the results of secondary data to promote policy change and bolster organizing. The authors explore how their research approach has sought to transform traditional scientific approaches to studying community environmental health. They conclude with a discussion of some of the challenges they have faced and the lessons learned from their work.

This book ends with sixteen appendixes that give the readers examples of the process methods tools, procedural documents, and data collection instruments discussed by some of the chapter authors. The intent of these appendixes is to provide further detail on methods for conducting CBPR and the instruments developed as a result of the process. Among the process methods and procedural documents included are an informed consent form, guidelines for establishing research priorities, and dissemination guidelines. The data collection instruments include a key informant in-depth interview protocol, the Neighborhood Observational Checklist, open-ended and closed-ended questionnaires for evaluating partnership functioning, and a group dialogue interview protocol. The appendixes are intended to further assist researchers, practitioners, and community partners in developing and implementing strategies and methods that strengthen the use of community-based participatory research.

CONCLUSION

As is evident throughout this volume, there is no one approach to community-based participatory research, and there are no process methods or data collection methods that are applicable to all CBPR efforts. Rather, community-based participatory research is a fluid, iterative approach to research, interventions, and policy change that draws from a wide range of research designs and methods and pays particular attention to issues of trust, power, cultural diversity, and equity. Furthermore, CBPR is one of many different approaches to research and action. The case examples throughout this book illustrate methods used by various CBPR partnerships whose goal has been to move the public health field forward by generating new knowledge (such as better information on the ways social and physical environmental factors influence health), identifying the factors associated with intervention success, and determining actions (based on partnership findings and co-learning) that will effect social and behavioral change in order to eliminate health disparities.

References

Altman, D. G. (1995). Sustaining interventions in community systems: On the relationship between researchers and communities. *Health Psychology, 14*(6), 526–536.

Argyris, C., Putnam, R., & Smith, D. M. (1985). *Action science: Concepts, methods and skills for research and intervention.* San Francisco: Jossey-Bass.

Balcazar, F. E., Taylor, R. R., Keilhofner, G. W., Tamley, K., Benziger, T., Carlin, N., et al. (2004). Participatory action research: General principles and a study with a chronic health condition. In L. A. Jason, C. B. Keys, Y. Suarez-Balcazar, R. R. Taylor, & M. I. Davis (Eds.), *Participatory community research: Theories and methods in action* (pp. 17–36). Washington, DC: American Psychological Association.

Blankenship, K. M., & Schulz, A. J. (1996, August 17). *Approaches and dilemmas in community-based research and action.* Paper presented at the annual meeting of the Society for the Study of Social Problems, New York.

Bronfenbrenner, U. (1990). *The ecology of human development: Experiments by nature and design.* Cambridge, MA: Harvard University Press.

Bruce, T. A., & McKane, S. U. (Eds.). (2000). *Community-based public health: A partnership model.* Washington, DC: American Public Health Association.

Butterfoss, F. D., Goodman, R. M., & Wandersman, A. (1993). Community coalitions for prevention and health promotion. *Health Education Research, 8*(3), 315–330.

Centers for Disease Control and Prevention. (1994). *Cooperative agreement program for Urban Center(s) for Applied Research in Public Health* (Program Announcement No. 515). Atlanta, GA: Author.

Centers for Disease Control and Prevention. (1999). *Racial and Ethnic Approaches to Community Health (REACH 2010)* (Program Announcement 00121). Atlanta: Author.

Chávez, V., Duran, B. M., Baker, Q. E., Avila, M. M., & Wallerstein, N. (2003). The dance of race and privilege in community-based participatory research. In M. Minkler & N. Wallerstein (Eds.), *Community-based participatory research for health* (pp. 81–97). San Francisco: Jossey-Bass.

Cheatham, A., & Shen, E. (2003). Community-based participatory research with Cambodian girls in Long Beach, California: A case study. In M. Minkler & N. Wallerstein (Eds.), *Community-based participatory research for health* (pp. 316–331). San Francisco: Jossey-Bass.

Collins, C., & Williams, D. (1999). Segregation and mortality: The deadly effects of racism? *Sociological Forum, 14*(3), 495–523.

Community-based participatory research. (2001). Special section of *American Journal of Public Health, 91*(12), 1926–1943.

Community-based participatory research—Addressing social determinants of health: Lessons from the Urban Research Center. (2002). Special issue of *Health Education & Behavior, 29*(3).

Community-based participatory research. (2003). Special issue of *Journal of General Internal Medicine, 18*(7).

Community-based participatory research. (in press). Special section of *Environmental Health Perspectives.*

Community Health Scholars Program. (2004). Community Health Scholars Program. Retrieved 2004 from www.sph.umich.edu/chsp

Cooper, R., Cutler, J., Desvigne-Nickens, P., Fortmann, S. P., Friedman, L., Havlik, R., et al. (2000). Trends and disparities in coronary heart disease, stroke and other cardiovascular diseases in the United States: Findings of the National Conference on Cardiovascular Disease Prevention. *Circulation, 102*(25), 3137–3147.

Cornwall, A. (1996). Towards participatory practice: Participatory rural appraisal (PRA) and the participatory process. In K. deKoning & M. Martin (Eds.), *Participatory research in health: Issues and experiences* (pp. 94–107). London: Zed Books.

Crampton, P., Dowell, A., Parkin, C., & Thompson, C. (2003). Combating effects of racism through a cultural immersion medical education program. *Academic Medicine, 78*(6), 595–598.

deKoning, K., & Martin, M. (Eds.). (1996). *Participatory research in health: Issues and experiences.* London: Zed Books.

Eng, E., & Blanchard, L. (1990–1991). Action-oriented community diagnosis: A health education tool. *International Quarterly of Community Health Education, 11,* 93–110.

Fals-Borda, O., & Rahman, M. A. (1991). *Action and knowledge: Breaking the monopoly with participatory action research.* New York: Intermediate Technology/Apex.

Farquhar, S., & Wing, S. (2003). Methodological and ethical considerations in community-driven environmental justice research: Two case studies from rural North Carolina. In M. Minkler & N. Wallerstein (Eds.), *Community-based participatory research for health* (pp. 221–241). San Francisco: Jossey-Bass.

Fetterman, D. M., Kaftarian, S. J., & Wandersman, A. (Eds.). (1996). *Empowerment evaluation: Knowledge and tools for self-assessment and accountability.* Thousand Oaks, CA: Sage.

Freire, P. (1973). *Education for critical consciousness.* New York: Seabury Press.

Gamble, V. N. (1997). The Tuskegee Syphilis Study and women's health. *Journal of the American Medical Women's Association, 52*(4), 195–196.

Gebbie, K. M., Rosenstock, L., & Hernandez, L. M. (Eds.). (2003). *Who will keep the public healthy? Educating public health professionals for the 21st century.* Washington, DC: National Academies Press.

Green, L. W. (2003). Tracing federal support for participatory research in public health. In M. Minkler & N. Wallerstein (Eds.), *Community-based participatory research for health* (pp. 410–418). San Francisco: Jossey-Bass.

Green, L. W., George, M. A., Daniel, M., Frankish, C. J., Herbert, C. J., Bowie, W. R., et al. (1995). *Study of participatory research in health promotion.* Ottawa: Royal Society of Canada.

Green, L. W., & Mercer, S. L. (2001). Can public health researchers and agencies reconcile the push from funding bodies and the pull from communities? *American Journal of Public Health, 91*(12), 1926–1929.

Hall, B. (1992). From margins to center? The development and purpose of participatory research. *American Sociologist, 23,* 15–28.

Hatch, J., Moss, N., Saran, A., Presley-Cantrell, L., & Mallory, C. (1993). Community research: Partnership in black communities. *American Journal of Preventive Medicine, 9*(6, Suppl.), 27–31.

Heron, J., & Reason, P. (2001). The practice of cooperative inquiry: Research "with" rather than "on" people. In P. Reason & H. Bradbury (Eds.), *Handbook of action research: Participative inquiry and practice* (pp. 179–188). Thousand Oaks, CA: Sage.

Higgins, D. L., Maciak, B. J., & Metzler, M. (2001). CDC Urban Research Centers: Community-based participatory research to improve the health of urban communities. *Journal of Women's Health and Gender Based Medicine, 10*(1), 9–15.

House, J. S., & Williams, D. R. (2000). Understanding and reducing socioeconomic and racial/ethnic disparities in health. In B. D. Smedley & S. L. Syme (Eds.), *Promoting health: Intervention strategies from social and behavioral research* (pp. 81–124). Washington, DC: National Academies Press.

Israel, B. A., Lichtenstein, R., Lantz, P., McGranaghan, R., Allen, A., Guzman, J. R., et al. (2001). The Detroit Community-Academic Urban Research Center: Development, implementation and evaluation. *Journal of Public Health Management and Practice, 7*(5), 1–19.

Israel, B. A., Schulz, A. J., Parker, E. A., & Becker, A. B. (1998). Review of community-based research: Assessing partnership approaches to improve public health. *Annual Review of Public Health, 19,* 173–202.

Israel, B. A., Schulz, A. J., Parker, E. A., Becker, A. B., Allen, A., & Guzman, J. R. (2003). Critical issues in developing and following community-based participatory research principles. In M. Minkler & N. Wallerstein (Eds.), *Community-based participatory research for health* (pp. 56–73). San Francisco: Jossey-Bass.

Jason, L. A., Keys, C. B., Suarez-Balcazar, Y., Taylor, R. R., & Davis, M. I. (Eds.). (2004). *Participatory community research: Theories and methods in action.* Washington, DC: American Psychological Association.

Kemmis, S., & McTaggart, R. (2000). Participatory action research. In N. K. Denzin & Y. S. Lincoln (Eds.), *Handbook of Qualitative Research* (pp. 567–605). Thousand Oaks, CA: Sage.

Kretzmann, J. P., & McKnight, J. L. (1993). *Building communities from the inside out: A path toward finding and mobilizing a community's assets.* Chicago: ACTA.

Krieger, N., Rowley, D. L., Herman, A. A., Avery, B., & Phillips, M. T. (1993). Racism, sexism, and social class: Implications for studies of health, disease, and well-being. *American Journal of Preventive Medicine, 9*(6, Suppl.), 82–122.

Labonte, R. (1994). Health promotion and empowerment: Reflections on professional practice. *Health Education Quarterly, 21,* 253–268.

Lantz, P., Viruell-Fuentes, E., Israel, B. A., Softley, D., & Guzman, J. R. (2001). Can communities and academia work together on public health research? Evaluation results from a community-based participatory research partnership in Detroit. *Journal of Urban Health, 78*(3), 495–507.

Lasker, R. D., Weiss, E. S., & Miller, R. (2001). Partnership synergy: A practical framework for studying and strengthening the collaborative advantage. *Milbank Quarterly, 79*(2), 179–205.

Maguire, P. (1987). *Doing participatory research: A feminist approach.* Amherst, MA: University of Massachusetts School of Education.

McKnight, J. L. (1994). Politicizing health care. In P. Conrad & R. Kern (Eds.), *The sociology of health and illness: Critical perspectives* (4th ed., pp. 437–441). New York: St. Martin's Press.

Minkler, M. (2004). Ethical challenges for the "outside" researcher in community-based participatory research. *Health Education & Behavior, 31*(6), 684–697.

Minkler, M., & Wallerstein, N. (Eds.). (2003). *Community-based participatory research for health.* San Francisco: Jossey-Bass.

Mittelmark, M. B., Hunt, M. K., Heath, G. W., & Schmid, T. L. (1993). Realistic outcomes: Lessons from community-based research and demonstration programs for the prevention of cardiovascular diseases. *Journal of Public Health Policy, 14*(4), 437–462.

Nardi, P. M. (2002). *Doing survey research: A guide to quantitative research methods.* Boston: Pearson Allyn & Bacon.

National Institute of Environmental Health Sciences. (1997). *Center for Children's Environmental Health and Disease Prevention Research Initiative* (RFA ES-97–004). Research Triangle Park, NC: Author.

Nyden, P. W., & Wiewel, W. (1992). Collaborative research: Harnessing the tensions between researcher and practitioner. *American Sociologist, 24*(4), 43–55.

O'Fallon, L. R., & Dearry, A. (2002). Community-based participatory research as a tool to advance environmental health sciences. *Environmental Health Perspectives, 110*(2), 155–159.

Park, P. (1993). What is participatory research? A theoretical and methodological perspective. In P. Park, M. Brydon-Miller, B. Hall, & T. Jackson (Eds.), *Voices of change: Participatory research in the United States and Canada* (pp. 1–19). Westport, CT: Bergin & Garvey.

Park, P., Brydon-Miller, M., Hall, B., & Jackson, T. (Eds.). (1993). *Voices of Change: Participatory Research in the United States and Canada.* Westport, CT: Bergin & Garvey.

Parker, E. A., Israel, B. A., Brakefield-Caldwell, W., Keeler, G. J., Lewis, T. C., Ramirez, E., et al. (2003). Community Action Against Asthma: Examining the partnership process of a community-based participatory research project. *Journal of General Internal Medicine, 18*(7), 558–567.

Patton, M. Q. (2002). *Qualitative Evaluation and Research Methods* (3rd ed.). Thousand Oaks, CA: Sage.

Peters, M., & Robinson, V. (1984). The origins and status of action research. *Journal of Applied Behavioral Science, 29*(2), 113–124.

Ramsden, I. (1997). Cultural safety: Implementing the concept: The social force of nursing and midwifery. In P. T. Whaiti, M. McCarthy, & A. Durie (Eds.), *Mai I Rangiatea* (pp. 113–125). Auckland: Auckland University Press, Bridget Williams Books.

Reason, P. (1994). Three approaches to participative inquiry. In N. K. Denzin & Y. S. Lincoln (Eds.), *Handbook of qualitative research* (pp. 324–339). Thousand Oaks, CA: Sage.

Reason, P., & Bradbury, H. (Eds.). (2001). *Handbook of action research: Participative inquiry and practice.* London: Sage.

Ribisl, K. M., & Humphreys, K. (1998). Collaboration between professionals and mediating structures in the community: Towards a third way in health promotion. In S. A. Shumaker, J. Ockene, E. Schron, & W. McBee (Eds.), *The handbook of health behavior change* (2nd ed., pp. 535–554). New York: Springer.

Rossi, P. H., Freeman, H. E., & Lipsey, M. W. (1999). *Evaluation: A systematic approach* (6th ed.). Thousand Oaks, CA: Sage.

Sabol, B. (2002). Innovations in collaboration for the public's health through the Turning Point Initiative: The W. K. Kellogg Foundation perspective. *Journal of Public Health Management and Practice, 8*(1), 6–12.

Schulz, A. J., Israel, B. A., & Lantz, P. (2003). Instrument for evaluating dimensions of group dynamics within community-based participatory research partnerships. *Evaluation and Program Planning, 26,* 249–262.

Schulz, A. J., Israel, B. A., Selig, S. M., Bayer, I. S., & Griffin, C. B. (1998). Development and implementation of principles for community-based research in public health. In R. H. MacNair (Ed.), *Research strategies for community practice* (pp. 83–110). New York: Haworth Press.

Schulz, A. J., & Northridge, M. E. (2004). Social determinants of health and environmental health promotion. *Health Education & Behavior, 31*(4), 455–471.

Schulz, A. J., Williams, D. R., Israel, B. A., & Lempert, L. B. (2002). Racial and spatial relations as fundamental determinants of health in Detroit. *Milbank Quarterly, 80*(4), 677–707.

Sloane, D. C., Diamant, A. L., Lewis, L. B., Yancey, A. K., Flynn, G., Nascimento, L. M., et al. (2003). Improving the nutritional resource environment for healthy living through community-based participatory research. *Journal of General Internal Medicine, 18*(7), 568–575.

Sofaer, S. (2000). *Working together, moving ahead: A manual to support effective community health coalitions.* New York: Baruch College School of Public Affairs.

Steuart, G. W. (1993). Social and cultural perspectives: Community intervention and mental health. *Health Education Quarterly,* Suppl. 1, S99–S111.

Stokols, D. (1996). Translating social ecological theory into guidelines for community health promotion. *American Journal of Health Promotion, 10*(4), 282–298.

Stringer, E. T. (1996). Action research: A handbook for practitioners. Thousand Oaks, CA: Sage.

Stringer, E. T., & Genat, W. (2004). *Action research in health practice.* Upper Saddle River, NJ: Prentice Hall.

Suarez-Balcazar, Y., Davis, M. I., Ferrari, J., Nyden, P., Olson, B., Alvarez, J., et al. (2004). University-community partnerships: A framework and an exemplar. In L. A. Jason, C. B. Keys, Y. Suarez-Balcazar, R. R. Taylor, & M. I. Davis (Eds.), *Participatory community research: Theories and methods in action* (pp. 105–120). Washington, DC: American Psychological Association.

Tandon, R. (1996). The historical roots and contemporary tendencies in participatory research: Implications for health care. In P. Reason & H. Bradbury (Eds.), *Participatory research in health: Issues and experiences* (2nd ed., pp. 19–26). London: Zed Books.

Tervalon, M., & Murray-Garcia, J. (1998). Cultural humility vs. cultural competence: A critical distinction in defining physician training outcomes in medical education. *Journal of Health Care for the Poor and Underserved, 9*(2), 117–125.

Torbert, W. R. (2001). The practice of action inquiry. In P. Reason & H. Bradbury (Eds.), *Handbook of action research: Participative inquiry and practice* (pp. 250–260). Thousand Oaks, CA: Sage.

Viswanathan, M., Ammerman, A., Eng, E., Gartlehner, G., Lohr, K., Griffith, D., et al. (2004). *Community-based participatory research.* RTI International-University of North Carolina Evidence-Based Practice Center, Contract No. 290-02-0016. Rockville, MD: Agency for Healthcare Research and Quality.

Wallerstein, N. (1999). Power between evaluator and community: Research relationships within New Mexico's healthier communities. *Social Science & Medicine, 49*(1), 39–53.

Wallerstein, N., & Duran, B. M. (2003). The conceptual, historical, and practice roots of community-based participatory research and related participatory traditions. In M. Minkler & N. Wallerstein (Eds.), *Community-based participatory research for health* (pp. 27–52). San Francisco: Jossey-Bass.

Wallerstein, N., Polacsek, M., & Maltrud, K. (2002). Participatory evaluation model for coalitions: The development of systems indicators. *Health Promotion Practice, 3*(3), 361–373.

Wang, C., & Burris, M. A. (1994). Empowerment through photo novella: Portraits of participation. *Health Education Quarterly, 21*(2), 171–186.

Weiss, E. S., Anderson, R. M., & Lasker, R. D. (2002). Making the most of collaboration: Exploring the relationship between partnership synergy and partnership functioning. *Health Education & Behavior, 29*(6), 683–698.

Whyte, W. F. (1991). *Participatory action research.* Thousand Oaks, CA: Sage.

Williams, D. R., & Collins, C. (1995). US socioeconomic and racial differences in health: Patterns and explanations. *Annual Review of Sociology, 21,* 349–386.

PART TWO

PARTNERSHIP FORMATION AND MAINTENANCE

Partnership formation and maintenance is a fundamental component of all community-based participatory research efforts. Many of the guiding principles for conducting CBPR focus on the role of partners and partnerships in the process. As described in the Introduction to this volume and elsewhere (Israel, Schulz, Parker, & Becker, 1998; Israel et al., 2003), these principles include an emphasis on developing collaborative, equitable partnerships; promoting capacity building and co-learning among all partners; disseminating results to all partners and involving all partners in the dissemination process; and supporting a long-term process and commitment. At the same time, community-researcher partnerships are complex and multidimensional and range from community driven and community initiated on one end of the partnership continuum to outside researcher initiated and controlled on the other end (Minkler & Wallerstein, 2003). Although numerous benefits result from partners working together successfully across diverse backgrounds, values, priorities, and expertise (Israel et al., 1998; Northridge et al., 2000; Schulz et al., 2003), developing and maintaining successful partnerships is considered one of the most challenging aspects of CBPR efforts (Green et al., 1995; Israel et al., 2001; Sullivan et al., 2003).

In Part Two (Chapters Two and Three), we focus on a range of *process methods* for forming and maintaining research partnerships, regardless of the specific focus of the project and the data collection methods used. As discussed in these two chapters, although it is essential to pay attention to partnership-related issues during the initial phases of a CBPR endeavor, continual attention to maintaining the partnership over time is equally essential.

In Chapter Two, Wallerstein, Duran, Minkler, and Foley draw upon their experiences working directly with American Indian tribes and urban and rural community-based organizations in New Mexico and California. They provide answers to the question, How do we start? and offer an in-depth discussion of four broad strategies that they recommend university or other institutionally based researchers consider during the initial phase of a CBPR partnership and beyond. These strategies are to assess and reflect on each member's personal capacities as well as each member's institution's capacities to participate in a partnership; to work with existing social networks, organizations, and community leaders in identifying potential partners and partnerships; to negotiate with community partners in determining each health issue that will be a focus of the research; and to engage in constituency building and organizational development in order to create and support structures to sustain the partnership. The authors' case examples reflect diverse conceptualizations of community partners, making their recommended strategies relevant to the diversity of the settings in which we all work. The authors stress throughout the need for critical self-reflection and ongoing attention to deeply rooted issues, such as historical legacies and current identities and contexts, as they affect the members' ability to effectively develop and maintain their CBPR partnership.

In Chapter Three, Becker, Israel, and Allen draw on the literatures on evaluation of CBPR partnerships and on group dynamics to make a convincing argument that CBPR partnerships must attend to group processes in order to achieve the goals and objectives of their research and action projects. This chapter is organized around twelve elements of group dynamics that are relevant to CBPR partnerships (such as ensuring equitable participation and open communication, establishing norms for working together, developing goals and objectives, addressing power and influence, resolving conflicts, and working in culturally diverse groups). For each of these elements the authors provide concrete examples of numerous strategies, techniques, and specific exercises that they have used for developing and maintaining effective CBPR partnerships in their work in Michigan and Louisiana. The strategies and techniques described in this chapter are useful in multiple contexts for strengthening CBPR partnerships through appropriate attention to group dynamics.

References

Green, L. W., George, M. A., Daniel, M., Frankish, C. J., Herbert, C. J., Bowie, W. R., et al. (1995). *Study of participatory research in health promotion.* Ottawa: Royal Society of Canada.

Israel, B. A., Lichtenstein, R., Lantz, P., McGranaghan, R., Allen, A., Guzman, J. R., et al. (2001). The Detroit Community-Academic Urban Research Center: Development, implementation and evaluation. *Journal of Public Health Management and Practice, 7*(5), 1–19.

Israel, B. A., Schulz, A. J., Parker, E. A., & Becker, A. B. (1998). Review of community-based research: Assessing partnership approaches to improve public health. *Annual Review of Public Health, 19,* 173–202.

Israel, B. A., Schulz, A. J., Parker, E. A., Becker, A. B., Allen, A., & Guzman, J. R. (2003). Critical issues in developing and following community-based participatory research principles. In M. Minkler & N. Wallerstein (Eds.), *Community-based participatory research for health* (pp. 56–73). San Francisco: Jossey-Bass.

Minkler, M., & Wallerstein, N. (Eds.). (2003). *Community-based participatory research for health.* San Francisco: Jossey-Bass.

Northridge, M. E., Vallone, D., Merzel, C., Greene, D., Shepard, P. M., Cohall, A. T., et al. (2000). The adolescent years: An academic-community partnership in Harlem comes of age. *Journal of Public Health Management & Practice, 6*(1), 53–60.

Schulz, A. J., Israel, B. A., Parker, E. A., Locket, M., Hill, Y., & Wills, R. (2003). Engaging women in community-based participatory research for health: The East Side Village Health Worker Partnership. In M. Minkler & N. Wallerstein (Eds.), *Community-based participatory research for health* (pp. 293–315). San Francisco: Jossey-Bass.

Sullivan, M., Chao, S., Allen, C. A., Koné, A., Pierre-Louis, M., & Krieger, J. (2003). Community-research partnerships: Perspectives from the field. In M. Minkler & N. Wallerstein (Eds.), *Community-based participatory research for health* (pp. 113–130). San Francisco: Jossey-Bass.

CHAPTER TWO

Developing and Maintaining Partnerships with Communities

Nina Wallerstein, Bonnie Duran, Meredith Minkler, and Kevin Foley

M ost of the guiding principles for conducting community-based participatory research reflect the work of partners and the concept of partnership. CBPR is described as supporting "collaborative, equitable partnerships in all phases of the research," which will "promote co-learning and capacity building among partners," "disseminate findings and knowledge gained to all partners and involve all partners in the dissemination process." Finally, it will "involve long-term process and commitment" (Israel et al. 2003, pp. 56–58).

CBPR *is* dependent on partnerships, yet the skills and methods we need to develop and maintain research partnerships often are not taught or explored in academic settings. In addition, those of us who are trained researchers based in universities, health and social service agencies, and other institutions may read about the importance of partnerships yet may neglect to engage in ongoing self-reflection about the inevitable challenges and dilemmas we face in initiating, nurturing, and maintaining partnerships. Finally, our community partners may

Acknowledgments: We wish to honor our tribal partners in the Southwest and our other urban community partners for their collaboration in the research discussed in this chapter. We acknowledge partial funding by grants K01MH02018, National Institute of Mental Health; U01 AA14926, National Institute on Alcohol Abuse and Alcoholism; and PO30 ES012072-01 National Institute of Environmental Health Sciences. Points of view in this article are those of the authors and do not represent the views of the funding agencies.

not be sufficiently aware of the imperatives of university and other institutional settings, which may inhibit the development of mutually beneficial partnerships.

Research partnerships are multidimensional and range across a continuum, with partnerships initiated and driven by communities at one end and collaborations initiated and controlled by universities or other "outside experts" at the other (Minkler & Wallerstein, 2003). Traditionally, universities or health and social service agencies have identified funding sources, responded to requests for proposals, and approached communities for their involvement. Increasingly, however, ongoing partnerships are being developed in which multiple groups of stakeholders raise concerns that are parlayed into mutual research pursuits. Most often relationships evolve in the course of a CBPR project, with projects that may have been initiated by one partner becoming more collaborative in their decision-making structure.

It is still rare, however, for communities to control the research process, as the expertise and structures of research most often reside in the institutional settings, such as universities, that have the benefit of methodological expertise, resources to execute grant proposals, human research review committees, and the explicit scholarly mission of the academy. Although some important exceptions exist (for example, the research structures being instituted in some tribal nations and discussed later in this chapter), the control that universities and other partners from outside the community continue to exert over most CBPR efforts underscores the importance of paying careful attention to the development of relationships with community partners that can work to redress such power imbalances and promote mutually satisfying collaborations.

Those of us who are professionally trained researchers may be fortunate in that we are able to build on existing relationships with communities through groundwork laid by our academic colleagues, our community colleagues, or our own personal connections with the community. Some of us may share common identities with the community, or we may be *insider outsiders:* insiders because of our bonds with the community owing to race, gender, or disability, for example; yet at the same time outsiders for other reasons, such as educational attainment. We may have to start de novo and therefore face challenges in being accepted. We may face failure and have to leave a community. These relationships are never static and may ebb and flow over time. If our partnership relationships are less than optimal during a certain period, we may be tempted to blame our institutions or our community partners, yet we also need to reflect on our own roles. In all cases we need to ask ourselves such questions as: Why do we want to work with a particular community? What are the benefits to us? What are the benefits to the community? and, What is the mutual benefit?

Those of us who have engaged in CBPR to bring about change will recognize that the process is fluid, dynamic, at times fast-paced and at times slow, and always requires long-term commitment. The old axiom "plan and then implement the plan" is too simplistic. To succeed, CBPR processes must be open to permutations and reformulations. Unexpected obstacles can surface, such as staff turnover or changes in leadership. Partnership means spending the time to develop trust and, most important, to develop the structures that support trust, so that moves in unexpected directions or setbacks can be seen as part of a long-term process that will continue.

The purpose of this chapter is to describe the how-to methods and the challenges of partnership development and maintenance, primarily for academic and other outside research partners. We expect, however, that all readers, including community partners and those new to CBPR, will benefit from the self-reflection and dialogue presented. We will discuss strategies and various starting points for developing partnerships, methods for developing and incorporating collaborative principles that support an effective partnership, means of addressing the dilemmas that are inherent in the coming together of the various contexts represented by outside researchers and communities, and issues in maintaining partnerships over the long haul.

In this chapter we draw on our own research experience and that of colleagues in working directly with Native American tribes and rural and urban community-based organizations (CBOs). Although we often use the shorthand of referring to *university* and *community* partners and although most of the examples we share reflect community-university partnerships, the reader is reminded here that researchers may be housed in any number of institutions and settings, such as health and human service departments, governmental and private nonprofit agencies, and integrated care systems. Community members and partners may be the staff and members of CBOs, including professionals with research expertise, or they may be residents of a shared neighborhood or members of a community of identity, such as gay or bisexual men who are HIV positive or teen mothers drawn together by common concerns. In the discussion that follows, we have purposely chosen case examples that reflect and employ various conceptualizations of community partners as we illustrate questions for critical reflection by researchers, regardless of the settings in which we work.

HOW DO WE START?

There is no one starting place, no single technique, no magic bullet for the development of relationships and partnerships with communities. As suggested earlier, this chapter defines a *community* as people who have a shared identity, whether that identity is based on geography, political affiliation, culture, race or ethnicity, faith or religion, sovereign tribal nationhood, institutional connections such as schools or workplaces, or other shared identification with a group

(Minkler & Wallerstein, 2003). Particularly when outside researchers are attempting to partner with geographical communities, there is a tendency to accept traditional definitions and boundaries, such as census or zip code tracts used for data collection. It is critical, however, that researchers begin by recognizing that residents within a geographical area may have their own designations and set of boundaries, for example, the neighborhood across the tracks or the location of a historically important event. It is shared identity and the institutions and associations that grow up within shared identity that allow the development of partnerships, and outside research partners must begin by getting to know how "the community" is in fact defined by those with whom they hope to partner.

Getting to know the community in all its complexity and in ways that are consistent with the principles of CBPR also means looking at the community through new sets of lenses. For several decades, Kretzmann and McKnight (1993) have admonished health and social service professionals to place far more attention on looking for community assets and strengths rather than simply for community needs and concerns. These strengths may reside within individual community members and leaders and within those community-based organizations that give the community a voice. At the neighborhood level these groups may be parent-teacher organizations, safety watch groups, or coalitions that have developed around community-identified concerns. When we develop academic-community partnerships or coalitions that do not come directly from the community, it is important that they not be window dressing, put together at the last minute because of a grant mandate. We need to consider how to make a partnership reflect the culture of the community and not simply replicate a *professional culture,* which may make participants uncomfortable. By respecting the community's expert knowledge concerning its assets as well as its needs and concerns, we will be in a much better position to forge egalitarian CBPR partnerships. (See Chapter Four for a discussion of the use of key informant interviews and focus groups to assess community strengths and resources as well as challenges and problems.)

Starting a research relationship for a specific project is always easier when we have a previous positive connection with the community, through, for example, services our agency or university provides, previous research collaborations, or referrals from trustworthy sources or through reputation. Students often will have facilitated trust and rapport through previous community projects or through their roles as research assistants. University reputations and previous institutional collaborations may also be problematic, however, which adds challenges to developing trust. Most often, we face both positive and negative existing connections.

When we have no previous connections, we need to rely on hard work and time to build the relationships. Public health professor and CBPR partner Mary

Northridge (2003) appropriately admonishes university faculty who desire to engage in CBPR to listen, show up, be yourself, and believe in social justice. One of the most important strategies in developing or strengthening relationships is to physically "show up" in the community, turning out for community events and demonstrating respect through our willingness to meet on the community's turf, rather than expecting residents to come to the university. Just showing up may make the situation worse, however, if outside researchers are arrogant or inflexible about their research agenda or if they underestimate the knowledge and grant-writing experience of community partners. Respect is an earned quality; it involves developing a mutually beneficial relationship and being responsive to the diverse needs of different constituents and partners. For example, Galen el-Askari and Sheryl Walton, former health department employees in West Contra Costa County, California, write that for gaining credibility it was important not merely to show up but also to help cook for a community memorial service after a drive-by shooting. The Healthy Neighborhood Project they helped create went on to become an effective community and health department collaboration through which CBPR frequently is conducted (el-Askari & Walton, 2004; el-Askari et al., 1998). This partnership might never have achieved this level of success had not the health department staff literally and figuratively shown up for and been part of numerous occasions of importance to local residents.

Four strategies are helpful for us as university or other institution-based researchers as we seek to begin a community partnership:

1. Self-reflecting on our capacities, resources, and potential liabilities as health professionals or academics interested in engaging with the community; this includes reflecting on our institution's capacities, resources, and potential liabilities as well and identifying historical and current relationships between the institution and the community.

2. Identifying potential partners and partnerships through appropriate networks, associations, and leaders.

3. Negotiating the health issue(s) for research; even if initiated by the university, issues and research questions can be reframed through the partnership.

4. Creating and nurturing structures to sustain partnerships through constituency building and organizational development.

These strategies are not sequential and may take place simultaneously, with strategies 3 and 4 in particular lending themselves to interchangeability in terms of time sequence. Yet all of these strategies require continual attention, and those carried out early in a partnership need to be revisited, especially when new partners join a long-standing relationship.

Strategy 1: Reflect on Our Capacities and Our Institution's Capacities to Engage in Partnership

To assess our capacities and resources as researchers working with communities, it is important to think about our own strengths as individuals and as the institutions we represent, our weaknesses as individuals and institutions, the benefits we might gain, and the dangers or concerns we might face. This assessment should include reflection about our own position of power in relation to the community, including the historical and current relationship of our institution to the community (Wallerstein, 1999; Israel et al., 2003).

One of the most important skills in this assessment of our own capacities is the ability to listen to ourselves as well as to and with our community partners. Such active and introspective listening requires patience, silence, and an attitude of openness, discovery, and nondefensiveness (Chávez, Duran, Baker, Avila, & Wallerstein, 2003; Freire, 1982; Wallerstein, 1999). There is much to learn from all sides of the partnership, from the community members working with the university to the university researchers working with the community.

For CBPR researchers in academic settings, part of listening to our history involves reflecting on and learning from the activist scholar traditions that reemerged in the 1960s, when many researchers moved out of the academy to participate in social movements and in local struggles to improve economic conditions (Macdonnel, 1986). For activist scholars these historical roles included helping to shine a spotlight on everyday forms of resistance among marginalized communities; the role of culture in everyday practices; the local, regional, and national context of social issues; and the reality of community partners with agency to define their agenda and identities as decision-makers (Ong, 1987).

In the 1970s and '80s, a key innovation of the new social movements was the shift from a predominantly Marxist analysis to analyses that combined economic analysis with an examination of the multiple ways people were oppressed owing to culture, race, sexual orientation, and other identities (Laclau & Mouffe, 1985). Academics engaged in CBPR began to see themselves as giving voice to people's lived experiences, with the belief that "only those directly concerned can speak in a practical way on their own behalf" (Macdonnel, 1986, p. 16). Yet beyond giving voice, the role of the academic intellectual could also shift in its academic discourse in order to "weaken the existing links between power and knowledge" and prevent local knowledge from being devalued and undermined (Macdonnel, p. 16). Our task, then, has become to extend beyond our legacy of "ventriloquism," or speaking *for* community members, to work in union with others to create multiple spaces (such as meetings and publications) in which the lived experience of our partners can be heard and validated (Spivak, 1990).

A second process of listening involves making explicit historical abuses (for example, the academic invention of "primitive societies," in part as a justification for colonization; Pierpont, 2004; Said, 1979). Such abuses may be relived and can reverberate in contemporary CBPR work with communities. New stories of alleged abuse (as in the Havasupai tribe's multimillion dollar lawsuit against Arizona State University for using tribal blood samples in ways for which research participants had not given consent [Potkonjak, 2004]) take on added potency in the face of such historical realities. One strategy to reduce such mistrust involves what Foucault has termed *effective history*—a critique of the universities' definition of the "other" and a retelling of the past that refutes the dominant perspective (Dean, 1994). One use of effective history is for researchers to create space for community partners to retell their histories of previous relationships with universities that contribute to mistrust and misunderstanding. This offers an opportunity for university and community CBPR partners to uncover previous inequalities and to choose a new approach that is not an inevitable outcome of the past.

A third process of listening is to uncover the role of power dynamics in our own collaborative processes. As researchers we have the power base of being perceived as having expert or scientific knowledge, and this may inadvertently prevent community knowledge from being viewed as equally legitimate. Many of us who are white or middle-class academics working in communities of color may fail to recognize the ways in which "unearned privilege" may foster stereotyping (McIntosh, 1989) or may maintain internalized oppression among community members who assume they have less to offer.

In addition, as principal investigators or as institution-based researchers we often have the power of resources. We may, for example, choose to engage in a re-granting mechanism, distributing subcontracts to community partners, but this may be potentially problematic if community members become interested in the jobs or resources primarily as economic benefit rather than as means to investigate the research questions. The Native American Research Centers for Health (NARCH), established in 2001 and funded by the National Institutes of Health and the Indian Health Service (IHS), has provided one strategy to alter the power imbalance (IHS, 2004); the NARCH request-for-proposal process allows only tribes or tribal entities to be principal investigators, with the tribes then negotiating subcontract agreements with their university partners.

Finally, as part of self-reflection, we should encourage each researcher who has privilege to consider how best to be an ally to research colleagues of color and to the communities with which he or she works. All of us have intersecting contexts, being in the dominant group in terms of power in some domains (for example, race or ethnicity, class, sexual orientation, or ability or disability) but not others (for example, gender or religion) (Stewart & McDermott, 2004; also see Arnold, Burke, James, Martin, & Thomas, 1991, for an exercise dealing with one's own power constellations). For example, university junior minority faculty may lead research projects but not have the power to influence their institutions' priorities for hiring, promotion, or student recruitment toward diversity. Public health faculty doing CBPR within schools of medicine can also become marginalized because of the higher status accorded to biomedical research.

Although we may face formidable obstacles to changing power imbalances within our institutions and with our community partners (such as funding mandates and norms that support giving superior validity to expert knowledge), as Foucault (1980) reminds us, power is inherently unstable and therefore can be challenged. In their review of the literature on institutional factors that facilitate community-university research partnerships, Seifer and colleagues (Community-Campus Partnerships for Health, 2003) note the importance of centers that support partnerships, interdisciplinary values, and faculty and student involvement in the community (Calleson, Seifer, & Maurana, 2002). Some universities are moving toward models that reward faculty who emphasize the scholarship of engagement, including CBPR (Seifer, 2003). Individual faculty can also change power dynamics, for example, by assisting their community partners to be principal investigators.

As Anne Bishop points out, however, oppressions are not all the same. In her book on becoming an ally, she describes an international visitor talking to a group of low-income, single mothers. They tell "her about some of their organizing work. 'Poverty?' the visitor says. 'What do you know about poverty? This is nothing'" (Bishop, 2002, p. 16). It is important to learn to live with the contradiction of finding that we have similarities with all people, including our own experiences of oppression, and yet at the same time refuse to take advantage by claiming the same level of marginalization. By recognizing our privilege, our power bases, we can have the integrity to create authentic partnerships (Labonte, 2004), which honor the strengths and knowledge each partner brings to the table.

Strategy 2: Identify Potential Partners and Partnerships Through Appropriate Networks, Associations, and Leaders

An important CBPR task is to identify potential community partners, and consider the practical, political, and personal implications of partnership choices. Ideally, the CBPR research topic comes from the community, and a concerned CBO may approach the university, health department, or other research organization about partnering to explore this topic. Frequently, however, it is a university faculty member or other outside researcher who wishes to initiate a partnership, and in such situations several steps should be taken.

First, outside researchers should plan to spend considerable time getting to know the community before they approach individuals, groups, or organizations about their interest in partnering. This process is important not only for gaining local credibility (Lewis & Ford, 1990) but also for getting a better sense of the groups that may be the most appropriate collaborators.

One of the authors of this chapter (Meredith Minkler) and her primary research partner (a graduate student with a disability) had each been independently involved with a local disability community for many years before they began discussing the possibility of engaging in a CBPR project with that community. Because the topic and proposed goal of the study was controversial (broadening the dialogue within the disability community about attitudes toward "death with dignity" legislation), meeting with key community stakeholders in advance and assessing their interest and concerns was imperative. Minkler and her research partner agreed that they would not proceed unless community buy-in could be achieved. Their existing status, one as an able-bodied ally and one as a member of the community, helped them know which stakeholders to approach for initial guidance, which organizations to approach about potential partnering, and once an agreement was achieved, how to form a diverse advisory committee whose membership reflected the differences of opinion about this topic in the larger disability community (Fadem et al., 2003).

For university faculty and other researchers not as familiar with the community with which they hope to partner, a variety of tools may be useful. Action-oriented community assessment and methods for identifying "movers and shakers" can help researchers find community partners and learn a community's perceived assets and concerns (Eng & Blanchard, 1990–1991; Hancock & Minkler, 2004; also see Chapter Four in this volume). Such techniques, however, are best used with the advice of community collaborators who can help determine which methods will function best in the unique context of their community. Again, although this chapter uses the shorthand of *the community*, it should be recalled at this point that the communities with which researchers partner are not monolithic and often a wide range of perspectives are present. Tribal communities, for example, have an official sovereign government, often a combination of traditional precolonization leadership and western bureaucratic forms dating from the Indian Reorganization Act of 1925. In addition to these political leaders, tribal communities have spiritual, cultural, and other leaders. CBPR efforts may start with official government representatives but may not stay there.

In a project in which chapter authors Bonnie Duran and Kevin Foley were involved, a progressive and farsighted division of a tribal health department applied for and received a large federal grant aimed at developing and integrating HIV services for a large tribe in the Southwest. The tribal council health committee, however, was the official lead agency, responsible for oversight of the research work and all other contract obligations. The health committee had factions that were very opposed to this work; some members even felt people with HIV should be quarantined. After the depth of the stigma was uncovered in the official body, the partners involved in this effort deliberately chose to work only with a small division of the official governmental agency and with a nongovernmental agency (NGO) on the reservation. They steered clear of more contentious governmental elements.

The need to recognize the multiple voices of a single community highlights the challenges of community participation. It is often a lot easier to attract service providers, professionals, and policymakers to board meetings than to get community members such as parents, low-wage workers, and the elderly to attend regularly. Service providers, especially staff of locally initiated CBOs, may also be community members. Ideally, community partners will emerge from previous collaborative work and the building of mutual respect; however, when university partners must actively seek new community partners, identification and selection criteria for people and organizations might include being well respected in the community, being knowledgeable about the community, having a long-standing history of working on community issues, and having a prior positive history of working in partnerships. Community partners may consider their own criteria for academic partners, looking for qualities such as commitment to the community beyond the funding period and flexibility in regard to university mandates.

An effective partnership clearly is dependent on the ability of people possessing diverse community and university perspectives to meet and actively participate. Some of the most obvious barriers to attendance for community members can be overcome by providing food, transportation, and child care and by holding meetings at the facilities of community partner organizations. Community members face many other barriers to attendance, however, such as job demands, other time commitments, and lack of official recognition for their work with the partnership. In the Healthy Neighborhoods Project, the health department began granting flextime to program employees. Once they were able to work from noon to 9 P.M. and on weekends, they were better able to engage in CBPR efforts at times that worked best for community residents. As the partnerships in this project matured, this show of respect was reciprocated, as community members began arranging their schedules so they could attend daytime events at the health department (el-Askari & Walton, 2004).

Encouraging active participation in CBPR activities also requires the use of methods and approaches that can reduce the intimidation community members may feel in groups characterized by major status differences. These methods may include nominal group processes (Delbecq, Van de Ven, & Gustafson, 1975); collaborative mapping of community indicators, risks, and assets (Hancock & Minkler, 2004); and support for bringing community voices to the table. (For a full discussion of these approaches, see Chapter Three in this volume; Minkler & Wallerstein, 2003; Sharpe, Greany, Lee, & Royce, 2000.)

Although the importance of constantly working to deepen the participation of our community partners cannot be overstated, outside researchers, particularly those of us who enjoy the "unearned benefits" of "white privilege" (McIntosh, 1989), also need to be aware of the impacts of racism on both the context in which we work and the process of the work itself. In our own CBPR work, we have identified various ways in which the levels of racism (institutional, interpersonal, and internalized) identified by Camara Jones (2000) have impeded our ability to authentically partner and identify the best networks. Community members may have differential access to knowledge and representation in institutions that affects their ability to connect as community partners. They may feel uncomfortable with the potential for stereotyping and believe they do not have opinions to offer. Or they may want to protect the community's hidden voices from perceived threats (Scott, 1990). To avoid such situations, and to confront them more honestly and openly when they do arise, outside researchers need to enter the community and the partnership with what Tervalon and Murray-Garcia (1998) have termed *cultural humility*. These authors make a distinction between this concept and the more popular term *cultural competence,* which describes an end point none of us can truly achieve because we cannot truly be competent in another's culture. The term *cultural humility* refers instead to "a lifelong commitment to self-evaluation and self-critique" to redress power imbalances and "develop and maintain mutually respectful and dynamic partnerships with communities" (Tervalon & Murray-Garcia, p. 118). Achieving cultural humility might involve a willingness to acknowledge institutional racism and an openness to changing organizations, through training in how to work effectively across cultures, for example.

Strategy 3: Negotiate or Reframe the Ultimate Health Issue(s) for Research

Ideally, all CBPR research projects become a negotiated process between community and outside research partners. In a newly formed partnership or an existing partnership where there is flexibility in choosing the research agenda, one of the first strategies is to gather information on community needs, concerns, resources, and strengths. Out of a data-gathering and prioritization strategy, research ideas will emerge. Even when the health issues to be investigated are determined by the university or other outside research partners, issues and research questions can be reframed through the partnership, as new needs and concerns emerge over time or as community concerns become clarified through increased trust and communication. Beyond the typical participatory data collection and prioritization methods used to identify needs and strengths (Wallerstein & Sheline, 1998; Eng & Blanchard, 1990–1991; Duran & Duran, 2000;

Hancock & Minkler, 2004; also see Part Four of this volume), a CBPR partnership will also benefit from identifying the culturally defined etiological theories and culturally specific mechanisms for change. No true prioritization can happen without the community's perspective being paramount.

Typically, universities have privileged empirically derived knowledge and empirically supported interventions (ESIs); yet increasingly there is a recognition of another valuable source of research, that of culturally supported interventions (CSIs), the indigenous theories and practices that emerge from communities (Hall, 2001). Many of the practices of community programs have never been formally studied or evaluated, nor have they been subject to rigorous exploration of their effectiveness for the specific population. Yet they are widespread and well utilized (consider, for example, Native American and Hispanic traditional healers and community-level and explanatory models such as cultural revitalization approaches). Recognizing these streams of knowledge is helpful for legitimizing the community perspective in a partnership.

For example, the case study that follows highlights the use of a culturally supported intervention by a CBPR partnership involving a tribal CBO treatment center, a tribal health department, and the University of New Mexico. The culturally supported intervention was the integration of traditional medicine into HIV/AIDS and substance abuse treatment, alongside medical care and other mainstream services provided by the Indian Health Service. Traditional healers are able to integrate the healing of diseases with attention to the psychological, physical, and emotional impact of genocide, or "historical traumas" (Brave Heart & DeBruyn, 1998; Duran, Duran, & Brave Heart, 1998; Duran, 1996; Duran & Walters, in press). Recently, historical trauma has emerged in Native American communities as an important theory of etiology for many social and medical problems. In this partnership the university supported the use of a culturally supported theory and made it a key component of the intervention, even though there is as yet no empirical evidence base to support its use. For outside researchers engaged in CBPR, understanding and appreciating concepts like historical trauma may prove critical to their ability to function effectively in and with oppressed communities.

The Community-Based Organization Perspective

From a community-based organization (CBO) perspective, universities, local health departments, and other research institutions need to understand a range of concerns: the possible draining of resources, talent, or money from the community; the potential competition and different, sometimes conflicting, regulations that exist between agencies; the distinct relationships agencies and community members have with the outside institution; and the possibility that outside institution guidelines might not reflect the needs of collaborative relationships. All these issues were present in one community-initiated research project in the Southwest.

In 2001, the clinical director of a Native American alcohol treatment CBO (Kevin Foley, one of the authors of this chapter) contemplated the possibility of applying for support for an integration of services research project, and called another community-based agency serving Native clients that provided HIV case management services. The executive director of the case management agency was interested, so a meeting was arranged with medical providers, social services providers, and researchers from the university (led by Bonnie Duran, also one of the authors of this chapter) to discuss forming a collaborative to apply for the grant. From the outset there was an agreement to start with culturally appropriate interventions and to make traditional healers central.

Concerns, however, remained among the partners. The HIV case management agency, with the Indian Health Service and the tribal government, had worked for five years on the first round of funding with Duran and wanted her as evaluator on the next five-year submission. Foley expressed his concern that his board might not buy into contracting for evaluation services. The CBO's board had a policy of not hiring outside contractors because in the past outside contractors had not been invested in the organization; the board's preference was to hire local evaluators to develop local capacity. Foley and Duran had known each other for several years, however, and trust had already been established. Hence Foley was able to convince his board to participate with this new collaborative and to contract with the university. In support of the board's agreement to work with the university, Duran assisted in making arrangements for training CBO staff in motivational interviewing at no cost. The training was offered to all agency members of the collaboration, providing an immediate service as part of the research project.

University guidelines however made it difficult to view Foley as an equal partner. Although he was principal investigator for the federal funding, the university's institutional review board (IRB) refused to allow his name to be placed on the participant consent form. The research collaborative was forced to accept this IRB condition, although it dishonored the community partner. Because of the long-standing relationship between Duran and Foley and the evolving relationships with other partners, the partnership has continued and has been able to openly reflect on and negotiate such issues as they emerge.

Strategy 4: Create and Nurture Structures to Sustain Partnerships Through Constituency Building and Organizational Development

The success of a CBPR partnership is heavily dependent on outside researchers' ability to develop strong personal relationships with communities, in part through showing up, demonstrating cultural humility, and showing a willingness to share power and resources. In addition, however, the ability to sustain lasting partnerships rests on careful attention to the development of new joint institutional structures, including new ways of working collaboratively based on mutually agreed-upon principles.

Although Israel and her colleagues (2003) have articulated a common set of principles that are widely used in the field, they also advise each new and ongoing partnership to develop its own principles to ensure local appropriateness and local ownership. The Oakland Community Health Academy, which grew out of the W. K. Kellogg Foundation–funded Community-Based Public Health Initiative, provides one example of collaborative development of principles and related goals (Brown & Vega, 1996). Located in the heart of an economically depressed but culturally vibrant urban area, the academy comprised local residents and representatives of the health department and of the School of Public Health at the University of California, Berkeley. Together, they crafted a research protocol designed to be a starting point for wider dialogue on the question, "How relevant is academic research to the health needs of our community?" The protocol asks such questions as, "How will research processes and outcomes serve the community?" and, "Are the research methods sufficiently rigorous yet true to community-based principles that incorporate perspectives and beliefs of community residents?" (Brown & Vega, pp. 4–5).

Such questions and sets of principles can become even more codified when working with American Indian tribes, as tribal codes tend to expand the general principles of respect and collaboration to emphasize the need to recognize government-to-government relationships in the research specifics, addressing such issues as who controls the data (see, for example, Turning Point, 2003). The Navajo Nation, which has its own institutional review board, articulates a research process for all researchers interested in conducting research with Navajo people on or near the reservation. The first phase calls for developing local ownership. This involves designating a Navajo tribal member or other "local" individual as a coinvestigator and seeking resolutions of support from at least 3 of the 110 Navajo Nation chapters (local community governing bodies) or from other local entities, such as school boards or health advisory boards, that may have responsibility over the study sites. The IRB research protocol must state how the tribe will benefit and how the results will be turned into community education or other technical assistance. Quarterly reports of progress are required, as are in-person reports to the IRB. The final report and dissemination plan for sharing the data with chapter houses and tribal programs must be submitted to the board, which has final approval. All outside dissemination, such as conference presentations, journal articles, and other products such as videos and photographs, is subject to board review and approval. Ultimately, the data are owned by the tribe and housed in the Navajo Nation Data Resource Center.

In addition to collaboratively developing working principles and guidelines as a basis for research partnerships, the work of sustaining partnerships means continuing to challenge institutional bureaucracies that have a stake in policies and practices that may militate against authentic partnerships. Change needs to be a process that takes place on all sides of a partnership rather than being focused solely on the community.

For example, in an adaptation of the Healthy Neighborhoods Project in Berkeley, California, health department staff successfully made their own agency a target for systems change. By holding monthly staff meetings on topics such as the different forms of racism and by working to address civil service restrictions that had often precluded the hiring of resident community organizers whom staff had trained, project staff demonstrated a commitment to institutional change as an often necessary condition for growing authentic partnerships (el-Askari & Walton, 2004). In another example, tribes and one of the chapter authors (Nina Wallerstein) successfully challenged a university IRB to reduce its boilerplate survey consent form from four pages to a single page. By mobilizing letters of support from tribal leaders, the university partner was able to convince her institution's IRB to adopt a more community-accessible product.

In addition to starting from a base of principles and agreements and viewing outside institutions as potential systems change targets, several other organizational strategies are helpful for developing early success. They include providing an immediately recognizable service to community partners; developing a vision statement, a mission statement, and a partnership agreement on leadership and decision making; and giving time to relationship building.

In partnering with communities it is crucial to establish the benefit of working with the outside institution and to provide mechanisms for feedback to the community in the short as well as the long term. Thinking in terms of short action research cycles is important because traditional epidemiological or intervention research is a multiple-year endeavor, where findings are often not returned to the community until well over a year after data are collected. Potential shorter-term benefits for communities might include training provided by outside researchers, help with writing grants, or technical assistance, which may or may not be directly related to the research. In a collaboration between West Harlem Environmental Action (WE ACT) and its research partners at the Columbia University Children's Environmental Health Center, a faculty member has offered sessions in environmental health issues for WE ACT's ambitious community leadership training program at the same time that WE ACT staff continue to be invaluable research partners with the center (Peggy Shepard and Patrick L. Kinney, personal communications, March 2004).

A key structural issue is the need to recognize that each partner has its own imperatives and needs, which may overlap but will be different from those of the other partners. Time, for example, is a dimension in which there will be key differences between academic and community partners. Academic calendars are driven by grant deadlines, student research assistant availability during semesters, or faculty needs to produce for tenure and promotion. Community calendars are driven by a desire for research results that can be disseminated quickly in support of action objectives. Community member participation in partnerships is often driven by members' other political or cultural commitments and will likely not be in sync with an academic calendar.

In addition to attending to time in terms of schedules, partners need to honor the time required for relationship building. For example, during the recent development of a substance abuse intervention center that required a community advisory board, researchers at the University of New Mexico sought to bring in traditional healers, from both the Latino/Hispanic and American Indian communities. It took an intermediary at the university, a Native research associate with strong ties to the practitioner community, to insist that participants spend the first community advisory board meeting just getting to know each other. Each person took time to talk about the community he or she came from, his or her family, and his or her own history of engagement in alcohol prevention or treatment. Participants simply listened to each other, rather than relying on the dominant culture instrumental approach of following an agenda packed with multiple tasks.

The structural challenges faced by university faculty who engage in CBPR are especially acute for junior faculty, who need to develop a productive research agenda in a timely manner. Time-intensive relationship building must occur before research projects can actually begin data collection, and questions of who has authority to use the data may threaten a junior faculty member's ability to publish in time for tenure and promotion review. Although Native American tribes may be more likely to have formal approval processes for publication of data, other communities of color deserve the same respect, and honoring this principle (through including community members as coauthors of publications, for example) can lengthen considerably the time before publication and in some cases may inhibit release of data. The Council on Practice of the Association of Schools of Public Health has recognized that promoting CBPR may require changes in tenure and promotion guidelines to accommodate these issues (Council on Practice, personal communication with Nina Wallerstein, September 2003).

Building in structures to deal with conflict is an important organizational development strategy, one that promotes proactive decision making and improves the partnership's ability to deal with difficult situations. Conflicts are inevitable; however, effective resolutions of conflict may strengthen the partnership as partners demonstrate commitment to each other and to mutual goals. As Gutierrez and Lewis (2004) suggest, particularly in situations where the researchers and community members are of different racial or ethnic or other groups, recognizing and embracing "the conflict that characterizes cross-cultural work" (pp. 243–244) can be a critical step in the development of respectful and effective collaborative work. (See Chapter Three for a discussion of strategies for addressing conflict in CBPR partnerships.)

Several CBPR assessment instruments have been developed to help academic researchers clarify the depth of involvement among community partners (Green et al., 1995, 2003; Brown & Vega, 1996, 2003). The questions ask about community partner involvement in such aspects of research as setting the research agenda and collecting and analyzing data and also whether there is community capacity building of research skills. These instruments can be used more than once, as partnerships may change throughout a project. Another tool has been developed to evaluate the capacity of health departments for engaging community partners (Parker, Margolis, Eng, & Renriquez-Roldan, 2003). Issues that have been identified as important include agency and employee skills in working with minority populations, the agency's networking with CBOs, and community participation in health department planning.

Although such tools are helpful, they do not fully capture such core issues in partnerships as the role of members' self-reflection about personal and institutional relationships; the ability to create new, interdependent partnering structures and policies; and the ability to create internal change in each participating member's institution. CBPR can be used to challenge the barriers within universities and other research partner institutions to collaborating with communities as well as to challenge the barriers within communities to working with universities and other institutions.

CONCLUSION

In this chapter we have provided principles and methods for developing and maintaining collaborative partnerships with communities for the purpose of better research and improved public health outcomes. This work demands interdependence, with all partners being open to change. The challenge for all outside researchers is to uncover and keep working to address our historical legacies and current identities and contexts as they affect our ability to successfully engage in community-based participatory research. Some excellent guidelines, protocols, and other tools now exist for assessing and supporting community–outside researcher collaboration in CBPR. As this chapter has suggested, however, without the necessary self-reflection and continued attention to many of the deeply rooted issues outlined here, such partnerships may have a difficult time thriving and achieving their goals. In the final analysis, as Maurana, Wolff, Beck, and Simpson (2000) suggest, two of the most important questions for assessing CBPR may well be, "Would the community work with the scholar again?" and, "Would the scholar work with the community again?" Through continued reflection and cultural humility, beginning in the critical early stages of laying the groundwork and developing the partnership, we may strengthen our ability to answer these questions in the affirmative.

References

Arnold, R., Burke, C., James, C., Martin, D., & Thomas, B. (1991). *Educating for a change.* Toronto: Between the Lines.

Bishop, A. (2002). *Becoming an ally: Breaking the cycle of oppression in people.* London: Zed Books.

Brave Heart, M.Y.H., & DeBruyn, L. (1998). The American Indian holocaust: Healing historical unresolved grief. *American Indian Alaska Native Mental Health Research, 8*(2), 56–78.

Brown, L., & Vega, W. A. (1996). A protocol for community based research. *American Journal of Preventive Medicine, 12*(4), 4–5.

Brown, L., & Vega, W. (2003). A protocol for community-based research. In M. Minkler & N. Wallerstein (Eds.), *Community-based participatory research in health* (pp. 407–409). San Francisco: Jossey-Bass.

Calleson, D., Seifer, S. D., & Maurana, C. (2002). Forces affecting community involvement of academic heath centers: Perspectives of institutional and faculty leaders. *Academic Medicine, 77*(1), 72–81.

Chávez, V., Duran, B., Baker, Q., Avila, M., & Wallerstein, N. (2003). The dance of race and privilege in community-based participatory research. In M. Minkler & N. Wallerstein (Eds.), *Community-based participatory research in health* (pp. 81–97). San Francisco: Jossey-Bass.

Community-Campus Partnerships for Health. (2003). *Developing and sustaining community–university partnerships for health research: Infrastructure requirements.* Community-Campus Partnerships for Health, National Institute of Health Report. Retrieved August 18, 2004, from http://www.ccph.info

Dean, M. (1994). *Critical and effective histories: Foucault's methods and historical sociology.* New York: Routledge.

Delbecq, A., Van de Ven, A. H., & Gustafson, D. H. (1975). *Group techniques for program planning: A guide to nominal group and Delphi processes.* Glenview, IL: Scott, Foresman.

Duran, B. (1996). Indigenous versus colonial discourse: Alcohol and American Indian identity. In E. Bird (Ed.), *Dressing in feathers: The construction of the Indian in American popular culture* (pp. 111–128). Boulder: Westview Press.

Duran, B., & Duran, E. (2000). Applied postcolonial research and clinical strategies. In M. Battiste (Ed.), *Reclaiming indigenous voice and vision* (pp. 86–100). Vancouver: UBC Press.

Duran, B., Duran, E., & Brave Heart-Yellow Horse, M. (1998). Native Americans and the trauma of history. In R. Thornton (Ed.), *Studying Native America: Problems and prospects in Native American studies* (pp. 60–76). Madison: University of Wisconsin Press.

Duran, B., & Walters, K. (in press). HIV/AIDS prevention in "Indian country": Current practice, indigenist etiology models and postcolonial approaches to change. *AIDS Education and Prevention.*

el-Askari, G., Freestone, J., Irizarry, C., Kraut, K. L., Mashiyama, S. T., Morgan, M. A., et al. (1998). The Healthy Neighborhoods Project: A local health department's role in catalyzing community development. *Health Education and Behavior, 25*(2), 146–159.

el-Askari, G., & Walton, S. (2004). Local government and resident collaboration to improve health: A case study in capacity building and cultural humility. In M. Minkler (Ed.), *Community organizing and community building for health* (2nd ed., pp. 254–271). New Jersey: Rutgers University Press.

Eng, E., & Blanchard, L. (1990–1991). Action oriented community diagnosis: A health education tool. *International Quarterly of Community Health Education, 11*(2), 96–97.

Fadem, P., Minkler, M., Perry, M., Blum, K., Moore, L., & Rogers, J. (2003). Ethical challenges in community-based participatory research: A case study from the San Francisco Bay Area disability community. In M. Minkler & N. Wallerstein (Eds.), *Community-based participatory research in health* (pp. 242–262). San Francisco: Jossey-Bass.

Foucault, M. (1980). Two lectures. In M. Foucault (Ed.), *Power/knowledge: Selected interviews and other writings, 1972–1977* (pp. 78–108). New York: Pantheon Books.

Freire, P. (1982). Creating alternative research methods: Learning to do it by doing it. In B. Hall, A. Gillette, & R. Tandon (Eds.), *Creating knowledge: A monopoly? Participatory research in development* (pp. 29–40). New Delhi: Society for Participatory Research in Asia.

Green, L. W., George, M. A., Daniel, M., Frankish, C. J., Herbert, C. P., Bowie, W. R., et al. (1995). *Study of participatory research in health promotion.* Ottawa: Royal Society of Canada.

Green, L. W., George, A., Daniel, M., Frankish, C. J., Herbert, C. P., Bowie, W. R., et al. (2003). Guidelines for participatory research in health promotion. In M. Minkler & N. Wallerstein (Eds.), *Community-based participatory research in health* (pp. 419–428). San Francisco: Jossey-Bass.

Gutierrez, L. M., & Lewis, E. (2004). Education, participation, and capacity building in community organizing with women of color. In M. Minkler (Ed.), *Community organizing and community building for health* (2nd ed., pp. 240–253). New Brunswick: Rutgers University Press.

Hall, G. C. (2001). Psychotherapy research with ethnic minorities: Empirical, ethical, and conceptual issues. *Journal of Consulting & Clinical Psychology, 69*(3), 502–510.

Hancock, T., & Minkler, M. (2004). Community health assessment or healthy community assessment. In M. Minkler (Ed.), *Community organizing and community building for health* (2nd ed., pp. 138–157). New Brunswick, NJ: Rutgers University Press.

Indian Health Service. (2004). *Indian Health Service research program: Native American Research Centers for Health.* Retrieved August 18, 2004, from http://www.ihs.gov/medicalprograms/Research/NARCH/narch.cfm

Israel, B. A., Schulz, A., Parker, E., Becker, A., Allen, A., & Guzman, J. R. (2003). Critical issues in developing and following community-based participatory research principles. In M. Minkler & N. Wallerstein (Eds.), *Community-based participatory research in health* (pp. 53–76). San Francisco, Jossey-Bass.

Jones, C. (2000). Levels of racism: A theoretic framework and a gardener's tale. *American Journal of Public Health, 8,* 1212–1215.

Kretzmann, J. P., & McKnight, J. L. (1993). *Building communities from the inside out: A path toward finding and mobilizing a community's assets.* Chicago: ACTA.

Labonte, R. (2004). Community, community development, and the forming of authentic partnerships: Some critical reflections. In M. Minkler (Ed.), *Community organizing and community building for health* (2nd ed., pp. 88–102). New Brunswick, NJ: Rutgers University Press.

Laclau, E., & Mouffe, C. (1985). *Hegemony and socialist strategy: Towards a radical democratic politics.* New York: Verso.

Lewis, E., & Ford, B. (1990). The network utilization project: Incorporating traditional strengths of African Americans into group work practice. *Social Work with Groups, 13*(3), 7–22.

Macdonnel, D. (1986). *Theories of discourse: An introduction.* Oxford: Basil Blackwell.

Maurana, C., Wolff, M., Beck, B. J., & Simpson, D. E. (2000). *Working with our communities: Moving from service to scholarship in the health professions.* San Francisco: Community-Campus Partnerships for Health.

McIntosh, P. (1989). White privilege: Unpacking the invisible knapsack. In M. McGoldrick (Ed.), *Re-visioning family therapy: Race, culture, and gender in clinical practice* (pp. 147–152). New York: Guilford Press.

Minkler, M., & Wallerstein, N. (Eds.). (2003). *Community-based participatory research in health.* San Francisco: Jossey-Bass.

Northridge, M. E. (2003). Partnering to advance public health: Making a difference through government, community, business, and academic vocations. *American Journal of Public Health, 93*(8), 1205–1206.

Ong, A. (1987). *Spirits of resistance and capitalist discipline: Factory women in Malaysia.* Albany: State University of New York Press.

Parker, E., Margolis, L. H., Eng, E., & Renriquez-Roldan, C. (2003). Assessing the capacity of health departments to engage in community-based participatory public health. *American Journal of Public Health, 93*(3), 472–476.

Pierpont, C. R. (2004, March 8). The measure of America: The anthropologist who fought racism. *The New Yorker,* pp. 48–63.

Potkonjak, M. (2004, March 17). Havasupai tribe files $50 M lawsuit against Arizona State University. *East Valley Tribune.* Retrieved July 4, 2004, from www.irbforum.com/forum/read/2/54/54

Said, E. (1979). *Orientalism.* New York: Vintage Books.

Scott, J. (1990). Domination and the arts of resistance: Hidden transcripts. New Haven, CT: Yale University Press.

Seifer, S. (2003). Documenting and assessing community-based scholarship: Resources for faculty. In M. Minkler & N. Wallerstein (Eds.), *Community-based participatory research for health.* San Francisco: Jossey-Bass.

Sharpe, P. A., Greany, M. L., Lee, P. R., & Royce, S. W. (2000). Assets-oriented community assessment. *Public Health Reports, 113,* 205–211.

Spivak, G.C. (1990). The problem of cultural self-representation. In S. Harasym (Eds.), *Post-colonial critic: Interviews, strategies, dialogues* (pp. 50–58). New York: Routledge.

Stewart, A. J., & McDermott, C. (2004). Gender in psychology. *Annual Review of Psychology, 55,* 519–544.

Tervalon, M., & Murray-Garcia, J. (1998). Cultural humility vs. cultural competence: A critical distinction in defining physician training outcomes in medical education. *Journal of Health Care for the Poor and Underserved, 9*(2), 117–125.

Turning Point. (2003). Thirteen policy principles for advancing collaborative activity among and between tribal communities and surrounding jurisdictions. In M. Minkler & N. Wallerstein (Eds.), *Community-Based participatory research in health* (pp. 436–437). San Francisco: Jossey-Bass.

Wallerstein, N. (1999). Power between evaluator and community: Research relationships within New Mexico's healthier communities. *Social Science & Medicine, 49*(1), 39–53.

Wallerstein, N., & Sheline, B. (1998). Techniques for developing the community partnership in community-oriented primary care. In R. Rhyne, R. Bogue, G. Kukulka, & H. Fulmer (Eds.), *Health care for the 21st century* (pp. 88–116). Washington, DC: American Public Health Association Press.

CHAPTER THREE

Strategies and Techniques for Effective Group Process in CBPR Partnerships

Adam B. Becker, Barbara A. Israel, and Alex J. Allen III

The development of equitable partnerships among members of a diverse set of communities and institutions is a central component of community-based participatory research (CBPR). CBPR partnerships consist of members of a community with a shared identity, representatives of organizations that work with the community, and academic researchers—all interested in exploring and addressing issues relevant to the community (Israel, Schulz, Parker, & Becker, 1998). CBPR initiatives that focus on health involve a process in which diverse groups of people become partners in a collaborative approach to research that integrates learning with action to increase knowledge about community health while improving the health of community members (Israel et al., 1998). The

Acknowledgments: The authors acknowledge the following groups (and the individuals involved with them) for their commitment to the development of effective CBPR partnerships and for contributing to the co-learning environments from which the examples and lessons described here have emerged: East Side Village Health Worker Partnership; Detroit-Community Academic Urban Research Center; Stress and Wellness Project; Broome Team of the Detroit-Genesee County Community-Based Public Health Initiative; SIP23/24 Research Group, and Project BRAVE. We thank the following organizations for supporting this work: U.S. Centers for Disease Control and Prevention, National Institute on Alcohol Abuse and Alcoholism, United Auto Workers/General Motors National Joint Committee on Health and Safety, W. K. Kellogg Foundation, and Students at the Center in New Orleans. We would especially like to acknowledge Rose M. Hollis for her ability to facilitate groups and help partnerships to work across difference and her contributions to the development of some of the activities and strategies described in this chapter.

ability of CBPR partnerships to address mutually defined priorities depends in part on effective collaboration among these diverse partners.

Key principles of and critical issues in CBPR have been reviewed elsewhere (see, for example, Chapter One in this volume; Israel et al., 1998, 2003) and will not be presented here. A number of principles and issues, however, are related to partnership development among diverse groups and are useful in making explicit the connection between group process and effective CBPR partnerships. Key partnership-related principles identified by Israel and colleagues (1998) include facilitating collaborative partnerships in all phases of the research, integrating knowledge and action for mutual benefit of all partners, and promoting a co-learning and empowering process that attends to social inequalities. Israel and colleagues (1998) also describe a number of challenges that are relevant to the development of successful partnerships. These include lack of trust and respect among potential partners; inequitable distribution of power and control; and conflicts associated with differences in perspectives, priorities, assumptions, values, beliefs, and language. These partnership-related issues in CBPR are also elements of group dynamics that are relevant to the effectiveness of any decision-making or problem-solving group (Forsyth, 1999; Johnson & Johnson, 2003).

Researchers, practitioners, and community partners who have participated in CBPR projects have noted the benefits that emerge when all partners successfully integrate their different backgrounds, expertise, values, and priorities (Israel et al., 1998; Lantz, Viruell-Fuentes, Israel, Softley, & Guzman, 2001; Northridge et al., 2000; Schulz, Israel, Parker, et al., 2003). Many have also noted, however, that the development and maintenance of successful partnerships can be one of the most challenging aspects of CBPR endeavors (Green et al., 1995; Israel et al., 2001; 2003; Sullivan et al., 2003). A body of literature on the evaluation of the CBPR partnership process has pointed to the importance of attending to group dynamics to increase the likelihood of partnership success (Eisinger & Senturia, 2001; Freudenberg, 2001; Israel et al., 2001; Lantz et al., 2001; Schulz, Israel, & Lantz, 2003). CBPR evaluation studies have noted that democratic leadership that attends to task goals and relationship maintenance and to equitable participation and open communication contributes to the effectiveness of a diverse collaborating group, as does a climate that supports group cohesion (Israel et al., 2001; Lantz et al., 2001; Schulz, Israel, & Lantz, 2003).

These integral factors in effective CBPR partnerships are elements that have been well examined by group dynamics researchers (Forsyth, 1999; Johnson & Johnson, 2003). Johnson and Johnson (2003) list a number of characteristics of effective groups that have been identified through group dynamics research: clear and operational group goals that emphasize cooperation but reflect individual interests; open communication; equitably distributed participation and leadership; and influence and power that is derived from members' capacities. In addition, effective groups use decision-making procedures that match specific situations; create an environment that encourages the creative use of conflict; emphasize group members' skills, and endorse individuality while advancing cohesion through high levels of inclusion, support, and trust. Processes and strategies for helping groups to develop these characteristics are critical for effective CBPR partnerships.

In this chapter we describe group process methods and facilitation strategies for establishing and maintaining effective partnerships. These approaches are based on findings from the field of group dynamics. We discuss specific techniques and activities that we have used in facilitating CBPR partnerships. Our examples are drawn from a number of CBPR initiatives in which we have been involved. All three authors have been active partners in the Detroit Community-Academic Urban Research Center (Israel et al., 2001; Lantz et al., 2001) and its original demonstration project, the East Side Village Health Worker Partnership (Parker, Schulz, Israel, & Hollis, 1998; Schulz et al., 2002). The majority of techniques and strategies presented here were and continue to be used in that work. Additional examples come from the Stress and Wellness Project (Israel, Schurman, & House, 1989), the Detroit-Genesee County Community-Based Public Health initiative (Schulz, Israel, Parker, et al., 2003), a multisite study to develop effective measures of community-level social protective factors, (Goodman & Becker, 2003; Becker, Willis, Joe, Baker, & Shada, 2002), and a CBPR project aimed at understanding and addressing youth violence, Project BRAVE (Becker & Randels, 2003).

ELEMENTS OF GROUP DYNAMICS RELEVANT TO CBPR PARTNERSHIPS

This chapter is organized around twelve elements, or dimensions, of group dynamics that are pertinent to CBPR partnerships. For each element, we briefly review the relevant group dynamics literature, and describe strategies and techniques we have used to establish these dimensions. The dimensions we discuss are group membership, equitable participation and open communication, establishing norms for working together, developing trust, selecting and prioritizing goals and objectives, identifying community strengths and concerns, leadership, power and influence, addressing conflict, decision making, specific strategies for working in diverse partnerships, and the importance of partnership assessment. We conclude with some broad lessons learned through applying group dynamics techniques to CBPR partnership development and maintenance.

Group Membership

Most definitions of an effective group refer to mutual recognition among members and a sense of belonging to the group (Forsyth, 1999; Johnson & Johnson, 2003). Definitions also refer to shared norms and values, goal interdependence (members recognize that group goals cannot be met by any one individual acting alone), mutual influence, a sense of shared purpose, and the ability of members to act in a unitary manner. Sufficient attention to relationship building and to fostering a sense of membership early in a CBPR partnership's development is needed to increase the likelihood of success (Schulz, Israel, & Lantz, 2003). Chapter Two describes in depth the issues relevant to partnership development. In this chapter we describe a number of activities that can help partners get acquainted and identify common ground. These activities can be equally useful when new partners join established partnerships.

Initial meetings among partners that focus on introductions and the sharing of ideas are beneficial. In the early stages of partnerships, meetings can include activities that help group members learn about each other and develop effective working relationships. For example, in a study involving four community-based research projects (Becker et al., 2002), a subcommittee charged with group process issues facilitated this activity to help partners get to know each other. Members brought to a meeting one object that reminded them of home. Each object was given a number, and each partner's nametag was given a number. After partners described their objects to the group, each partner gave her or his item as a gift to the individual with the matching number, so that each partner left the meeting with something that another had brought. Other activities that may be used involve members pairing up, conducting brief interviews of each other, and then introducing each other to the group, and a *human bingo* activity in which partners have to identify and obtain the signatures of other partners who have specific characteristics (for example, partners who are able to speak two languages). Activities such as these can help group members connect on a personal level. Other partnership-building activities can be found in *A Handbook of Structured Experiences for Human Relations Training, Vols. 1–10* (Pfeiffer, 1975–1985).

Equitable Participation and Open Communication

Equitable participation and open communication are at the crux of all other group processes (Schwarz, 1994). Effective groups are those in which all members' knowledge and skills are used fully to accomplish tasks and maintain productive relationships (Forsyth, 1999; Johnson & Johnson 2003; Schwarz, 1994). For this to occur, all members must have opportunities to participate in group discussion and action and must be able to communicate openly. Appropriate patterns, or *networks,* of communication can help a group achieve this goal

(Forsyth, 1999). A communication network may be centralized (so that one or a few members receive information from and give information to all other members) or decentralized (so that all members freely share information with all other members) (Forsyth, 1999; Johnson & Johnson, 2003). Different types of networks may be needed, depending on the complexity of a task. When a task is simple (for example, informing partners of a meeting date), a centralized network may be more effective in terms of efficiency and accuracy. When a task requires multiple perspectives or broad-based support, decentralized networks may be more appropriate—particularly if the decentralized network means that all members are present when the information is transmitted and discussed (Forsyth, 1999). Here are a number of techniques that can help CBPR partnerships to foster equitable participation and open communication.

Establish Appropriate Group Size. Group dynamics research suggests that smaller group size is better for effective communication (Johnson & Johnson, 2003), with some authors suggesting groups of no more than eight or nine members (Watson & Johnson, 1972). Most research acknowledges, however, that decisions about group size should be based on the purpose of the group (Johnson & Johnson, 2003). There are several reasons to keep groups relatively small. Studies have shown that the larger the group is, the less members will be actively involved in discussion and decision making, the less members will see their participation as essential for success, and the less effective the group will be (Kerr, 1989; Olson, 1965). If a group is too large, members may feel that they are not integral and may not commit to take action to support group goals. In addition, the greater the complexity of the group's structure and the more effort it takes to coordinate the group, the less effective the group will be (Johnson & Johnson, 2003).

Keeping CBPR partnerships to a manageable size, however, can be challenging. Inclusion is an important value of CBPR, and partners often want to engage as many stakeholders as possible. The Detroit Community-Academic Urban Research Center (URC), for example, has consisted of as many as ten partner organizations, a few with as many as three or four representatives participating in meetings. Large partnerships often set up structures that minimize the numbers of participants in some decision-making or problem-solving tasks. For example, a steering committee may be responsible for overall project management and decision making, with subcommittees that carry out specific tasks. When large numbers of people must be present at meetings, a number of techniques and strategies can be used to facilitate effective communication, as discussed in the following sections.

Use Individual and Small-Group Work. One technique for maximizing participation is to give members time to consider the issue at hand, so they can organize and write down their thoughts before participating in discussion.

Another strategy is to break the initial group into small groups that discuss an issue or generate ideas and then come back together for large-group discussion. Small groups give more people the opportunity for input. Small-group work also enables the participation of members who may be uncomfortable speaking in large groups or who are in "low-power" positions relative to others who are present (for example, a staff member in relation to a supervisor, a junior in relation to a senior faculty member, a community resident in relation to an academic or public health partner).

Employ the Nominal Group Technique. Another technique that can be used is the *nominal group technique* (NGT) (Delbecq, Van de Ven, & Gustafson, 1975). Members form one or more groups of approximately five to fifteen persons. Each individual writes out a list of points or items in response to a particular question, and then, one at time, group members share one idea from their lists with the rest of their group. A facilitator writes each idea out verbatim where it is visible to all members (on sheets of newsprint, for example). Others are asked to raise their hand if they have written exactly the same idea. This number is tallied and recorded next to the idea. This process continues around the group, without discussion, until all individuals' lists have been exhausted. Discussion for clarification then occurs, with the option to collapse very similar ideas into one. The facilitator must be careful at this stage not to eliminate ideas in an attempt to reduce the number of responses posted. Members must be in agreement that one idea is similar enough to another that integrating them will not result in loss of meaning. If two or more small groups engage in this process simultaneously, they share their results, followed by discussion and integration of ideas by the entire partnership. Studies have shown that "groups produce more ideas and members report feeling more satisfied with the process" when NGT is used (Forsyth, 1999, p. 276).

Apply Facilitation Strategies. Facilitators can use a number of strategies to encourage participation. A facilitator may encourage nonparticipating members to participate by asking if anyone else has a comment to make or by explicitly noting that not everyone has been heard from. Facilitators should be careful, however, not to pressure members to participate or put them on the spot by referring to them individually. After a meeting, members who have not participated may be approached individually to make sure that they are satisfied with their level of participation or to get their suggestions about strategies that would help them to participate more freely. The group may also engage in evaluation activities that elicit partners' feelings about participation and communication in the group (see the section on partnership assessment later in this chapter).

A number of groups and organizations use the process known as Robert's Rules of Order, in which members are formally recognized, one at a time, to discuss a proposed motion. Following discussion, they cast a binding vote.

Although many groups use this approach because the rules are concrete and provide a structure for getting through a meeting's agenda, we suggest that this system be used with caution as it may inhibit open communication in CBPR partnerships. When this process is strictly applied, group members do not have the opportunity to ask questions freely, negotiate and jointly problem solve, or engage in a free-flowing discussion. In addition, the principle that the "majority rules" may make it difficult for the "minority" to commit to the outcome of a vote. Finally, the formality of the process may be intimidating to partners who prefer less formal approaches or who are not comfortable speaking in front of the whole group. We encourage CBPR partnerships to use other approaches. If they do consider using Robert's Rules of Order as a process, they should discuss the benefits and challenges, try the approach, and be willing to move to alternative processes if the group is not comfortable with the results.

Use Agendas and Take Minutes. Equally important as communication during meetings is communication between meetings. Effective communication and decision making require consideration of such issues as who sets the agenda, who takes minutes, and when minutes will be distributed. Although these activities are often seen simply as logistical tasks of partnership coordination, they may actually transfer power to those who take them on. For example, those responsible for creating the agenda have more control than other members over what gets discussed at a meeting and for how long. The individual or group in charge of minutes has control over what gets entered into the official record of the partnership. Sharing these responsibilities may distribute control more equitably. It is important to recognize, however, that these tasks do require some degree of resources (for example, the time and personnel to type agendas and minutes and distribute them by mail or fax).

In the various CBPR partnerships in which we have been involved, the academic partners have typically had the responsibility for physically creating and distributing agendas and minutes, due to their greater access to administrative support and to their formal role as evaluators documenting the CBPR process. We have used a number of procedures, however, to ensure that these processes are carried out equitably and do not constitute undue control by the academic partners. One approach is to reserve time at the end of each meeting to brainstorm ideas for the next meeting's agenda. Another is to include "new business" or "other" as a permanent agenda item and allow sufficient time during every meeting for new issues to be raised and discussed. A third is to distribute ahead of time a draft agenda to which partners may add items. A combination of these strategies may also be useful.

Similarly, before the minutes of a particular meeting are distributed to all partners, draft minutes can be distributed for revisions to those who were present at that meeting. Some groups take time at the beginning of a meeting to review minutes and make changes as appropriate. This may not be effective, however, if the process is rushed or members have not seen the minutes beforehand. A technique that may be used during a meeting to jointly develop minutes is for the facilitator to summarize each discussion and the decisions made before moving on to the next point. With this process, partners who are present have an opportunity to clarify a decision and make sure that all members have the same understanding. This technique also gives the note taker guidance by identifying the aspects of the discussion that are most important and that should be recorded.

Establishing Norms for Working Together

One way to increase the likelihood of effective communication is for the partnership to develop a set of norms for working together. Different from the CBPR principles that guide the overall work (Israel et al., 1998, 2001, 2003; Schulz, Israel, Selig, Bayer, & Griffin, 1998), group norms guide day-to-day functioning of the partnership and often include guidelines for communication, decision making, addressing conflict, and group climate. For example, a group might "agree to disagree" or might prefer decision making by consensus. Group norms have been defined as "emergent consensual standards that regulate group members' behaviors" (Forsyth, 1999). Once accepted and regulated by the group, norms help group members to behave consistently (Johnson & Johnson, 2003).

Norms can be explicitly written and adopted, or they can emerge gradually as members work together (Johnson & Johnson, 2003). We recommend that CBPR partnerships, because they consist of diverse members and have explicit values pertaining to equity and openness, discuss norms jointly and explicitly decide upon those to which they will adhere, although the degree of formality of these norms will depend on the interests of the group. Regardless of their degree of formality, norms are most effective when the group develops them together. In developing CBPR partnerships we have used what we call the *norming exercise* (Israel et al., 2001). In this exercise, the facilitator asks group members to take several minutes to independently complete the following task:

> Think about groups in which you have been a member that have been positive experiences—groups in which you enjoyed participating. . . . Considering these groups, write down the three to five factors that contributed to this being a positive experience. . . . That is, what was it about the group that made it successful? If you have not had any such experiences working with groups, then think about groups in which you were a member that you did not think were effective and consider what are three to five factors that would have needed to change in order to have made it a more effective group [Israel et al., 2001, p. 5].

Using NGT or some other process for sharing their ideas with the group, partners then share the factors that they think contribute to effective and satisfying groups. The facilitator writes down all factors and the group then discusses which ones they will adopt as their norms for working together.

Developing Trust

Another important element of successful group process is trust among the partners. This is especially important in CBPR partnerships where there may be a history of negative relationships among community members and researchers. Mistrust may be present from the outset in a partnership's development not because of specific experiences that partners have had with each other but because partners carry with them the histories of the institutions they represent. Community-based organization representatives, for example, have described feeling an initial need to be "gatekeepers" in a CBPR partnership, to keep researchers from doing harm in the communities in which their organizations are involved (Israel et al., 2001). Researchers may also mistrust community partners, fearing, for example, that community members will act to limit, rather than facilitate, the research process or that community influence will result in a decrease in scientific rigor. Developing trust among CBPR partners is a time-consuming process but is among the most important aspects of creating effective partnerships. Partners in CBPR efforts, particularly academic partners, have to demonstrate trustworthiness throughout the life of the partnership; in keeping with the principle of addressing social inequalities, higher-power partners must demonstrate trustworthiness rather than simply expecting trust from lower-power partners (Israel et al., 1998). There are a number of ways partners can display trustworthiness and gain each other's trust.

Show Respect. Partners can display trustworthiness by seriously considering the ideas and opinions of others. Feeling heard and respected can be as important as being agreed with (Becker, 1999), and members who feel they have been listened to will be able to better support the final decision, even if it did not go the way they had initially hoped (Johnson & Johnson, 2003). In our work, partners have set group norms that foster showing respect through listening—agreeing, for example, that partners will allow other partners to finish their statements before interjecting or will change the subject only when all partners agree to move on.

Follow Through. Trustworthiness can also be demonstrated by doing what one commits to. Although lack of follow-through may not be intentional, it can lead to a lack of confidence among partners. Taking accurate minutes can help with follow-through, as partners can see in writing and be reminded of what they committed to do. When a partner agrees to take on a particular task, it can be entered in the minutes as an *action item.* At subsequent meetings progress on the action item is checked, and adjustments are made as needed. Partners should be careful to follow through on anything to which they commit and not to commit to anything they cannot follow through on.

Respect Confidentiality. Demonstrating respect for confidentiality is another dimension of trustworthiness. CBPR partners may share with each other the institutional challenges they face in their individual work environments. Knowing that such comments will not go beyond the partners present helps partners to trust each other. Numerous other issues may arise within a partnership for which respecting confidentiality is of utmost importance (for example, events going on in the community or challenges related to funding institutions). Again, the adoption of group norms explicitly requesting that all partners respect confidentiality helps to support this dimension of trustworthiness.

Attend to Each Other's Interests and Needs. Acting as allies can help CBPR partners to establish trustworthiness and gain trust. Partners may be asked to participate in activities that are not directly related to their work together. In our experiences, academic research partners have written grant proposals and participated in activities organized by community and practice partners that are beyond the specific work of the CBPR partnership. Community and practice partners have interviewed candidates for university positions and worked with students on class projects not related to the specific CBPR effort. Attending significant events in each other's nonwork lives (such as birthday celebrations or other important family events) has helped us to develop trust and friendship among partners. These activities help to solidify trusting relationships (Israel et al., 2001) and may help keep the partners together even without specific funding.

Selecting and Prioritizing Goals and Objectives

To be effective, groups must set goals to which all members can agree and commit and to which all partners are willing and able to contribute (Johnson & Johnson, 2003). When partners operate under different understandings of the partnership's goals, success can be diminished. Although it is appropriate for groups to have goals that are different from those of individual members, conflicts can arise when individual goals are not made explicit (that is, when people have hidden agendas) (Johnson & Johnson, 2003). Even though the revealing of individual goals may happen only over time, with the building of trust and the development of effective communication, a number of activities can be used to set goals cooperatively and give partners the opportunity to express their individual interests and motivations for participating and perhaps have those interests incorporated into the overall goals of the group.

CBPR partnerships often start with brainstorming activities, using nominal group technique or small- and large-group discussion, to develop a *wish list* of priority activities within the parameters of the partnership. For example, starting with a phrase such as, "by the end of our first five years we will have accomplished . . .," partners list all of the goals they would like to see the partnership attain. These lists can then be narrowed down and prioritized according to a number of criteria (for example, resources available, skills and interests of partners and organizations, health statistics in the community) and these become the goals for the partnership. Specific theoretical frameworks (a conceptual model of the stress process, for example) may be used to structure brainstorming, as was done in the URC (see Israel et al., 2001; also Chapter Five in this volume). Theoretically guided brainstorming can help to ensure that CBPR projects and activities will contribute to the partnership's overall research and action agendas. The use of a force field analysis, a group-process activity, can help partnerships to identify both facilitating factors and barriers and their potential impact on achieving the goals identified in brainstorming (Lewin, 1944; Johnson & Johnson, 2003; also see Appendix A). Identifying forces for and forces against accomplishing a goal can help partnerships to prioritize goals and subsequent action steps according to their viability.

Partnerships can also engage in goal-setting and prioritizing exercises that help the group to think creatively. Partners may use *visioning* activities to describe, for example, the ideal community or accomplishments that the partners would like to achieve. Creative exercises that move away from verbal lists and toward visual images and products can give partners with diverse backgrounds and experiences a common set of tools to work with. In the East Side Village Health Worker Partnership training, for example, Village Health Worker trainees, working in small groups, used craft materials to "build" their ideal community—discussing its elements while representing them visually.

Identifying Community Strengths and Concerns

CBPR seeks to identify and mobilize the strengths and resources available in the community and among partners to address research questions and communal health concerns (Israel et al., 1998, 2003). All communities possess strengths, such as the knowledge and skills of individuals, the positive contributions of organizations and other resources, and desirable features of the physical environment (green space, for example). Identifying strengths can help community members feel more valued and respected, as partners recognize the strengths in a community rather than emphasize problems to be solved (Steuart, 1993; Minkler & Hancock, 2003). Acknowledging strengths can also help CBPR partners to make their own work more effective. For example, one of the partners in the URC was a city-owned multipurpose center. This center was identified in the early stages of partnership development as an important community resource and invited to join the effort during the proposal-writing stage. Once the project was funded, the center's director provided office and meeting space. This centrally located physical space in the community was a critical factor in the project's success.

A number of exercises can help CBPR partnerships identify and mobilize strengths and resources. For example, the first author of this chapter and a

Detroit-based colleague adapted a skills inventory activity (Kretzmann & McKnight, 1993) to train lay health advisors in the East Side Village Health Worker Partnership about the importance of personal strengths and community assets and approaches for asset assessment. Facilitators listed, on separate pieces of newsprint around the training room, numerous skills (for example, can drive a van) and experiences (for example, organized a party of twenty guests or more) that people might have. Trainees signed their names under the skills and experiences that they had. The facilitated discussion then focused on the community-organizing and community-building activities that the group of trainees could accomplish given the skills that they each possessed. Other partnerships have used mapping to identify and categorize organizational and institutional resources (for example, schools and health care facilities) that are available to the partnership and the community (Kretzmann & McKnight, 1993). (See Chapter Nine for a discussion of mapping social and environmental influences on health.) *Windshield tours,* in which partners familiar with the community educate other partners about its history, culture, and environment (Minkler & Hancock, 2003; Parker et al., 1998); in-depth interviews with key informants; and a review of historical documents can also help CBPR partnerships learn about the strengths and resources available in the community in which they are working (Warren & Warren, 1977; Eng & Blanchard, 1990–1991; also see Chapter Four in this volume).

Leadership

Shared leadership has been identified as an important element of CBPR approaches that seek to create an equitable partnership among diverse individuals and groups (Israel et al., 2001; Lantz et al., 2001; Schulz, Israel, & Lantz, 2003). One theory of leadership that is particularly relevant for CBPR partnerships is the *distributed-actions* theory. This theory posits that any member of a group can provide leadership functions by taking actions that help the group to achieve its goals and maintain effective working relationships (Johnson & Johnson, 2003). Forsyth (1990, p. 114) notes that "a group generally requires the services of both a task specialist to help it work in the direction of its goals and a socioemotional specialist who intervenes regularly to reduce interpersonal strains and stresses within the group." These roles may be filled by group members who undertake task leadership and maintenance leadership functions. Examples of task leadership actions include asking for or giving opinions or information and summarizing discussions. Examples of maintenance leadership actions (less common in working groups) include encouraging participation, relieving tension, and supporting and praising group members. Task and maintenance leadership actions can and should be distributed among CBPR partners in keeping with the principles of equity and shared ownership (Israel et al., 2001).

Although we do not use specific exercises to foster distributed leadership, we have used a number of strategies to assist CBPR partnerships to distribute task and maintenance leadership throughout their groups. Having community and academic partners share facilitation tasks is one strategy that emerged from a partnership assessment. Not all partnerships are interested, however, in sharing facilitation. The URC board, for example, stated its preference for an academic partner who had substantial experience in group facilitation and could maintain this role (Israel et al., 2001). Nonetheless, leadership actions can and should go beyond the particular person facilitating meetings.

Strategies for distributing task and maintenance leadership functions include modeling by those who are comfortable with these leadership actions until others begin to take on leadership roles within the group, specifically integrating task and leadership actions into the working norms of the group, and reflecting periodically on how group members are feeling after discussions or at the end of a meeting until this type of maintenance leadership action becomes part of the working norms of the group (partnership assessment strategies are discussed later in this chapter).

Power and Influence

Balancing power and influence is challenging in CBPR partnerships (Israel et al., 2003; Wallerstein, 1999; Chávez, Duran, Baker, Avila, & Wallerstein, 2003), which by definition consist of diverse partners who represent multiple levels of social hierarchy (Israel et al., 1998). CBPR partnerships may include leaders of community-based organizations and community residents, leaders and frontline staff or clients of public health departments, and senior and junior faculty. CBPR members represent not only different power levels *within* each system represented (community, practice agency, or university) but also levels *across* systems in terms of perceived status and access to and control over resources.

Group process literature states that principles of equity, mutual influence, co-learning, and maintaining a balance of power and influence are critical for successful group efforts. Most studies in group dynamics have found that a group's effectiveness is improved when "power is relatively balanced among its members, and power is based upon competence, expertise, and information" (Johnson & Johnson, 2003, p. 246). Power and influence in a group can come from expertise, personal attraction, access to information, the ability to reward or punish, legitimate role-based authority, verbal skill, or even self-confidence (Johnson & Johnson, 2003; Mansbridge, 1973). Mansbridge maintains that "in groups committed to the ideal that all members have an equal influence on decisions, continuing inequalities can be disastrous" (Mansbridge, 1973, p. 361). Mansbridge recommends beginning group initiatives and activities with "more than one task or with a task that depends on the skills of many members"

(p. 362) in order to ensure a better balance of power and influence from the outset.

Balanced power and influence are related to equitable participation, and we described earlier a number of strategies and techniques that may encourage participation among all partners. Influence and power imbalances may not be solved, however, by simply encouraging equal participation in group discussion. Mansbridge (1973) makes several suggestions that may be helpful. If influence is skill based, skilled members can transfer those skills to other members through training. If verbal fluency is a source of influence, members can interact in small groups in order to develop verbal skills and confidence. If information results in power, all members can be given the same information as soon as possible.

A number of other strategies can help to balance power differences among partners. Small-group work, as described previously, may enable lower-power members to participate more freely than they might in a large-group discussion. Partnerships might also have discussions up front about issues of equity in power and influence, or about hypothetical situations in which power imbalances occur, to bring out the issues and then develop solutions that partners might use if these imbalances begin to play out in the partnership.

Decentralized decision making is another strategy that we have used to balance power in CBPR partnerships in which we have been involved. We have established subcommittees with representation from community, practice, and academic contexts to make proposals to the larger group on, for example, policies and procedures for writing manuscripts, content and methods of partnership evaluation, and hiring staff. Multiple subcommittees give a greater number of members the opportunity to shape decisions, thus balancing power and influence among partners.

Addressing Conflict

Conflict is often one of the most challenging issues for a group to address. Some group members may believe that conflict should always be avoided. Group dynamics literature proposes, however, that conflict is a necessary part of group development (Bales, 1965; Tuckman, 1965). Many group dynamics experts believe that when conflict is welcomed by a group and addressed effectively, decisions are more creative and effective (Johnson & Johnson, 2003). Forsyth categorizes conflict according to what he calls "the roots of conflict" (1999, p. 237). He posits that conflict among group members may be personal (individuals' personalities conflict), substantive (members disagree over opinions or ideas), or procedural (members' strategies or preferred operating methods clash) or may be caused by competition among members. Some types of conflict contribute more than others to overall group goals and effectiveness. For example, when members disagree over substantive or procedural issues, the use of clear communication, effective negotiation, and norms that support working through conflict effectively can lead to stronger relationships among members and better decisions and outcomes for the group (Johnson & Johnson, 2003). All types of conflict, however, when not appropriately addressed, can be damaging to a group temporarily or permanently.

One group process we have used early on in partnership development to address conflict is to establish norms for conflict. Discussing conflict explicitly before it occurs is one way to encourage group members to see conflict as something that most surely will occur but that can lead to positive results if handled effectively. One norm that has been common in our work is to "agree to disagree." This norm sets the tone that conflicts do not have to end with one position winning out over the other. When supported by appropriate decision making, such as consensus as opposed to unanimous agreement (as discussed later), agreeing to disagree can help a group resolve a particular conflict and reach a decision that all members can support.

Johnson and Johnson (2003, pp. 361–363) describe the "constructive controversy" process for addressing conflict. First, group members who disagree over a substantive or procedural issue each present their case clearly, using all available supporting information. Each member agrees to keep an open mind and listen carefully to the others' cases. Members then work to understand, first, and challenge, second, each other's cases. Members clarify the differences in their ideas and integrate where possible so that aspects of all ideas are included in the final decision. This approach to conflict helps to ensure that the best-informed and most appropriate solutions come out of different points of view.

Other types of conflict may not be as systematically addressed. Personality conflict, for example, may need to be addressed outside the group setting, perhaps with a mediator working with the parties. Conflict that stems from competition may be reduced by setting up a cooperative goal structure in which any success is a group success, all members have opportunities to contribute, and members are assigned tasks and roles according to their interests and capacities.

Decision Making

Groups that sufficiently address the dimensions of group process described thus far have the best chance of making effective decisions. The use of specific decision-making methods further helps to ensure effective decision making. Johnson and Johnson (2003) present several decision-making methods, including decision by authority, expert member decision making, averaging members' opinions, majority or minority control, and consensus.

We suggest that groups engage in discussion to develop processes for decision making. In some of our partnerships this process has been referred to, with some degree of humor, as "deciding how to decide." Too often groups enter into a decision-making process before determining how the decision will be made (for example, by consensus or by the leadership). Partners may set one process for all decisions, or they may take time before each decision to discuss how it will be made. When all members know what the process will be, they can engage in the process with more appropriate contributions and expectations.

Decision making may also be hindered if all members do not know ahead of time what will be up for discussion during each meeting. Distributing the agenda before each meeting, reviewing it at the beginning of the meeting, and following it as the meeting progresses may help members prepare for decision making. Members will know in advance the issues to be discussed and can formulate opinions. Before a new topic is opened for discussion, the previous agenda item can be closed with a decision and agreement on an action step to be taken in light of that decision.

Group dynamics researchers agree that different types of decisions may need different methods (Forsyth, 1999; Johnson & Johnson, 2003). Using a time-consuming consensus-building process to make a decision in which partners have a low emotional stake (for example, determining the color of a publicity flyer) would be a frustrating experience. Conversely, having a high-stakes decision (how to cut a jointly developed budget, for example) made unilaterally by partners from one organization is likely to have far-reaching negative implications. Decentralized decision making, with subcommittees assigned to make certain decisions, is a common way to distribute decision-making responsibility among group members. Well thought out subcommittee membership that is agreed to by the group (rather than appointed by the leaders) may be an effective method for making decisions that do not require everyone's input.

For complex decisions, however, consensus decision making may be useful. Consensus is a "collective opinion arrived at by a group of individuals working together under conditions that permit communications to be sufficiently open and the group climate to be sufficiently supportive for everyone in the group to feel that he or she has had a fair chance to influence the decision" (Johnson & Johnson, p. 220). Consensus does not necessarily mean unanimity. The URC, for example, has agreed to use a 70 percent rule as their form of consensus. This means that "everyone still has to support a decision but they do not have to be behind it 100 percent. Rather, if all members can buy into a decision with at least 70 percent of their support, then an overall consensus has been reached" (Israel et al., 2001, p. 5).

Specific Strategies for Working in Diverse Partnerships

CBPR partnerships are diverse by definition, including partners with different educational backgrounds and areas of expertise and usually having diverse gender, racial, ethnic, and class backgrounds as well. Partners may also be of different religions, sexual orientations, generations, political affiliations, or ability or disability status. A number of activities carried out in the early partnership development stages can help diverse partners identify and respect differences. Similar to the gift exchange exercise described earlier, Culture Box, developed by the University of Michigan's Program on Intergroup Relations, is one such exercise. In this exercise, partners share items that they believe represent aspects of their identity (for example, their cultural heritage, religious beliefs, or gender). Through discussion of these items, members can begin to understand and value the personal diversity among them.

To deal with diversity of affiliation (community, practice, or academia), the Detroit-Genesee County Community-Based Public Health initiative developed an exercise that enabled partners to express their hopes and concerns for working with partners from different perspectives. Partners divided first into the three groups (community, practice, academia). Each group was asked to complete the following task:

> List separately for each of the other two groups the things that you hope they
> will contribute to our work together, based on your understanding of their skills,
> knowledge, backgrounds, and resources. Next, list the things you believe will be
> challenges in working with each of the other two groups because of who they
> are and the contexts they represent.

In the second step of the activity, the groups shared and discussed their lists in the large group, asking for clarification when necessary but not debating the issues. In the third step, the same groups worked together to complete the following task:

> Each group take with you the contributions and challenges that the other two
> groups thought you would bring to our work. Discuss strategies that your group
> or the entire partnership can use to increase the likelihood that your group will
> be able to contribute the things listed and decrease the likelihood that your
> group will present the challenges listed.

Again working in the large group, the partners discussed the strategies each small group had developed, in some cases establishing group norms to support particular strategies. This exercise helped the partners engage more effectively with diversity in terms of the context that each one represented.

Importance of Partnership Assessment

Partnership effectiveness is influenced in part by whether or not groups reflect on how well they are functioning (Johnson & Johnson, 2003). Hanson (1975) proposes feedback as "a technique that helps members of a group achieve their goals" (p. 147). CBPR partnerships can benefit from devoting time to evaluating their process and reviewing their progress (Israel et al., 2001; Lantz et al., 2001; Schulz, Israel, & Lantz, 2003). Acting expediently on such feedback can help a CBPR partnership make adjustments and improve functioning. Participation of all members in the assessment process should be encouraged so that all points of view are considered. Such evaluation can take a number of forms, and partnerships may engage in one or several over the course of their work together. In this section we describe a number of techniques to evaluate the *process* through which partnerships work together, as distinct from the health-related or social outcomes they are trying to achieve.

There are a number of approaches groups can take to evaluate and improve group process at specific meetings. Meeting evaluations are usually conducted by means of a brief questionnaire that asks participants to rank on a scale from least to most effective a number of the process dimensions reviewed earlier (for example, communication and trust). Responses to these anonymous questionnaires can be tallied and distributed and discussed at a subsequent meeting, with revisions of meeting agendas and procedures carried out as indicated by the findings. Another method asks those present to answer three open-ended questions in writing: "What was the most helpful aspect of this meeting?" "What was the least helpful aspect of this meeting?" and, "What should we do differently next time?" Here again, these written responses can be summarized and distributed subsequently, or they can be provided verbally and discussed at the next meeting. Again, the key is that members have an opportunity to offer input based on their experience in one meeting in order to make improvements in subsequent meetings. In both of these approaches it is important for the group to review members' input and make appropriate changes as soon as possible.

Approaches to evaluating group dynamics that are more formal and that go into greater depth are also useful; they employ both qualitative and quantitative data collection methods. The overall approach we use is described in Chapter Twelve (also see Schulz, Israel, & Lantz, 2003) and will not be repeated here. All groups are different, and each evaluation method may be more or less appropriate for any one CBPR partnership. For individuals as well as groups, however, reflection and subsequent feedback form a significant stage in an experiential learning cycle (Johnson & Johnson, 2003).

CONCLUSION

We have briefly reviewed key principles and common challenges related to the successful functioning of CBPR partnerships. We have drawn from evaluation literature on CBPR partnerships and from group dynamics literature to demonstrate and emphasize that CBPR partnerships need to attend to group process in addition to achieving goals and completing research and action projects. We find Johnson and Johnson's (2003) book on group process particularly useful for understanding and addressing group dynamics and for describing activities that can foster effective group dynamics within CBPR partnerships. We have reviewed and described a number of strategies, techniques, and specific exercises that we have used in CBPR partnerships to support effective partnership development. We recognize that group dynamics are not always viewed as equally important by all partners. At various stages in all of our partnership work, partners have mentioned as a frustration or challenge the time and attention spent on group process, which is sometimes perceived as delaying action (Israel et al., 2001; Schulz, Israel, & Lantz, 2003). However, evaluation and assessment in CBPR partnerships have indicated that in the long run, attention to group process is valued and seen as worthwhile (Schulz, Israel, & Lantz, 2003; Israel et al., 2001; Lantz et al., 2001). Partners often point to the up-front and ongoing group processes in which their partnership engages as factors that contribute to the group's accomplishments and to the strong relationships the partners enjoy, not only as colleagues but also as friends. For optimal goal attainment, however, it is important for this ongoing attention to group process to be balanced with continual attention to tasks. It is our hope that the strategies provided in this chapter will be useful to other CBPR partnerships, helping them develop mechanisms for further strengthening their own partnerships through careful attention to group dynamics. We encourage others who develop strategies and techniques for effective group process in CBPR to share their experiences through writing and other forms of dissemination, in order to further advance the field of CBPR and the development of effective CBPR partnerships.

References

Bales, R. (1965). The equilibrium problem in small groups. In A. Hare, E. Borgatta, & R. Bales (Eds.), *Small groups: Studies in social interaction* (pp. 444–476). New York: Knopf.

Becker, A. B. (1999). *Perceived control as a partial measure of empowerment: Conceptualization, predictors, and health effects.* Unpublished doctoral dissertation, University of Michigan, Ann Arbor.

Becker, A. B., & Randels, J. (2003, October). *Project BRAVE: A community-based participatory approach to understanding youth violence.* Paper presented at the Social Determinants of Health Forum, Centers for Disease Control and Prevention, Atlanta, GA.

Becker, A. B., Willis, M., Joe, L., Baker, E. A., & Shada, R. E. (2002, November). *A multi-site CBPR experience: Layers of collaboration and participation.* Paper presented at the annual meeting of the American Public Health Association, Philadelphia.

Chávez, V., Duran, B., Baker, Q. E., Avila, M. M., & Wallerstein, N. (2003). The dance of race and privilege in community-based participatory research. In M. Minkler & N. Wallerstein (Eds.), *Community-based participatory research for health* (pp. 81–97). San Francisco: Jossey-Bass.

Delbecq, A., Van de Ven, A., & Gustafson, D. (1975). *Group techniques for program planning.* Glenview, IL: Scott, Foresman.

Eisinger, A., & Senturia, K. (2001). Doing community-driven research: A description of Seattle Partners for Healthy Communities. *Journal of Urban Health, 78*(3), 519–534.

Eng, E., & Blanchard, L. (1990–1991). Action-oriented community diagnosis: A health education tool. *International Journal of Community Health Education, 11,* 93–110.

Forsyth, D. R. (1990). *Group dynamics* (2nd ed.). Pacific Grove, CA: Brooks/Cole.

Forsyth, D. R. (1999). *Group dynamics* (3rd ed.). Belmont, CA: Wadsworth.

Freudenberg, N. (2001). Case history of the Center for Urban Epidemiologic Studies in New York City. *Journal of Urban Health, 78*(3), 508–518.

Goodman, R., & Becker, A. B. (2003, November). *How four universities and their respective community partners collaborated in developing participatory assessments of community capacity and social capital.* Paper presented at the annual meeting of the American Public Health Association, San Francisco.

Green, L. W., George, M. A., Daniel, M., Frankish, C. J., Herbert, C. P., Bowie, W. R., et al. (1995). *Study of participatory research in health promotion.* Ottawa: Royal Society of Canada.

Hanson, P. G. (1975). What to look for in groups. In J. W. Pfeiffer & J. E. Jones (Eds.), *1975 annual handbook of group facilitators* (pp. 147–154). San Diego, CA: University Associates.

Israel, B. A., Lichtenstein, R., Lantz, P., McGranaghan, R., Allen, A., Guzman, R., et al. (2001). The Detroit Community-Academic Urban Research Center: Lessons learned in the development, implementation, and evaluation of a community-based participatory research partnership. *Journal of Public Health Management and Practice, 7*(5), 1–19.

Israel, B. A., Schulz, A. J., Parker, E. A., & Becker, A. B. (1998). Review of community-based research: Assessing partnership approaches to improve public health. *Annual Review of Public Health, 19,* 173–202.

Israel, B. A., Schulz, A. J., Parker E. A., Becker, A. B., Allen, A. J., III, Guzman, J. R. (2003). Critical issues in developing and following community-based participatory research principles. In M. Minkler & N. Wallerstein (Eds.) *Community-based participatory research for health* (pp. 53–76). San Francisco: Jossey-Bass.

Israel, B. A., Schurman, S. J., & House, J. S. (1989). Action research on occupational stress: Involving workers as researchers. *International Journal of Health Services, 19*(1), 135–155.

Johnson, D. W., & Johnson, F. P. (2003). *Joining together: Group theory and group skills* (8th ed.). Boston: Allyn & Bacon.

Kerr, N. (1989). Illusions of efficacy: The effects of group size on perceived efficacy in social dilemmas. *Journal of Experimental Social Psychology, 35,* 287–313.

Kretzmann, J. P., & McKnight, J. L. (1993). *Building communities from the inside out: A path toward finding and mobilizing a community's assets.* Chicago: ACTA.

Lantz, P. M., Veruell-Fuentes, E., Israel, B. A., Softley, D., & Guzman, J. R. (2001). Can communities and academia work together on public health research? Evaluation results from a community-based participatory research partnership in Detroit. *Journal of Urban Health, 78*(3), 495–507.

Lewin, K. (1944). Dynamics of group action. *Educational Leadership, 1,* 195–200.

Mansbridge, J. J. (1973). Time, emotion and inequality: Three problems of participatory groups. *Journal of Applied Behavioral Science, 9*(2–3), 351–368.

Minkler, M., & Hancock, T. (2003). Community-driven asset identification and issue selection. In M. Minkler & N. Wallerstein (Eds.), *Community-based participatory research for health* (pp. 135–154). San Francisco: Jossey-Bass.

Northridge, M. E., Vallone, D., Merzel, C., Greene, D., Shepard, P., Cohall, A. T., et al. (2000). The adolescent years: An academic-community partnership in Harlem comes of age. *Journal of Public Health Management and Practice, 6*(1), 53–60.

Olson, M. (1965). *The logic of collective action: Public goods and the theory of groups.* Cambridge, MA: Harvard University Press.

Parker, E. A., Schulz, A. J., Israel, B. A., & Hollis, R. M. (1998). Detroit's East Side Village Health Worker Partnership: Community-based lay health advisor intervention in an urban area. *Health Education & Behavior, 25*(1), 24–45.

Pfeiffer, J. W. (1975–1985). *A handbook of structured experiences for human relations training* (Vols. 1–10). San Francisco: Jossey-Bass/Pfeiffer.

Schulz, A. J., Israel, B. A., & Lantz, P. (2003). Instrument for evaluating dimensions of group dynamics within community-based participatory research partnerships. *Evaluation and Program Planning, 26,* 249–262.

Schulz, A. J., Israel, B. A., Parker, E. A., Lockett, M., Hill, Y. R., & Wills, R. (2003). Engaging women in community-based participatory research for health: The East Side Village Health Worker Partnership. In M. Minkler & N. Wallerstein (Eds.), *Community-based participatory research for health* (pp. 293–315). San Francisco: Jossey-Bass.

Schulz, A. J., Israel, B. A., Selig, S. M., Bayer, I. S., & Griffin, C. B. (1998). Development and implementation of principals for community-based research in public health. In R. H. MacNair (Ed.), *Research strategies for community practice* (pp. 83–110). New York: Haworth Press.

Schulz, A. J., Parker, E. A., Israel, B. A., Allen, A., DeCarlo, M., & Lockett, M. (2002). Addressing social determinants of health through community-based participatory research: The East Side Village Health Worker Partnership. *Health Education & Behavior, 29*(3), 326–341.

Schwarz, R. M. (1994). *The skilled facilitator.* San Francisco: Jossey-Bass.

Steuart, G. W. (1993). Social and cultural perspectives: Community intervention and mental health. *Health Education Quarterly,* Suppl. 1, S99–S111.

Sullivan, M., Chao, S. S., Allen, C., Kone, A., Pierre-Louis, M., & Krieger, J. (2003). Community-researcher partnerships: Perspectives from the field. In M. Minkler & N. Wallerstein (Eds.), *Community-based participatory research for health* (pp. 113–130). San Francisco: Jossey-Bass.

Tuckman, B. W. (1965). Developmental sequence in small groups. *Psychological Bulletin, 63,* 384–399.

Wallerstein, N. (1999). Power between evaluator and community: Research relationships within New Mexico's healthier communities. *Social Science & Medicine, 49,* 39–53.

Warren, R. B., & Warren, D. I. (1977). *The neighborhood organizer's handbook.* Notre Dame, IN: University of Notre Dame Press.

Watson, G., & Johnson, D. W. (1972). *Social psychology: Issues and insights* (2nd ed.). Philadelphia: Lippincott.

PART THREE

COMMUNITY ASSESSMENT AND DIAGNOSIS

I n Part Three (Chapter Four), we focus on *how to* acknowledge a community as a social and cultural unit of identity, which is a CBPR principle, and *how to* conduct a community assessment that is as much a process of community organizing and relationship building as it is a research process, which is a specific phase of CBPR. The objectives for this phase are to gain entry to a community, observe and record the collective dynamics and functions of relationships in the community, observe and record the interactions between the community insiders and the outsiders who represent other structures, and promote the conditions and skills required for both insiders and outsiders to enlarge their roles and representation as research partners and program planners (Eng & Blanchard, 1991).

For a community to function as a full partner in community-based participatory research, all involved must view the community as a social and cultural unit of identity, *not* as a setting (Steuart, 1985; Israel, Schulz, Parker, & Becker, 1998). People within a community associate through multiple and overlapping networks, with diverse linkages based on diverse interests (Cornwall & Jewkes, 1995; Israel et al., 1998; O'Fallon & Dearry, 2002). Community partners might be members of a local community, residents of a neighborhood or hamlet, or members of community-based organizations (Green, Fullilove, Evans, & Shepard, 2002; Anyanwu, 1988; Seeley, Kengeya-Kayondo, & Mulder, 1992; Wang, Burris, & Ping, 1996; Wing, 2002). For these members, it is their collective community that has the strongest potential to be the source of the power they will need to negoti-ate the production and use of knowledge with the institutions and systems that govern the research enterprise (O'Fallon & Dearry, 2002; Boston et al., 1997; Freudenberg, 2001). Institutions and systems might be represented by university faculty, elected officials, or professional staff at a workplace, such as managers, supervisors, medical practitioners, and other health and human services workers (Chesler, 1991; Ivanov & Flynn, 1999; Kovacs, 2000; Giesbrecht & Ferris, 1993; McQuiston, 2000).

Enlarging the role and representation of communities as full research part-ners in taking action for social change and health status improvement is the particular emphasis of CBPR (Israel et al., 1998; O'Fallon & Dearry, 2002; Freudenberg, 2001). Two primary reasons that researchers need community part-ners are, first, to gain entry into the world of the people who are experiencing the issue being studied and, second, to instill accountability and responsibility for what researchers learn to see, hear, and experience (Chesler, 1991; Kovacs, 2000; VanderPlaat, 1997). By examining the multiple worldviews that commu-nity partners can provide, researchers can maximize insider-outsider reciproc-ity during study design, the construction and validation of instruments, the planning of the intervention, and the interpretation and dissemination of findings (Badger, 2000; VanderPlaat, 1997).

Chapter Four, written by Eng, Moore, Rhodes, Griffith, Allison, Shirah, and Mebane, describes an approach for completing the CBPR community assess-ment phase that meets the CBPR principle of acknowledging community as a social and cultural unit of identity. The purpose of the *action-oriented commu-nity diagnosis* (AOCD) that they discuss is to identify the collective dynam-ics and functions of relationships within a community, and also the interactions between insiders and outsiders, in order to promote the conditions and skills that will assist community members in taking action for social change and health status improvement (Eng & Blanchard, 1991). The authors trace the origins of AOCD to South Africa and the work of Guy Steuart, to whom this book is dedicated. They describe the details of AOCD's application of CBPR competencies, research assumptions, case study design, and use of multiple methods (participant observation, use of secondary data, key informant one-on-one interviews, key informant focus-group interviews, and a community forum to interpret findings and move toward action). The authors present an AOCD case example involving United Voices of Efland-Cheeks, Inc. (UVE), a community-based organization, and its decade-long CBPR partnership with the University of North Carolina at Chapel Hill and with local agencies. The authors discuss the history and structure of the partnership, its goals and objectives, and its various funding streams in order to provide a vivid picture of the partnership context in which the AOCD occurred. They then describe in detail the CBPR approach to engaging insiders and outsiders in formulating the AOCD case study research design, selecting and using multiple data collection methods, analyzing data, and interpreting the findings and determining action steps to address them. They also offer an insightful examination of the limitations encountered and lessons learned.

References

Anyanwu, C. N. (1988). The technique of participatory research in community development. *Community Development Journal, 23,* 11–15.

Badger, T. G. (2000). Action research, change and methodological rigour. *Journal of Nursing Management, 8,* 201–207.

Boston, P., Jordan, S., MacNamara, E., Kozolanka, K., Bobbish-Rondeau, E., & Iserhoff, H. (1997). Using participatory action research to understand the meanings aboriginal Canadians attribute to the rising incidence of diabetes. *Chronic Disease in Canada, 18,* 5–12.

Chesler, M. A. (1991). Participatory action research with self-help groups: An alternative paradigm for inquiry and action. *American Journal of Community Psychology, 19,* 757–768.

Cornwall, A., & Jewkes, R. (1995). What is participatory research? *Social Science & Medicine, 41,* 1667–1676.

Eng, E., & Blanchard, L. (1991). Action-oriented community diagnosis: A health education tool. *International Journal of Community Health Education, 11*(2), 93–110.

Freudenberg, N. (2001). Case history of the Center for Urban Epidemiologic Studies in New York City. *Journal of Urban Health, 78,* 508–518.

Giesbrecht, N., & Ferris, J. (1993). Community-based research initiatives in prevention. *Addiction, 88*(Suppl.), S83–S93.

Green, L., Fullilove, M., Evans, D., & Shepard, P. (2002). "Hey, Mom, thanks!": Use of focus groups in the development of place-specific materials for a community environmental action campaign. *Environmental Health Perspectives, 110*(Suppl. 2), S265–S269.

Israel, B. A., Schulz, A. J., Parker, E. A., & Becker, A. B. (1998). Review of community-based research: Assessing partnership approaches to improve public health. *Annual Review of Public Health, 19,* 173–202.

Ivanov, L. L., & Flynn, B. C. (1999). Utilization and satisfaction with prenatal care services. *Western Journal of Nursing Research, 21,* 372–386.

Kovacs, P. J. (2000). Participatory action research and hospice: A good fit. *Hospice Journal of Physical and Psychosocial Pastoral Care and Dying, 15,* 55–62.

McQuiston, T. H. (2000). Empowerment evaluation of worker safety and health education programs. *American Journal of Industrial Medicine, 38,* 584–597.

O'Fallon, L. R., & Dearry, A. (2002). Community-based participatory research as a tool to advance environmental health sciences. *Environmental Health Perspectives, 110*(Suppl. 2), S155–S159.

Seeley, J. A., Kengeya-Kayondo, J. F., & Mulder, D. W. (1992). Community-based HIV/AIDS research: Whither community participation? Unsolved problems in a research programme in rural Uganda. *Social Science & Medicine, 34,* 1089–1095.

Steuart, G. W. (1985). Social and behavioral change strategies. In H. T. Phillips & S. A. Gaylord (Eds.), *Aging and public health.* New York: Springer.

VanderPlaat, M. (1997). *Emancipatory politics, critical evaluation and government policy.* Washington, DC: American Sociological Association.

Wang, C., Burris, M. A., & Ping, X. Y. (1996). Chinese village women as visual anthropologists: A participatory approach to reaching policymakers. *Social Science & Medicine, 42,* 1391–1400.

Wing, S. (2002). Social responsibility and research ethics in community-driven studies of industrialized hog production. *Environmental Health Perspectives, 110,* 437–444.

CHAPTER FOUR

Insiders and Outsiders Assess Who Is "The Community"

Participant Observation, Key Informant Interview, Focus Group Interview, and Community Forum

Eugenia Eng, Karen Strazza Moore, Scott D. Rhodes,
Derek M. Griffith, Leo L. Allison, Kate Shirah, and Elvira M. Mebane

Researchers who study groups or communities different from themselves have been called *professional strangers* (Merton, 1970). They differ in social status, a status frequently characterized by race or ethnicity, age, gender, social class, sexual orientation, or some combination of these characteristics. Being different in social status from the communities they study can impede researchers from getting into a community, getting along with community members, and gaining an *emic,* or insider's, view on how people live (Cassel, 1976; Kauffman, 1994; Steuart, 1985). An insider's view is privileged knowledge that is born through membership in a particular group, culture, and society and is socialized by position in that group, culture, and society (Merton, 1970; Steuart, 1985).

Acknowledgments: The authors deeply appreciate the considerable support, commitment, and contributions of the following individuals and groups with whom we serve as coinvestigators and co-learners. We thank the graduate students in health behavior and health education at the University of North Carolina at Chapel Hill School of Public Health who have set a high standard for following CBPR principles: the Efland-Cheeks Action-Oriented Community Diagnosis (AOCD) Team of Felicity Aulino, Jennifer Farnsworth, Jaimie Hunter, Julia Martin, Theresa Jackson, and Danielle Spurlock, and the AOCD teaching assistants Molly Loomis and Lauren Shirey. We express our sincere gratitude to our CBPR partners of thirteen years, from whom we continue to learn lessons about what a community is: the Orange County Health Department, the United Voices of Efland-Cheeks, Inc., and the Efland-Cheeks community. And we recognize our good fortune in receiving continued support from the W. K. Kellogg Foundation for preparing public health professionals to take a CBPR approach to addressing the major health problems and challenges facing society.

As professional strangers, researchers do not have direct access to the insider's view, and in some communities with prior negative experiences with and cultivated resentment of professional strangers, researchers may be excluded from access to the insider's view (Kauffman, 1994). At the same time, researchers can provide an *etic,* or outsider's, view of how people live, a view that is not complicated by membership in or socialization by the community being studied and therefore is relatively "objective." In addition, researchers can raise questions and seek new understanding about the ways people live that a community's insiders would be unlikely to recognize without outsider assistance (Kauffman, 1994; Merton, 1970; Steuart, 1985).

Understanding how people live is fundamental to the mission of public health in the United States, which is to ensure that the conditions exist in which people can be healthy (Institute of Medicine, 1988). As the Institute of Medicine concluded in *The Future of Public Health* (1988), achieving this mission will require public health agencies to join forces with organizations and communities to generate new learning for health status improvement. Through new learning about the conditions necessary for people to be in good health, each participating organization and each community will be changed. And through such mutual change, participating organizations and communities will have developed new models for community-based education, research, and service. The public health aim "is to generate organized community effort to address the public interest in health by applying scientific and technical knowledge to prevent disease and promote health. The mission of public health is addressed by private organizations and individuals as well as by public agencies. But the governmental public health agency has a unique function: to see to it that vital elements are in place and that the mission is adequately addressed" (p. 7).

This statement has three important implications for the field of public health in general and community-based participatory research (CBPR) in particular. First, the conditions required for people to be in good health are multidimensional—rooted in determinants that are not only biomedical and behavioral but also social, political, economic, and cultural (Cassel, 1970; Krieger, 2003; Taylor, 2002; Williams, 2003). Second, a community assessment is essential if service agencies, community-based organizations, and academic institutions are to pool their resources to gain the views of both insiders and outsiders on the multiple dimensions of health *and* are to succeed in organizing collective action to improve these dimensions (Butterfoss, Goodman, & Wandersman, 1996; Eng & Blanchard, 1991; Fetterman, 1989; Green & Kreuter, 1991; Parker et al., 1998; Steuart, 1985). Third, the procedures for conducting such a community assessment combine the principles and methods of scientific research with those of community organizing (Eng & Blanchard, 1991).

In this chapter we describe such a community assessment procedure, the *action-oriented community diagnosis* (AOCD). The purpose of AOCD is to understand the collective dynamics and functions of relationships within a community and the interactions between community members and broader structures that promote the conditions and skills required to assist community members in taking action for social change and health status improvement (Eng & Blanchard, 1991). Here, we explain the origins of AOCD and describe its research assumptions and methods and its link with CBPR. We follow that discussion with a case example. The example begins with a brief historical summary of United Voices of Efland-Cheeks, Inc. (UVE), a community-based organization, and its decade-long CBPR partnership with the University of North Carolina at Chapel Hill and local agencies. The structure of the partnership, its goals and objectives, and its various funding streams are also described to provide a vivid picture of the partnership context in which the AOCD occurred. We then describe in detail the CBPR approach to engaging insiders and outsiders in

- Formulating the AOCD case study research design
- Selecting and using multiple data collection methods
- Analyzing data
- Interpreting the findings and determining action steps to address them

In concluding, we highlight the limitations uncovered and the lessons learned from the Efland-Cheeks AOCD.

ORIGINS OF AOCD

The origins of action-oriented community diagnosis can be traced to the pioneering work of a small group of South African researchers at the Institute of Family and Community Health in South Africa from 1945 to 1959 (Kark & Steuart, 1962). Their methodology and their broad inclusion of social factors, such as poverty and discrimination, as determinants of health have been acknowledged as the fundamental work of the twentieth century in social epidemiology (Trostle, 1986). The group's leader, Sidney Kark, credited Guy Steuart, the psychologist in the group, with calling the researchers' attention to the importance of social networks and primary groups as community strengths and assets on which to build their work in community health education (Israel, Dawson, Steckler, & Eng, 1993).

Steuart trained health center staff in conducting a community assessment and using the findings to inform and incorporate new techniques into their daily practice at the health centers. The staff found that by engaging social groupings of people in a ten-week mutual exchange of discussion and decisions, as a natural extension of the staff's patient education activities, infant feeding practices changed in the desired direction (Kark & Steuart, 1962). Moreover, staff increased their own understanding of individuals within their own family situations, families within their communities, and what it is like to live in a community in relation to the social structure of South Africa (Kark & Steuart, 1962).

This group of South African researchers, trained as epidemiologists and behavioral scientists, considered gaining an insider's view from communities and blending it with their own outsider's view to be among the institute's most important work (Kark & Steuart, 1962). Their work, however, came to an abrupt end in 1959, when a new South African government began to apply apartheid policy to the medical professions. The group members dispersed to Israel, Kenya, and the United States.

From 1970 to 1984, Steuart chaired the Department of Health Education at the University of North Carolina at Chapel Hill (UNC-CH) School of Public Health, where he refined his community assessment procedure. He called it an *action-oriented community diagnosis* to indicate that when public health professionals engage communities in assessing their own strengths and problems, they are ethically bound to take action to address the problems, as physicians are ethically bound to ensure medical treatment for patients they diagnose with an illness or disability (Steckler, Dawson, Israel, & Eng, 1993). Steuart (1969) considered AOCD to be a critical first step in program planning and evaluation because it provides the foundation for

- The establishment of baselines from which objectives, intended outcomes, and measures of change are derived

- The selection of intervention methods and "units of practice" that are most appropriate to the natural networks of communication and influence

- A collaborative relationship between professionals and communities, who can begin "closing the gap between what we do not know and what we ought to know" (Steckler et al., 1993)

Since 1971, the Department of Health Behavior and Health Education at UNC-CH has been training students in its master's degree in public health program to acquire the competencies in community-based participatory research (CBPR) that are necessary for conducting AOCD. The competencies relevant to following CBPR principles (Israel et al., 2003) include proficiency in

- Discovering and articulating a conceptual foundation for defining community, community participation, community capacity, and community competence

- Adopting an ecological orientation to health promotion theories and interventions

- Facilitating groups in consensus decision making and conflict accommodation

- Gathering and interpreting secondary data sources
- Interviewing, participant observation, and other forms of primary data collection and analysis in community settings
- Using empowerment education techniques and conducting program planning

AOCD RESEARCH DESIGN AND METHODS

The following section provides a general description of the research paradigm, design, and methods applicable to conducting an AOCD. This is followed by a description and analysis of a case example.

Constructivist Research Paradigm

Every research design and its accompanying methods, such as the design and methods used in AOCD, reflect a specific research paradigm, that is, a set of basic beliefs about the nature of reality that can be studied and understood (Guba & Lincoln, 1994; Tashakkori & Teddlie, 1998). However well argued, these basic beliefs must be accepted simply on faith because there is no way to establish their ultimate truth. The *positivist* and *postpositivist* research paradigms, for example, hold that a single reality of how things really are and really work exists to be studied and understood. The *positivist* research paradigm holds that this single reality can be fully captured, and this paradigm is reflected in experimental research designs and methods (used most often in the basic sciences), whereas the *postpositivist* research paradigm holds that this single reality can be only approximated, and this view is reflected in quasi-experimental research designs and methods (used most often in the social and behavioral sciences). Both experimental and quasi-experimental methods require objective detachment between researchers and participants, so that any influence in either direction (that is, threats to validity) on what is being studied can be eliminated or reduced.

In AOCD, the set of basic beliefs derives from a *constructivist* research paradigm, which holds that multiple realities exist to be studied and understood (Guba & Lincoln, 1994; Tashakkori & Teddlie, 1998). Each reality is an intangible construction; rooted in people's experiences with everyday life and how they remember those experiences and make sense of them. Individual constructions of reality are assumed to be more or less *informed*, rather than more or less *true*, because they are always alterable. That is, as researchers and participants encounter and consider different perspectives, they will alter their own views. The result is a "consensus construction of reality" (Guba & Lincoln, 1994) that is informed by variations in predecessor constructions (including those of the researchers) and that can move both participants and researchers toward communicating about action and change (Habermas, 1984). The methods of constructivist research require researchers and participants to be interactively linked so that the consensus construction of reality is, literally, created as the study proceeds. AOCD researchers are cast, therefore, in the roles of participant and facilitator.

Case Study Research Design

AOCD researchers follow the case study research design, defined by Creswell (1998) as "an exploration of a 'bounded system' or case (or multiple cases) over time through detailed, in-depth data collection involving multiple sources of information rich in context, [which] include observations, interviews, audiovisual material, and documents and reports" (p. 61). The foundation of the case study design is purposeful sampling (Creswell, 1998), that is, the data to be collected are selected to represent what are considered to be the critical perspectives of the case. For AOCD, the case is a community, which is typically defined as geographically and locality based or identity based and in which members share a common culture or characteristics (Quinn, 1999). The critical perspectives to be represented in the data are those of insiders and outsiders. Insiders' views come from those who are members of the community of interest. Outsiders' views come from those who are not members but who provide services or otherwise exert external influence on the community, such as elected officials and academic researchers (Eng & Blanchard, 1991).

AOCD is conducted by a team of researchers and guided by one or two *preceptors* who are insiders, outsiders, or both. Preceptors work closely with the AOCD team through the important initial phase of entering a community and establishing rapport with its members. Being guided, accompanied, and introduced by preceptors is critical to the team's entry into the community. For the collection and analysis of primary and secondary data, preceptors connect the team with local agencies, community-based organizations, and special interest groups. Building relationships, developing trust, and fostering respect for the team's commitment to the community are important foundations of the data collection process. Finally, preceptors help the team coordinate and integrate tasks across institutional boundaries for interpreting and disseminating AOCD findings. In sum the interpersonal aspects of establishing a CBPR partnership with preceptors, agency professionals, and community members cannot be separated from AOCD research design, data collection and analysis, interpretation, and dissemination (Israel et al., 2003).

Data Collection and Analysis

It is important to note that one principle of the CBPR approach is to develop research systems, such as for data collection and analysis, that build research competencies among all partners by engagement in processes that are cyclical and iterative (Israel, Schulz, Parker, & Becker, 1998). Hence, with guidance from preceptors, the AOCD team collects and analyzes data iteratively, using the process of constant comparison (Strauss & Corbin, 1998). AOCD data sources are the following:

- Demographic data to describe population characteristics of the community

- Secondary data that represent professionals' perspectives on the community's social and health indicators

- Secondary data on the community's history and geography, including information on health and human service organizations serving the community

- Field notes containing each AOCD team member's observations of the community and of the agencies that serve community residents

- Transcripts from interviews with key informants for outsiders' views

- Transcripts from interviews with key informants for insiders' views

As data are collected the AOCD team members and their preceptors immediately analyze them to inform the next lines of inquiry.

Incidents, actions, and events reported by insiders are compared within and across data sources, using the qualitative research method of coding and retrieving (Huberman & Miles, 1994). A code is a category of meaning or a concept (for example, *voice in government and politics*) that is identified by reading through text from interview transcripts and secondary data. To develop a list of codes, at least two researchers independently read through the initial data, come to a consensus on the name and definition for each code, and present the list to the rest of the team and the preceptors for final refinement. All text lines representing the same concept are assigned the same code so that they can be retrieved and grouped to determine one or more patterns of meaning, or themes. The same is done with data sources that represent the perspectives of outsiders (for example, interview transcripts and secondary data), including those of individuals on the AOCD team (for example, field notes from participant observations). Convergent analysis of themes is conducted to examine similarities and differences between the perspectives of insiders and the perspectives of outsiders on the conditions needed for a community to be in good health.

Dissemination

As the findings are identified, the AOCD team and its preceptors select insiders and outsiders to serve on the AOCD *forum planning committee*. The purpose of this committee is to review, interpret, prioritize, and disseminate the themes that are identified from insiders' and outsiders' views on a community's assets, challenges, and needs for change. The committee then determines the content, format, and logistics for a forum to engage community residents and local service providers in interpreting the results, forging a *consensus construction* from the findings on the conditions necessary for a community to be in good health, and committing to the next action steps (Eng & Blanchard, 1991; Quinn, 1999; Shirah, Eng, Moore, Rhodes, & Royster, 2002). In addition, a written full report on the AOCD procedures, findings, and forum outcomes is produced by the team and approved by the preceptors. Hard copies and electronic files are distributed to local public libraries and other organizations determined by the AOCD team and the preceptors.

Duration

In short, both AOCD and CBPR are as much processes of relationship building and community organizing as they are research processes (Eng & Blanchard, 1991; Israel et al., 1998). Given the necessity of building relationships and research partnerships, it is important to realistically anticipate the time required to complete AOCD. Although the duration will vary according to the skills of the individuals on the team, the readiness of the community, travel distance, and other variables, it is realistic to estimate a *minimum* of six to nine months. This time period is needed to begin building relationships and, ultimately, to establish mutual commitment to the research as well as to taking action. Even when researchers are invited by a community to conduct AOCD, as described in the case example that follows, all involved should allow at least six months for the process.

APPLICATION OF AOCD METHODS WITH UNITED VOICES OF EFLAND-CHEEKS

In the following section we describe the application of AOCD methods with United Voices of Efland-Cheeks, Inc. (UVE). We describe the partnership background, the data collection methods used, and the steps involved in conducting this AOCD.

Partnership Background

UVE is a community-based organization operating with its own governing structure and by-laws. The North Carolina communities served by UVE are rural and largely African American separated historically and geographically from the health, business, educational, and financial resources of Chapel Hill, located in the same county fifteen miles away. UVE's mission is to improve the quality of life for children, youths, adults, and seniors in Efland-Cheeks, North Carolina, by providing a variety of educational, literary, scientific, and charitable activities. Since 1992, UVE has sustained a partnership with the UNC-CH School of Public Health, through the North Carolina Community-Based Public Health Consortium's governing structures and processes aimed specifically at engaging all partners in CBPR (Parker et al., 1998). UVE board members include concerned community members and representatives from the Orange County Health Department and other local health agencies and the UNC-CH School of Public Health. Through these collaborations, UVE has undertaken such activities as serving as a CBPR training site for three postdoctoral fellows in the W. K. Kellogg Foundation–funded Community Health Scholars Program, providing Community Voices Leadership Training for local residents, and serving as a community research partner for the CDC-funded Men As Navigators (MAN) for Health Project to increase informed decision making about prostate cancer screening among rural African American men.

Our focus is on the action-oriented community diagnosis conducted in Efland-Cheeks from October 2002 to April 2003 by a team of six graduate students while they were enrolled in a two-semester AOCD course sequence required for the MPH degree in the UNC-CH Department of Health Behavior and Health Education. Two were from North Carolina, five were white, and one was African American. All were women. In the classroom, they learned the concepts and practiced the skills for conducting AOCD from a teaching team (two instructors, two teaching assistants, and two postdoctoral fellows). In Efland-Cheeks, two preceptors simultaneously guided the students in applying their newly learned skills. These preceptors were African Americans born and raised in Efland-Cheeks: the UVE president at that time (a retired man) and a founding member of UVE (a woman employed as a records clerk at the Orange County Health Department).

The last community assessment of Efland-Cheeks had been conducted in 1990, as an important part of the activity associated with a planning year award to the UNC-CH School of Public Health for the Community-Based Public Health Initiative, funded by the W. K. Kellogg Foundation. This initiative led to the formation of UVE in 1992. Ten years later, UVE and two long-time UNC-CH partners, who teach the required AOCD course, agreed that the process and new knowledge to be generated through another AOCD would be mutually beneficial. UVE would be able to revitalize its agenda and membership, based on a new understanding of changes in the conditions within and surrounding Efland-Cheeks. New public health professionals being trained at UNC-CH would be guided by a community's insiders in gaining skills, through on-the-ground experience, in community-based practice and participatory research.

During the six-month AOCD period, the team members met weekly, and with their preceptors every two weeks, rotating the responsibilities for creating the meeting agenda, facilitating the meeting, and writing the minutes. To communicate with the preceptors by e-mail or telephone more frequently, the team designated a liaison. Hard copies of the minutes, along with other AOCD documents, were placed in a locked, central file. The teaching team also created a password-protected Web site for the AOCD team and the team preceptors to facilitate electronic file sharing. In addition, the teaching team held a lunch meeting every other month with the preceptors for the Efland-Cheeks team and the preceptors for seven other AOCD teams, and designated an instructor as the liaison who would communicate with the preceptors.

Gathering Secondary Data

Gathering secondary data provided the AOCD team with an initial broad brushstroke that revealed how the community was portrayed by outsiders in the health and human service professions, political arena, and elsewhere. The Efland-Cheeks team members used secondary data as background information to chart their entry into the community, identify gaps in existing data, and inform their interview guides. They collected statistics from secondary sources and qualitative data, including U.S. and North Carolina census data and data from the Web sites of North Carolina and Orange County governmental agencies (for example, health departments, planning departments, school boards, departments on aging, chambers of commerce, transportation departments, and the Environmental Protection Agency), and information from an earlier AOCD report on the Efland-Mebane Corridor (Roodhouse, Siegfried, & Viruell, 1990), an evaluation report on UVE's Teens In Power program (Bruning, Eastwood, Gerhard, & Reid, 1993), and a master's degree thesis on a photovoice study conducted with Efland-Cheeks youths (Tucker, 2000). In addition, during interviews, the team solicited brochures, newspaper articles, annual reports, and grant applications.

Efland-Cheeks is an unincorporated community with no legally defined boundaries. Hence geographical boundaries are approximate, statistical data have rarely been collected at the community level, and relevant data that are part of other data sets cannot be extracted easily, efficiently, or cost effectively from available sources. Efland-Cheeks' population size of 500 to 600 families, of whom about one-fourth are African American, is also just an estimate. "For some, Efland is a state of mind" (Aulino et al., 2003, p. 14). Consequently, the team had to extrapolate from county-level statistics and make interpretations, while avoiding generalizations about Efland-Cheeks, to prepare for entering the community.

Participant Observation and Gaining Entry

Participant observation is a primary data-gathering device used for an in-depth case study approach in which researchers are directly involved with people's lives. It is intended to "generate practical and theoretical truths about human life grounded in the realities of daily existence" (Jorgensen, 1989, p. 14). In preparing for their entry into Efland-Cheeks as a group of outsiders, the team members and their preceptors decided on the following honest, jargon-free way of introducing themselves and explaining why they were there (Bogdewic, 1992): "We are a group of six UNC students collaborating with community members in Efland-Cheeks to learn about the strengths and concerns of the Efland-Cheeks community."

The AOCD team's first participant observation was a *windshield tour* of Efland-Cheeks and the surrounding area, guided by the preceptors. The team members observed and recorded field notes on local names for back roads and landmarks such as churches, the community center, and a car wash; physical conditions of housing, other buildings, and roads; and distances to businesses, schools, and other service agencies. During the tour they stopped to enter places where people gathered to observe and participate in social exchanges. In addition, they used the opportunity of UVE's annual Octoberfest fundraiser to make initial contacts, and they volunteered in UVE's after-school program in order to see and be seen with residents and service providers. These direct interactions at local community events were essential for the AOCD team to begin gaining access to key people in the community and local agencies and to begin to be entrusted with information that was pertinent and dependable (Bogdewic, 1992). The team also identified local organizations and decision-making bodies to observe by reviewing the "community pages" of the local telephone directory. In consultation with the preceptors, the team selected the following for participant observation: the Efland-Cheeks Seniors Group's morning activities; the county health department's waiting room; board meetings of the county commissioners, the school board, the planning board, and the transportation board; PTA meetings; and UVE monthly meetings. To avoid being obtrusive, no more than two team members observed an event.

It was important for each team member to record field notes systematically on her reactions, thoughts, and feelings about what she saw and heard (Bogdewic, 1992). A participant observer consciously recording details can construct patterns and meanings from analyzing those field notes. Moreover, it is the team members' views that will have an impact on their data collection, interpretation, and next steps. Recording field notes and debriefing with other members of the team on their respective perceptions, thoughts, and feelings are critical sources of data. Each team member therefore transcribed her field notes and entered them into an electronic database for analysis by other members. To prepare to use the qualitative research method of coding and retrieving (Huberman & Miles, 1994), the team determined initial codes, which are categories of meaning, by having each team member code her own field notes. The team then convened with the preceptors to come to an agreement on an initial list of domains, associated code names, and definitions. For example, the domain of *potential key informants* included the code *service providers,* which was defined as *names or positions of staff at a local agency to be interviewed.* To aid in analyzing coded field notes, the team created an electronic table, using domains and code names as column headings, and entered extracted text from their field notes. During the team members' biweekly meetings with the preceptors, they reviewed the contents of this table to inform their decisions about key informants to be recruited for interviews and important issues to be explored during those interviews. (For further discussion of the use of field notes, see Chapter Ten and Appendix F.)

Key Informant Interviews

To represent the views of insiders and outsiders, it is important to interview knowledgeable community members and representatives from local agencies and institutions. Given the constraints of time and resources, however, AOCD researchers cannot cultivate relationships with every knowledgeable insider and outsider. Instead, AOCD researchers conduct in-depth interviews with *key informants* (Goetz & LeCompte, 1984; Spradley, 1979), those who have been in the community or institution for sufficient time to have accumulated special knowledge, relationships with people, and access to observations that are denied to researchers. Key informants who are thoughtful observers and informal historians are valuable to AOCD researchers (Bernard, 1988). Not only can they articulate important issues but they can explain why they see those particular issues as important. (See Chapter Twelve for a discussion of how to design and conduct in-depth interviews in a CBPR context.)

Key informants' views on the history and culture of the community, social groupings and relationships with institutions, and perceived barriers and facilitators for past and current health promotion efforts provide an indispensable foundation for interventions to promote good health. Their perspective and expertise, however, are often eclipsed by secondary data used to define where the problem areas are and what a community needs to ameliorate the problem. Nevertheless, once researchers connect with key informants, these individuals' investment in the AOCD and their expertise can increase the willingness of community members and local institutions to embrace, participate in, and sustain the process initiated by the AOCD team. Moreover, recognizing and valuing priorities identified by key informants is a major CBPR principle (Israel et al., 1998).

In Efland-Cheeks the team identified key informants through seeking referrals from the preceptors, looking in public domain listings of leaders in institutions and agencies, and asking questions like these at the end of each interview:

- Are there people or organizations with whom you think we should speak that you would be willing to gain permission for our team to contact?

- How would you describe this specific person or organization?

- Why would you think their opinion and views would be helpful for us to hear?

In addition the team gave copies of a fact sheet to preceptors and others to distribute to potential key informants. The fact sheet described the purpose of AOCD, data collection procedures, potential benefits and harms, and information for contacting the AOCD team. This fact sheet was reviewed and approved by the UNC-CH institutional review board (IRB) for the protection of human subjects. To ensure casting a wide net the team maintained a record of referrals to information sources and key informants in order to chart the diversity of views represented.

Receiving IRB approval in December 2002, the team recruited a total of forty-two key informants (twenty-eight community members and fourteen service providers). Of the twenty-eight community members, ten adults participated in face-to-face interviews, and twelve youths and six adults participated in the focus group interviews (described later). The fourteen service providers all participated in face-to-face interviews.

Key informant face-to-face interviews used an in-depth interview guide (see Appendix B). To develop this guide, the team members reviewed guides used in the past by other AOCD teams. They modified the issues covered by these previous interview guides in light of the findings from their own participant observations and review of secondary data sources. They modified the wording and the sequence of questions as a result of what they learned from practice interviews with each other and pretesting with the preceptors. After the pretesting they made final revisions to the interview guide and then conducted a debriefing session.

Each interview began with introductions and a brief explanation of the interviewing process that was guided by the fact sheet. The community key informant interview guide contained twenty-two open-ended questions that explored the following seven areas:

- General information about the Efland-Cheeks community

- Assets and needs of the community

- Problem-solving and decision-making patterns

- Services and businesses

- Recommended individuals to interview

- Recommendations for the community forum

- Additional information

The team members and their preceptors followed similar procedures to develop and pretest the service provider key informant interview guide.

It contained and explored the same areas and asked similar questions in all areas except the one for services and businesses, which asked the following seven questions:

1. How long have you worked in this community? Why did you choose to work in Efland-Cheeks?

2. What is your agency's role in the community? What is your source of funding?

3. What services do you provide to residents of Efland-Cheeks?

4. What services go underutilized?

5. Who in the community is in most need of your agency's services?

6. What are your biggest barriers/challenges?

7. Which community needs are not met by your agency or other organizations in Efland-Cheeks?

Each interview was conducted and audiotaped by two members of the AOCD team, and took from forty-five to ninety minutes to complete. A note taker accompanied the interviewer to record written verbal statements and nonverbal cues. After completing each interview, the two team members met to debrief the interview and discuss their written field notes on important points made by the key informant and their own personal reflections on the experience. The interviewer transcribed these debriefing notes and the note taker's written record of the interview itself, which were then reviewed for accuracy by the note taker.

To maintain the confidentiality of the interviewees, the team assigned an identification code to each respondent and kept this list, along with the audio-cassette, in a locked file. Moreover, to prepare the transcripts for analysis by the full team and their preceptors, they removed all identifiers. To determine initial codes for identifying and retrieving relevant text, each team member coded the same two transcripts (one service provider interview and one community member interview). Team members convened with the preceptors to come to an agreement on an initial list of domains, associated code names, and their definitions. For example, for the domain of *community strengths,* the code of *neighbors helping neighbors* was defined as *social support exchanged among residents.* For the domain of *community needs,* the code of *youth recreation* was defined as *inadequate facilities or activities for kids outside of school.* To code the transcripts, two team members (one present at the interview and one who was not) listened to the audio recordings three times: the first time all the way through; a second time to make notes on important points; and a third time to assign codes. To analyze coded transcripts, the team created two electronic matrices (one for service provider transcripts with accompanying debriefing notes and one for community member transcripts with accompanying debriefing notes). Row headings were each key informant's identification number, and column headings were the domains and code names for entering extracted text assigned a particular domain and code. This analytical method of coding and retrieving (Huberman & Miles, 1994) was done within a week after each interview by the note taker. During the team's biweekly meetings with the preceptors, they reviewed the text entered into each matrix to inform their decisions on additional key informants to be recruited, additional probes for future interviews, and additional codes.

By the end of March the team and its preceptors determined that the interviews were no longer generating new information, that is, team members could predict the responses. At this point three members were assigned the task of reading through the text entered into each cell of the matrices to identify themes or patterns of meaning, with representative quotes, from the perspectives of insiders and outsiders respectively. They brought these findings for review by the full team and preceptors, who then discussed how to present them to the forum planning committee (described later).

Key informant focus group interviews were conducted with one group of six adult community members and two groups of six youths each. The procedures followed for the adult focus group interview were identical to those described earlier for conducting key informant in-depth interviews with adult community members. The procedures for the youth focus group interviews, however, were different.

During a February meeting with the team to read through the matrices, the preceptors realized that the perspectives of youths in Efland-Cheeks were not being solicited through AOCD. They considered youths such an important part of UVE's mission that they asked the team to recruit and interview youths. The team submitted a modification to the IRB and received approval for youths to participate anonymously in focus group interviews.

The preceptors distributed a fact sheet to the youths and their guardians, which was similar to the fact sheet for key informant interviews described earlier. The focus group interview guide explored four topics with the youths:

1. Their satisfaction with Efland-Cheeks, and what they would change about it
2. What they do for fun and to make money
3. Interactions at school, and what they would change
4. Their recommendations for the community forum

The focus group interviews with both youths and adults took from forty-five to ninety minutes to complete. (For further discussion of focus group interview procedures, see Chapter Seven.) The analytical method of coding and retrieving, described earlier, was again used. In addition, youth members were added to the forum planning committee.

Community Forum

The desired outcome of AOCD is not only to produce a report but also to begin a process of action informed by and grounded in systematic analysis of and reflection on the findings. One of the most valuable means for generating this outcome is present when the AOCD process culminates in a community forum so that diverse community groups and those who serve them are able to gather, listen to, and discuss the results of the data collection process.

Facilitation of the community forum is critical, as the articulation of insider and outsider perspectives must be done equitably, with both insiders and outsiders discussing the health, needs, and resources of the community and prioritizing the next steps in an action plan. A community forum has three goals (Eng & Moore, 2003):

1. Arrive at a consensus on priority needs and motivations for change.

2. Examine possible causes and consequences of a priority problem.

3. Establish a partnership between communities and local agencies to develop a plan of action.

The session should not be spent merely identifying what is "wrong" in the community; time should be dedicated to articulating community strengths and resources as well. At the forum's culmination, it is intended that some of those attending will have identified themselves as willing to commit to accepting responsibility for planning a next meeting and following through with specific elements of the action plan. (See Chapter Thirteen for further discussion of dissemination methods.)

In anticipation of the need to enlist collaborators to plan the Efland-Cheeks Community Forum, the team and preceptors identified fifteen community residents and service providers from those interviewed. That is, at the conclusion of each interview, the interviewer explained that a gathering would be held to discuss the findings and asked if the key informant would be willing to be contacted again to assist with planning such an event. In early March, the fifteen who had agreed to help were invited to serve on the Efland-Cheeks Community Forum Planning Committee with the team and preceptors.

With the formation of this committee, the team and preceptors began an important transition: the preceptors assumed the role of UVE representatives and offered the resources of UVE for coordinating the work of the committee and ensuring follow-up, and the university members of the team assumed the role of staff to the committee for the forum and the role of participants for the first follow-up meeting. For the first planning committee meeting, in mid-March, one team member and one preceptor cofacilitated introductions, a brief description of AOCD, and a discussion of the goals of the forum and of the roles of the planning committee before, during, and after the forum. The committee agreed to meet once a week, to hold the forum in late April in the local elementary school cafeteria, and to title the forum "Showcase for the Future: Spotlight on Efland." During these weekly meetings, the team reviewed the fourteen themes found in the data for the committee to interpret, restate, and prioritize. In selecting themes with the highest priority, committee members considered the number of people affected and the role of agencies in contributing to causes and consequences. They also developed the following strategies to promote the forum:

- They posted flyers in prominent places throughout the community, such as the post office, barbershops, the car wash, a local convenience store, and the Efland-Cheeks Community Center. In addition, each child at the elementary school received a flyer to take home on the Wednesday before the forum. The school also posted a banner announcement outside the school the week before the forum.

- They delivered personal invitations to church leaders and announcements that these leaders could read to congregations on three consecutive Sundays before the forum.

- They delivered printed inserts to the Orange-Alamance Water System to be included with water bills mailed in April.

- To engage participation of local businesses in the forum they solicited pizzas and door prizes such as passes to sporting events, restaurant gift certificates, and movie tickets.

- To showcase local talent they arranged for performances by the local youth step team, a gospel singing group, and others.

Over one hundred people, including thirty youths, participated in the forum. Members of the planning committee welcomed attendees and explained the goals of the forum. The university-based team members then briefly described the purpose of AOCD and the methods used, presented the major themes that had emerged, and invited participants to choose a small group to discuss one of the four themes selected by the committee. Themes discussed were lack of recreational opportunities for youth, poor water and sewer infrastructure, lack of transportation, and the need for services located in the community. (For a more detailed discussion about each theme, see www.hsl.unc.edu/phpapers/ Efland2003.pdf.20)

Team members, trained in empowerment education techniques, used force field analysis (Lewin, 1997) and SHOWED (Wallerstein, 1992) to facilitate the small-group discussions. (See Chapter Fifteen for a description of the SHOWED technique and Appendix A for a description of the force field analysis procedure.). Small-group participants discussed the causes and consequences of their particular theme and then reflected on how this issue affected them personally and the community as a whole. They then formulated action steps that were summarized and presented back to the large group by a community representative from each of the small groups. In anticipation that some strong feelings might arise from the small-group discussions, the committee interspersed performances and door prizes throughout the forum's agenda. Finally, the action steps generated at the forum were incorporated into the AOCD final report (Aulino et al., 2003).

At the conclusion of the forum, a preceptor formally announced two important transitions. One was the transition from findings to action steps, formalized by announcing the date for a follow-up meeting that would be coordinated by UVE. The second was that although UVE and the committee would coordinate follow-up activities, the university members of the team would be exiting Efland-Cheeks after the next meeting. A team member then expressed, on the behalf of the entire team, the team members' appreciation to all participants and especially to planning committee members. To underscore the importance of moving from findings to next action steps, the team member requested participants to complete an interest form to indicate the action steps they would personally like to pursue at the follow-up meeting (Aulino et al., 2003). Finally, a committee member thanked the Efland-Cheeks AOCD team and its preceptors.

CHALLENGES AND LIMITATIONS

Although conducting a social diagnosis such as AOCD is considered an essential initial phase of program planning, it is too often skipped, for a variety of reasons (Green & Kreuter, 1991). As discussed earlier, if it is to follow CBPR principles, AOCD requires a substantial investment of time—a minimum of six months—for gaining entrée to a community and agencies, building relationships with preceptors and key informants, and engaging them in collecting, analyzing, and interpreting data, and also for planning and conducting a forum to transition from findings to action steps. Frequently, health professionals engage in AOCD as part of their job responsibilities, and researchers as part of their investigations. Their involvement in AOCD is governed by a clock imposed and paced by their institutions. The progress of the Efland-Cheeks AOCD, for example, was challenged by academic institution inflexibility in the form of the IRB's meeting schedule, semester breaks, and deadlines for submitting grades. Similarly, community members' ongoing obligations to jobs and families competed with the time required to collaborate with the AOCD team in such roles as preceptor, key informant, or forum planning committee member.

Another challenge is that the CBPR approach of AOCD requires co-learning from both insiders and outsiders. They must reconcile the new knowledge generated with their current understandings and experiences of the community (Perry, 1968; Israel et al., 1998); however, such co-learning can sometimes frustrate people. On the personal level, professionals engaged in AOCD often encounter and collaborate with people who differ from themselves in social status (Merton, 1970; Shirah et al., 2002). To make these differences explicit in the consciousness of students, the UNC-CH AOCD course organizes three required workshops, led by trained facilitators, on institutionalized racism, invisibility of persons with disabilities, and homophobia. Members of the Efland-Cheeks AOCD team, for example, wrote extensively in their field notes about being conscious of their internalized privilege resulting from their being white or being UNC-CH graduate students, or both. They speculated on how being different from rural, low-income, African Americans could limit their capacity to graft the cultural, historical, and experiential roots of Efland-Cheeks onto AOCD methods and findings. Similarly, reflections on invisible differences have been recorded by AOCD teams working with communities of persons with disabilities or lesbian, gay, bisexual, and transgender communities. In short, one important feature of co-learning is the discovery of "what we don't know and what we ought to know" about these differences. Such self-other awareness is critical to the CBPR approach for establishing research partnerships with communities.

AOCD also requires the application of a range of concepts and skills from the fields of anthropology, epidemiology, health education, political science, community psychology, and community organizing. Learning and applying all these ideas and abilities adeptly is impossible for a single person (Shirah et al., 2002). Hence using a partnership approach that builds synergistically on each partner's experiences and skill set can maximize the quality of each method and task used in completing AOCD. To ensure a range of skills among students assigned to each UNC-CH AOCD team, the teaching team used the information from a twenty-five-item *profile questionnaire* that is completed by each student to identify the assets she or he brings to AOCD. These assets included training in cultural competency or small-group facilitation; experience in conducting surveys, qualitative interviews, or focus group interviews; proficiency with computer software programs; exposure to populations and cultures different from one's own; ability to speak two or more languages; and having a driver's license and access to a car. Furthermore, the members of each team and their preceptors completed an *inventory of assets* to document their respective contributions, such as time, skills, resources, access to other resources and people, and vested interests.

A final challenge in applying AOCD is to exit the community and yet sustain movement from data collection, analysis, and interpretation to the action steps generated during the community forum. When an AOCD team is using a program planning procedure, such as Precede-Proceed (Green & Kreuter, 1991), the next phase would be for the team to engage the community forum planning committee and other forum participants in an epidemiological diagnosis of the identified priority need, which would be followed by several more phases of needs assessment, intervention design, implementation, and evaluation. However, when the team is an AOCD team of students, as it was in Efland-Cheeks, the team members could prepare for the process of exiting the community with their preceptors—agreeing on the goals, deadlines, and responsibilities for establishing a community forum planning committee that would ensure follow-up on the action steps generated during the AOCD forum and documented in the final report. The Efland-Cheeks team and its preceptors took this approach and had also asked a question earlier in the process about key informants' availability to serve on the forum planning committee. Finally, the Efland-Cheeks team and the preceptors were explicit with committee members about the committee's role in facilitating follow-up.

LESSONS LEARNED AND IMPLICATIONS FOR CONDUCTING AOCD

How a community is defined (as an entity that is relational, that is a geographical locality, or that has the potential for political power; Heller, 1989) can have an important impact on both CBPR and the AOCD process. When an AOCD team uses geographical boundaries to define a community, it may overlook the assets and needs of subcommunities whose membership is based on a common interest, history, or some other relational characteristic that is not geographically based. When an AOCD team defines a community as relational, the potential risk is that it will neglect the impact of the physical environment on the community's identity. When geographical boundaries are not clear and shared relationships are not clearly visible, a community-based intervention can be problematic to design, implement, and evaluate (Shirah et al., 2002). It is essential therefore that public health researchers attempt to identify and collaborate with existing communities of identity, as defined by community members (Steuart, 1985). Given the CBPR principle of recognizing community as a unit of identity in order to strengthen sense of community through collective engagement (Israel et al., 1998), AOCD is a viable option. In an ideal world, AOCD would be conducted by public health organizations that respect and recognize a community's shared ownership of research procedures, findings, and dissemination. Organizations, however, do not always recognize when their own priorities are in conflict with those of a community. They have administrative and policy mandates that are likely to differ from the historical traditions and cultural norms to which the community gives precedence. Funding organizations have expectations, which in most cases do not allow study focus flexibility, not even when the change is requested by the community being studied. Furthermore, organizations may place their professionals in the awkward position of negotiating on the behalf of a community or speaking for a community.

For these professionals, the pressures of competing interests are counterbalanced by the privilege of gaining entry to and developing trust with a community.

In this less-than-ideal world, AOCD offers public health organizations, universities, and communities a process for beginning a CBPR partnership—one that engenders a constant of open negotiation, co-learning, and reciprocity. Entering into such a relationship can be a difficult transition for well-intentioned professionals who have been trained to be in control and to perceive themselves as having a larger skill set than that of their community partners. Yet engaging in AOCD carries the long-term rewards of a CBPR partnership committed to understanding and addressing the conditions that support a community's good health.

CONCLUSION

The purpose of action-oriented community diagnosis is to understand the collective dynamics and functions of relationships in a community as well as the interactions between that community and broader structures. This understanding can promote the conditions and skills required to assist community members in taking action for social change and health status improvement (Eng & Blanchard, 1991). Drawing on the disciplines of anthropology, epidemiology, and community psychology, AOCD follows the assumptions of a constructivist research paradigm and combines both quantitative and qualitative methods to elicit and juxtapose the insiders' view and the outsiders' view.

Key to AOCD is its community-based participatory research approach that includes lay community members, community-based organization representatives, health department and other agency staff, and university personnel, especially student and faculty researchers (Israel et al., 1998). These individuals share control over all phases of the research process, including community assessment, issue definition, development of research methodology, data collection and analysis, interpretation of data, dissemination of findings, and application of the results to address community concerns (action). This approach recognizes that lay community members are the experts in understanding and interpreting their own lives.

AOCD is also an assets-oriented approach to understanding a community. Although identifying community needs and gaps is important in the quest to improve health outcomes, identifying assets that the community can build on or further develop is equally important. Building on social structures and existing networks, decision-making processes, and local resources and strengths can yield intervention strategies that are rooted in the community, develop local critical-thinking and problem-solving skills, and ensure sustained efforts.

Finally, like CBPR, AOCD is research committed to movement toward action. This action may be loosely defined and may involve community organizing and mobilization, the development of new and authentic community member and agency partnerships with concrete tasks, and measurable plans for action with assigned responsibilities and defined timelines. The actions may be focused on immediate changes to improve health-related conditions, such as revising public health department policies in order to increase access to services or improving lighting on an outdoor neighborhood running and walking track. Or the actions may be focused on bringing about long-term changes in social determinants of health, such as improving racial equality in political representation through community mobilization and organization.

References

Aulino, F., Farnsworth, J., Hunter, J., Jackson, T., Philpott, J., & Spurlock, D. (2003). *Efland, Orange County: An action-oriented community diagnosis: Findings and next steps of action.* Retrieved from http://www.hsl.unc.edu/phpapers/Efland2003.pdf.

Bernard, H. R. (1988). *Research methods in cultural anthropology.* Thousand Oaks, CA: Sage.

Bogdewic, S. P. (1992). Participant observation. In B. F. Crabtree & W. L. Miller (Eds.), *Doing qualitative research* (pp. 47–70). Thousand Oaks, CA: Sage.

Bruning, A., Eastwood, K., Gerhard, L., & Reid, A. (1993). *Teens in Power: A program for the prevention of illicit drug use by adolescents in the Efland-Cheeks Community.* Report prepared for PUBH246, Public Health Program Planning and Evaluation, University of North Carolina at Chapel Hill.

Butterfoss, F. D., Goodman, R. M., & Wandersman, A. (1996). Community coalitions for prevention and health promotion: Factors predicting satisfaction, participation, and planning. *Health Education Quarterly, 23*(1), 65–79.

Cassel, J. C. (1976). The contribution of the social environment to host resistance: The Fourth Wade Hampton Frost Lecture. *American Journal of Epidemiology, 104,* 107–123.

Creswell, J. W. (1998). *Qualitative inquiry and research design: Choosing among five traditions.* Thousand Oaks, CA: Sage.

Eng, E., & Blanchard, L. (1991). Action-oriented community diagnosis: A health education tool. *International Journal of Community Health Education, 11*(2), 93–110.

Eng, E., & Moore, K. S. (2003). *The community forum.* Lecture in HBHE 241, Action-Oriented Community Diagnosis, University of North Carolina, School of Public Health.

Fetterman, D. M. (1989). *Ethnography: Step by step.* Thousand Oaks, CA: Sage.

Goetz, J. P., & LeCompte, M. D. (1984). *Ethnography and qualitative design in educational research.* New York: Academic Press.

Green, L. W., & Kreuter, M. W. (1991). *Health promotion planning: An educational and environmental approach* (2nd ed.). Mountain View, CA: Mayfield.

Guba, E. G., & Lincoln, Y. S. (1994). Competing paradigms in qualitative research. In N. K. Denzin & Y. S. Lincoln (Eds.), *Handbook of qualitative research.* Thousand Oaks, CA: Sage.

Habermas, J. (1984). *The theory of communicative action.* Cambridge, MA: Polity Press.

Heller, K. (1989). The return to community. *Journal of Community Psychology, 17*(1), 1–15.

Huberman, A., & Miles, M. (1994). Data management and analysis methods. In N. K. Denzin & Y. S. Lincoln (Eds.), *Handbook of qualitative research* (pp. 179–210). Thousand Oaks, CA: Sage.

Institute of Medicine. (1988). *The future of public health.* Washington, DC: National Academies Press.

Israel, B. A., Dawson, L., Steckler, A. B., & Eng, E. (1993). Guy W. Steuart: The person and his works. *Health Education Quarterly* (Suppl. 1), S137–S150.

Israel, B. A., Schulz, A. J., Parker, E. A., & Becker, A. B. (1998). Review of community-based research: Assessing partnership approaches to improve public health. *Annual Review of Public Health, 19,* 173–202.

Israel, B. A., Shulz, A., Parker, E. A., Becker, A., Allen, A. J., & Guzman, R. (2003). Critical issues in developing and following community-based participatory research principles. In M. Minkler & N. Wallerstein (Eds.), *Community-based participatory research for health* (pp. 53–76). San Francisco: Jossey-Bass.

Jorgensen, D. L. (1989). *Participant observation: A methodology of human studies.* Thousand Oaks, CA: Sage.

Kark, S. L., & Steuart, G. W. (1962). *A practice of social medicine: A South African team's experiences in different African communities.* Edinburgh: Livingstone.

Kauffman, K. S. (1994). The insider/outsider dilemma: Field experience of a white researcher "getting in" a poor black community. *Nursing Research, 43*(3), 179–183.

Krieger, N. (2003). Does racism harm health? Did child abuse exist before 1962? On explicit questions, critical science, and current controversies: An ecosocial perspective. *American Journal of Public Health, 93*(2), 194–199.

Lewin, K. (1997). *Resolving social conflicts and field theory in social science.* Washington, DC: American Psychological Association. (Original work published 1948)

Merton, R. K. (1970). Insiders and outsiders: A chapter in the sociology of knowledge. *American Journal of Sociology, 7,* 9–45.

Parker, E. A., Eng, E., Laraia, B., Ammerman, A., Dodds, J., Margolis, L., Cross, A. (1998). Coalition building for prevention: Lessons learned from the North Carolina Community-Based Public Health Initiative. *Journal of Public Health Management and Practice, 4*(2), 25–36.

Perry, W. G. (1968). *Forms of intellectual and ethical development in the college years: A scheme.* Austin, TX: Holt, Rinehart and Winston.

Quinn, S. (1999). Teaching community diagnosis: Integrating community experience with meeting graduate standards for health educators. *Health Education Research 14*(5), 685–696.

Roodhouse, K., Siegfried, J., & Viruell, E. (1990). *Orange County community diagnosis, 1990: Needs assessment of Efland-Mebane Corridor.* Report prepared for the Department of Health Behavior and Health Education, University of North Carolina at Chapel Hill.

Shirah, K., Eng, E., Moore, K., Rhodes, S. D., & Royster, M. O. (2002). *Insider's view and outsider's view: Duality of cultural understanding and planned social change.* Paper presented at the meeting of the American Public Health Association, Philadelphia.

Spradley, J. P. (1979). *The ethnographic interview.* Austin, TX: Holt, Rinehart and Winston.

Steckler, A. B., Dawson, L., Israel, B. A., & Eng, E. (1993). Community health development: An overview of the works of Guy W. Steuart. *Health Education Quarterly* (Suppl. 1), S3–S20.

Steuart, G. W. (1969). Planning and evaluation in health education. *International Journal of Health Education, 2,* 65–76.

Steuart, G. W. (1985). Social and behavioral change strategies. In H. T. Phillips & S. A. Gaylord (Eds.), *Aging and public health* (pp. 217–247). New York: Springer.

Steuart, G. W. (1962). Community health education. In S. L. Kark & G. W. Steuart (Eds.), *A practice of social medicine: A South African team's experiences in different African communities* (pp. 65–90). Edinburgh and London: E. & S. Livingstone.

Strauss, A., & Corbin, J. (1998). *Basics of qualitative research* (2nd ed.). Thousand Oaks, CA: Sage.

Tashakkori, A., & Teddlie, C. (1998). Introduction to mixed method and mixed model studies in the social and behavioral sciences. In *Mixed methodology: Combining qualitative and quantitative approaches* (pp. 3–19). Thousand Oaks, CA: Sage.

Taylor, R. B. (2002). Fear of crime, social ties, and collective efficacy: Maybe masquerading measurement, maybe déjà vu all over again. *Justice Quarterly, 19*(4), 773–792.

Trostle, J. (1986). Anthropology and epidemiology in the twentieth century: A selective history of the collaborative projects and theoretical affinities, 1920–1970. In C. R. Janes, R. Stall, & S. M. Gifford (Eds.), *Anthropology and epidemiology: Interdisciplinary approaches to the study of health and diseases (culture, illness, and healing)* (pp. 59–94). Boston: Reidel.

Tucker, C. (2000). *The Efland Youth Photovoice Project: A participatory social assessment.* Unpublished master's paper, Department of Health Behavior and Health Education: University of North Carolina at Chapel Hill.

Wallerstein, N. (1994). *Empowerment education applied to youth.* In Matiella, A. C. Multicultural challenge in health education (pp. 153–176). Santa Cruz, CA: ETR Associates.

Williams, G .H. (2003). The determinants of health: Structure, context and agency. *Sociology of Health and Illness, 23,* 131–154.

PART FOUR

DEFINITION OF THE ISSUE

Part Four examines strategies used to define the issue to be addressed by a community-based participatory research effort. In this phase of the participatory research process, partners work to define the specific issue on which they will work together, building on the health concerns as well as the community history, resources, and assets identified in the community assessment phase. As partners work together to understand in greater depth the factors and processes that contribute to a given issue, and to identify potential points of intervention, they may draw on a variety of methods for systematic collection and analysis of information. Working collaboratively in this phase of the process allows partners not only to contribute their skills and understandings of the community but also to continue learning from each other, building mutual trust, and building their capacity as both individuals and as a partnership for identifying, understanding, and creating means to address local health concerns.

Each of the seven chapters (Chapters Five through Eleven) in this section describes the application of a particular data collection method within the context of a community-based participatory research effort. The methods described are both qualitative (for example, ethnography, focus groups) and quantitative (for example, survey, systematic social observation). The choice of data collection method is informed by the research questions being asked and, ideally, is made collectively by the members of the CBPR partnership. CBPR partnerships may choose to use multiple data collection methods at this phase of the process—for example, survey, focus group, mapping, and systematic social observation—in order to compensate for the limitations of any one method. An example of the use of multiple methods in a participatory effort is found in the work of Mullings and Wali (2001), which brought together participant observation, in-depth interviews, and survey and census data to conduct an in-depth assessment of the social context of African American women in Harlem and its influence on infant health.

The chapters in Part Four illustrate the application of CBPR to the collection of data intended to address basic research questions, such as questions about the relationship between aspects of the built environment and the risk of cardiovascular disease or about the ways in which economic and social conditions combine with cultural frameworks to influence the risk of acquiring HIV. Depending on the design and sample size, such data collection can also contribute to answering basic research questions with relevance beyond the boundaries of the particular community. The chapters in this section also illustrate the use of CBPR to guide intervention research, by, for example, identifying how local programs, policies, and new interventions might most effectively support women's efforts to eat a healthy diet and be physically active during and following pregnancy or by using community mapping as a tool for identifying strategies to address social and environmental influences on health. Several of the studies described in these chapters address both basic research questions and specific questions designed to inform the development of future interventions, demonstrating the potential for addressing multiple aims.

Together, these chapters illustrate the application of a wide range of data collection methods in the context of community-based participatory research efforts to contribute to both understanding community health challenges and developing solutions to address these challenges. They also demonstrate a range of partnership approaches and applications of underlying principles associated with CBPR. The mutual understanding that emerges from these processes contributes to each partnership's foundation and its capacity to make future decisions about priorities and actions. Despite the wide range of data collection methods and partnership processes, there are similarities that cut across these efforts. For example, each chapter describes processes through which community members as well as academically based researchers were engaged in developing measurement instruments, tailoring instruments to local communities and language groups, and interpreting and disseminating results.

In Chapter Five, Schulz, Zenk, Kannan, Israel, Koch, and Stokes describe the application of a population-based community survey in the context of a CBPR effort. The Healthy Environments Partnership, a CBPR effort funded by the National Institute of Environmental Health Sciences, examines the contributions of the social and physical environment to cardiovascular risk in Detroit, Michigan. Surveys, a widely used method of gathering public health information, can be used to describe and document the distribution of particular phenomena and also to test specific hypotheses or explanations (in this case hypotheses linking aspects of the social and physical environment to health outcomes). The survey was conducted to provide the communities involved with the partnership with data that documented both community concerns and strengths. This information helped to establish connections between those phenomena and the health of community residents and provided information to inform specific community-level interventions and policy change efforts.

The authors of this chapter provide a case study that describes the participatory process through which the Healthy Environments Partnership members worked together to design, implement, and analyze data from a stratified random sample of Detroit community residents. They describe four mechanisms established to ensure community participation and influence in the development and implementation of the community survey: a steering committee made up of representatives from each of the partner organizations, subcommittees with responsibility for specific aspects of the study, focus groups designed to elicit input from community members on specific topics, and pilot tests of data collection instruments with debriefings that engaged community members in resolving concerns. Furthermore, they provide an insightful description of several challenges encountered in this process, and offer concrete and useful suggestions for both structures and processes that can effectively facilitate collaborative working relationships. Their discussion of the challenge of determining what type of participation to seek, by whom, and in which decisions at various stages of the process is particularly instructive.

In Chapter Six, Christopher, Burhansstipanov, and Knows His Gun McCormick focus in some detail on one aspect of the process of conducting a community survey—one that, as they argue persuasively, has implications for every other aspect of the survey as well as for the broader work of the partnership effort. The authors describe the development of an interviewer training manual for survey interviewers in the context of a CBPR initiative. The project Messengers for Health, which took place on the Apsáalooke Reservation in Montana, was designed to decrease barriers to screening for cervical cancer and increase the participation of Apsáalooke women in that screening.

As this CBPR effort evolved and sought to gather survey information about women's perceptions of and participation in screening for cervical cancer, the authors found that existing training materials for survey interviewers were designed primarily for use in non-Native communities and had no sensitivity to this community's historical inequalities or cultural values. The description of the CBPR process used to adapt an interviewer training manual designed initially for non-Native communities so that it could be used effectively by interviewers on the Apsáalooke Reservation offers a model for partnerships seeking to improve the cultural acceptability of interview protocols and thus to increase the accuracy and reliability of survey data gathered. The specific modifications to the training process described by these chapter authors included changes in the manner in which participants were recruited and the interviews were conducted, changes in the language used in the context of the interviews, and changes in the dissemination and use of study findings. This chapter illustrates the profound implications of historical relations between dominant and dominated groups in shaping contemporary research efforts, and demonstrates both a process and practical strategies through which community-based partnerships may address these factors.

In Chapter Seven, Kieffer, Salabarría-Peña, Odoms-Young, Willis, Baber, and Guzman describe a multistage process that engaged community residents and policymakers in Detroit in focus groups to define and develop concrete strategies to intervene in challenges faced by women as they sought to maintain healthy diets and physical activity levels during and following pregnancy. This innovative use of focus groups in the context of a community-based participatory research effort offers a model for linking participation and action with research (Israel, Schulz, Parker, & Becker, 1998). As the chapter authors point out, the use of focus groups "allows groups and community members to become agents of change by telling their stories, articulating their perspectives on the health and social issues affecting them, and recommending strategies for addressing these issues that are grounded in the realities of their environment and experience."

By engaging community members in a first series of focus groups, and then sharing community concerns with policymakers to initiate discussion in a second series of focus groups, decision makers were able to consider how they might use resources at their disposal to address some of the women's concerns. Furthermore, involving pregnant women in the community allowed these women to provide input into the development of future interventions specifically designed to address their concerns. This is an important chapter in offering concrete strategies for building an action-oriented analysis of community factors that contribute to obesity while engaging community women, local organizations, and state decision makers in a problem-solving discussion of future potential action strategies.

In Chapter Eight, Zenk, Schulz, House, Benjamin, and Kannan describe a participatory approach to the design and implementation of a systematic observation instrument for documenting characteristics of neighborhoods that may be linked to health outcomes in Detroit. Building on a large body of research that demonstrates that living in impoverished neighborhoods is associated with poorer health, the Healthy Environments Partnership developed this instrument in an effort to move beyond measures available through census and administrative sources and to better identify neighborhood characteristics that affect health. This effort to systematically observe neighborhood characteristics was developed to document aspects of neighborhoods, such as the nature and quality of public space, that might be difficult for individual participants in the Healthy Environments Partnership survey (introduced in Chapter Five) to describe and quantify in a manner that allows comparisons across neighborhoods.

The authors describe how partners representing community-based organizations, health service providers, and academic institutions worked together to design the Healthy Environments Partnership Neighborhood Observational Checklist (NOC). They highlight a number of strategies the Healthy Environments Partnership used to obtain input from and to engage community residents—some of whom were and others of whom were not partnership members—in this process. Furthermore, the authors provide direct and concrete examples of specific contributions made through this participatory process to the development of this neighborhood observation tool. They offer a cogent discussion of the challenges they faced and the lessons they learned in the process of applying a CBPR approach to the design of this tool. Particularly useful here is the thoughtful discussion of the timing and sequencing of participation. This is an insightful and informative chapter for CBPR projects seeking to apply systematic social observation during their efforts to define community concerns.

In Chapter Nine, Ayala, Maty, Cravey, and Webb describe two partnerships in North Carolina that incorporated community-mapping techniques into the study designs as tools for defining health concerns. They examine the use of mapping in the context of two distinct community-based participatory research efforts—one that engaged African American youths and their parents and a second that engaged Latino families. Their goal is to illustrate ways of using mapping techniques in collaboration with community members to define community problems and, ultimately, to refine research questions and subsequent action steps. The partnerships differed in the length of time that the partners had worked together and in the mapping techniques applied, allowing the authors to examine variations in partnership characteristics, study communities, and mapping techniques as these contributed to variations in the process as well as in the outcome of social mapping. Their case studies of this innovative and important method and its application in two projects demonstrates its potential for engaging communities in discussions of the patterns, social relationships, and environmental features that shape health in particular settings.

In Chapter Ten, McQuiston, Parrado, Olmos, and Bustillo, coining the term *community-based ethnographic participatory research*, describe a community-based participatory approach to gathering ethnographic data toward the end of gaining a better understanding of the social context of health and illness in a population of recent immigrants in Durham, North Carolina. Focusing on culture and *cultural interpretation*, they examine culture as it emerges under local conditions and as it is influenced by, for example, gender ratios, opportunities for employment, and conditions of poverty. The process of cultural interpretation that they describe, which emphasizes within-group dialogue about how cultural frameworks and assumptions may influence interpretations, provides a model for conducting collaborative research that is critical and self-reflective.

They conclude with a cogent discussion of lessons learned about the conduct of community-based ethnographic participatory research in immigrant communities faced with multiple challenges, including health challenges. The skills gained by community members in conducting ethnography as well as in understanding research more broadly, the skills developed by academically based researchers in working with communities, the mutual trust and respect that emerged through this process, the insights contributed by community members, and the application of the findings to a proposal for intervention funds illustrate the collective benefits that can emerge from such community-based participatory processes.

In Chapter Eleven, the final chapter in Part Four, Krieger, Allen, Roberts, Ross, and Takaro describe a community-based participatory process used in the Seattle-King County Healthy Homes Project in the state of Washington to assess indoor environmental triggers of asthma as part of an intervention designed to reduce these triggers. Application in community assessment and intervention efforts of exposure assessment methods initially developed primarily by industrial hygienists to assess workplace hazards is an important development for community health interventions. These methods, however, come with their own set of challenges as they are adapted for use in community settings. This discussion of the application of a CBPR approach to collecting information on exposure to indoor environmental asthma triggers is an important one in illuminating both the challenges raised and the contributions made by combining the efforts of epidemiologists, toxicologists, community residents, and community health workers.

The descriptions in this chapter of a partnership's process and evolution over time are particularly useful in identifying challenges that arose and in outlining the partnership's response to them. The collaborative efforts of the partners as they worked to address challenges illustrate the emergence of trust and trustworthiness among the academic researchers and the community members involved as they learned to both understand and value the contributions that each partner made to the success of the project. The discussion of lessons learned offers insights for researchers as well as for community members who are seeking to adapt complex and sophisticated technologies to address public health concerns in community settings.

References

Israel, B. A., Schulz, A. J., Parker, E. A., & Becker, A. B. (1998). Review of community-based research: Assessing partnership approaches to improve public health. *Annual Review of Public Health, 19,* 173–202.

Mullings, L., & Wali, A. (2001). *Stress and resilience: The social context of reproduction in central Harlem.* New York: Kluwer Academic/Plenum.

CHAPTER FIVE

CBPR Approach to Survey Design and Implementation

The Healthy Environments Partnership Survey

Amy J. Schulz, Shannon N. Zenk, Srimathi Kannan,
Barbara A. Israel, Mary A. Koch, and Carmen A. Stokes

Population-based community surveys are a primary data collection method for epidemiologists, sociologists, health educators, and others interested in describing and documenting the distribution of health and disease within and across populations. Such surveys are useful for testing hypotheses or explanatory models that may establish pathways linking specific risk and protective factors to health outcomes (Fink & Kosecoff, 1998; Fowler, 2001; Nardi, 2002). Questionnaires used for this purpose generally include a range of closed-ended items that assess the health outcomes of interest and a wide range of variables

Acknowledgments: The Healthy Environments Partnership (HEP) is a community-based participatory research effort that includes representatives from the Brightmoor Community Center, Detroit Department of Health and Wellness Promotion, Friends of Parkside, Henry Ford Health System, Southwest Detroit Environmental Vision, Southwest Solutions, University of Detroit Mercy, and University of Michigan Schools of Public Health, Nursing, and Social Work, and the Survey Research Center (www.hepdetroit.org). HEP is funded by the National Institute of Environmental Health Studies, grant RO1 ES10936-0, and is a project of the Detroit Community-Academic Urban Research Center (www.sph.umich.edu/urc). We thank the additional members of the HEP Survey Subcommittee, without whom the work presented in this chapter could not have been accomplished: Indira Arya (Detroit Department of Health and Wellness Promotion), Alison Benjamin (Southwest Detroit Environmental Vision), James House (Survey Research Center and Department of Sociology, University of Michigan), Sherman James (Duke University), Edie Kieffer (University of Michigan School of Social Work), Paul Max (Detroit Department of Health and Wellness Promotion), Zachary Rowe (Friends of Parkside), Joan Shields (Henry Ford Health System), and Antonia Villaruel (University of Michigan School of Nursing). Finally, we thank Sue Andersen for her assistance with the preparation of this manuscript.

thought to be predictive of health. They are generally administered according to a sampling design constructed to allow the results to be generalized to a defined population. Furthermore, they emphasize consistency of administration, use of standardized items with established reliability (consistency) and validity (the extent to which they measure what they are intended to measure), and use of a large enough sample size to allow tests of statistical significance.

Despite the importance of community surveys in research endeavors, the literature contains very few examples of how to develop and conduct a population-based survey with community participation. In this chapter we draw on the experience of the Healthy Environments Partnership (HEP) with a community survey to illustrate collaboration among community and academic partners in jointly developing and implementing a survey administered to a stratified random sample of community residents. Specifically, we examine four mechanisms established to ensure community participation and influence in the development and implementation of the HEP community survey. Particular attention is given to processes through which representatives from diverse groups were actively engaged and to the contributions of various forms of engagement to survey conceptualization, identification of specific survey areas and items, selection of survey language and wording, and survey administration. We end with a discussion of challenges, lessons learned, and implications for community-based participatory research partnerships seeking to jointly develop and implement community surveys.

HEP PARTNERSHIP BACKGROUND AND DESCRIPTION

The Healthy Environments Partnership (HEP) is a community-based participatory research (CBPR) effort investigating the prevalence of physiological indicators of cardiovascular disease (CVD) risk and the contributions of social and physical environments to those risk factors in three areas of Detroit, Michigan (Schulz et al., under review).

HEP's specific aims are to

- Estimate relationships between racial and ethnic group status, socioeconomic position (SEP), and mental and physical health, particularly indicators of and risk factors for CVD among residents of Detroit

- Examine relationships between neighborhood sociodemographic context and aspects of the physical and social environments

- Investigate independent and cumulative effects of exposures in the social and physical environments on biological risk markers for CVD

- Test mediating and moderating effects of behavioral and psychosocial responses to stress and micronutrient intake on the relationships between physical and social environments and CVD risk

- Document the strength of the association between airborne particulate matter and selected proximate risk and protective factors for CVD

- Disseminate and translate findings to inform new and established intervention and policy efforts through HEP's Community Outreach and Education Program (COEP)

The three study areas (eastside, northwest, and southwest Detroit) were initially selected due to variations in air quality, a key component of the HEP study design. The selected communities differ in socioeconomic characteristics, racial and ethnic composition, and histories. A major hypothesis to be tested through HEP was that differences in stressors and protective factors associated with the physical and social environments contribute to variations in risk factors for heart disease across these communities.

HEP was initiated in October 2000 as a part of the Health Disparities Initiative of the National Institute of Environmental Health Sciences (NIEHS), and it is affiliated with the Detroit Community-Academic Urban Research Center (URC) (see Chapter Twelve for a description of the URC). The URC board, comprising representatives from community-based organizations, health service and public health institutions, and academic institutions, identified health disparities, with a particular focus on the contributions of the environment, as a priority. Members of the URC board conceptualized HEP's specific aims in addressing this priority as linking aspects of the social and physical environment to cardiovascular disease.

Researchers based in academic institutions (the University of Michigan and the University of Detroit Mercy), health service organizations (the Detroit Department of Health and Wellness Promotion and the Henry Ford Health System) and community-based organizations (Brightmoor Community Center, Friends of Parkside, Southwest Solutions, and Southwest Detroit Environmental Vision) developed the data collection instruments and were involved in all aspects of the implementation process. This initial team was subsequently joined by two additional community-based organizations: Boulevard Harambee and the Detroit Hispanic Development Coalition.

Because of the comprehensive nature of the study questions, HEP employed a wide range of data collection methods (Schulz et al., under review). In addition to the random sample community survey described in this chapter, which included a semiquantitative food frequency questionnaire, HEP collected biomarker data from a subgroup of survey respondents; monitored air quality in the three study communities over a three-year period; collected observational data on neighborhoods in which survey respondents lived (see Chapter Eight); and gathered a wide range of data from census and administrative sources (the city planning department, for example). (For a more complete discussion of HEP's overall research design and methods, see Schulz et al., under review.) Community-based organizations, health service providers, and academic partners involved with HEP worked together to develop each of these data collection instruments.

Board members of the Detroit URC decided to propose a survey as a component of the grant proposal submitted to NIEHS because it was thought this survey would improve understanding of the environmental determinants of cardiovascular disease in Detroit. The HEP Steering Committee (SC) was formally established once the grant proposal was funded. It included representatives from the Detroit URC board who were involved in putting the proposal together as well as representatives from the partner organizations from southwest, eastside, and northwest Detroit (as listed earlier). In the following pages, we describe several strategies used once the SC was established to facilitate the engagement of community members, academic partners, and health service providers in the design and implementation of the HEP survey. Material for this chapter is drawn primarily from field notes, review of documents (for example, minutes from the HEP SC and the HEP Survey Subcommittee meetings), and discussion among SC members.

THE ROLE OF PARTNERS AND COMMUNITY MEMBERS IN SURVEY DEVELOPMENT

HEP drew on several key structures and processes to ensure that multiple constituencies had opportunities for input and influence as the HEP survey was developed and implemented. In the following pages, we describe four such mechanisms:

- The HEP Steering Committee
- Focus groups with community residents
- The HEP Survey Subcommittee
- Pretest and discussion of survey instrument with community residents

We also give examples of the specific contributions made by each mechanism.

Creating a Framework for Participation and Influence: The Steering Committee

Community-based participatory approaches to research seek to equitably engage residents, community-based organizations, governmental and service-providing agencies, and academic institutions in the process of designing and implementing efforts to address factors that affect the health of community residents (Israel, Schulz, Parker, & Becker, 1998). Creating both a structure and a range of processes through which representatives from diverse organizations, with diverse sets of resources, skills, and perspectives, can not only participate in but also have influence over the research process is key to the implementation of CBPR.

The HEP Steering Committee provided the core structure for this collaborative work. The SC met monthly to discuss and make decisions about project activities. It was guided by a set of CBPR principles adapted from those used by the Detroit URC (see Chapter One in this volume for a discussion of CBPR principles). These principles were the topic of discussion during several SC meetings as the partnership began its joint work, and were finalized and adopted in November 2001. To facilitate participation and equitable influence in decision making, at the suggestion of an SC member, HEP adopted what has been termed the 70 percent consensus rule, which encourages consensus decision making by asking whether each group member can support a given decision by at least 70 percent (as opposed to seeking 100 percent support) (Israel et al., 2001).

In addition, building on the work of other Detroit URC-affiliated projects, the HEP SC discussed and adopted a set of guidelines for dissemination of the partnership's work (see Chapter Thirteen for a discussion of the development and implementation of dissemination guidelines in a CBPR project). These guidelines spell out processes for determining, for example, coauthorship on presentations and publications based on HEP's work, and processes to ensure equitable participation in HEP-related activities and decisions. They state clearly that whenever possible, presentations about HEP and its findings will be made jointly by academic and community or health service–providing representatives from the SC.

The steering committee structure and the agreed-on processes described here provided the framework for the partnership to build a common vision, develop and work toward shared goals, and ensure mutual accountability in the process.

Engaging Diverse Community Members: Focus Groups

As the HEP SC members developed the community survey, they considered variations in the environments in the three areas of the city in which the study was to be implemented. As mentioned earlier, these noncontiguous areas were initially selected due to variations in air quality. They also differed in socioeconomic characteristics, racial and ethnic composition, and histories. HEP sought to test the hypothesis that differences in stressors and protective factors associated with the physical and social environments across these communities would contribute to variations in risk factors for heart disease.

HEP conducted eight focus groups in the three study areas to identify a wide range of stressors and potential protective factors experienced by the residents of the different neighborhoods. Focus group participants represented various racial and ethnic identities and both genders, to ensure that the survey reflected a comprehensive set of experiences. Focus groups were organized by race, gender, and area of residence in the city: two with white residents of northwest Detroit (one with men and one with women); one with African American men from eastside Detroit; one with African American women from northwest Detroit; two with English-speaking Hispanic residents of southwest Detroit; and two with Spanish-speaking residents of southwest Detroit. Information collected through these focus groups was supplemented with data collected through an affiliated URC project, the East Side Village Health Worker Partnership, which examined stressors experienced by African American women on Detroit's east side (Schulz et al., 1998; Schulz, Parker, Israel, & Fisher, 2001).

The protocol for the focus groups built on prior work, including efforts conducted through the East Side Village Health Worker Partnership (Parker, Schulz, Israel, & Hollis, 1998; Schulz et al., 2001). This protocol, which has been termed the *stress process exercise* (Israel, Schurman, & House, 1989; Israel et al., 2001), asked focus group participants to respond to the following questions: What are the things that create stress for you? How do you feel when you experience those things? What do you do when you experience those things? When you experience those stressors, those feelings, and respond in those ways, day in and day out, week after week, month after month, year after year, what are the long-term effects? And finally, what are the things that make it not so bad? In response to concerns raised by a team member, the protocol was modified to include a question that ascertained the terms or phrases used by community members to refer to life circumstances and situations that might be considered "stressful."

The HEP SC organized focus groups, recruited participants, and helped to locate community sites, including their own organizations, at which to conduct the focus groups. Sites included churches, community centers, family centers, and housing developments in the study communities. Each focus group was supported by a team that included a facilitator, a note taker (who wrote on newsprint so the group could see the ideas being generated), and a third person who took field notes and managed the tape recorder. Team members were SC representatives from community-based organizations, health service organizations, and academic institutions; doctoral students; and in one case a study community resident. They were matched to focus group participants in terms of gender and language (Spanish or English). Facilitators, newsprint note takers, and field note takers completed an in-depth training sequence on administration of the informed consent statement, techniques for facilitating the groups and using follow-up probes, and strategies for addressing group dynamic issues and concerns that might arise in the context of the discussions. Each focus group meeting took approximately two hours.

HEP staff summarized themes from the focus group interviews and presented them for discussion at an SC meeting. Focus group participants identified multiple stressors that they had experienced (such as public disorder), some of which were associated with neighborhood contexts. In addition, participants described a number of things (such as social support) that reduced the negative effects of those stressors on their health. Some issues were raised across multiple groups (for example, concerns about safety, worries about children, problems with city services), whereas others were specific to a subset of groups (for example, in the Spanish-speaking Hispanic groups, some stressors were associated with language). SC members provided input as HEP staff developed a resource guide in both Spanish and English and mailed copies to all focus group participants along with a letter thanking them for their participation and a summary of the results across all the focus groups.

The focus groups helped to identify stressors and protective factors that might be associated with health outcomes. They suggested multiple potential determinants of health within and across the three study areas. The HEP Survey Subcommittee, described in the following section, used themes from the focus groups as it identified topics to be covered in the HEP community survey.

Creating a Structure for Focused Collaborative Work: The Survey Subcommittee

Recognizing the challenges involved in having all members of the steering committee involved in each aspect of the project, the HEP SC decided to divide into five subcommittees to work on the various components of the study described earlier: air quality, biomarkers, the survey, and (later) the neighborhood observation checklist and community outreach and education. The survey subcommittee comprised three SC representatives from community-based organizations, three from health service organizations, and four from academic institutions. In addition, several researchers with specific survey expertise who were coinvestigators for HEP but who did not actively participate in the SC, were active members of the survey subcommittee. This group, with critical support from a doctoral student research assistant, was responsible for the detailed development of the survey questionnaire.

The survey subcommittee met (either face-to-face or via conference call) for over a year (December 2000 to January 2002). They reviewed results from the focus groups, discussed the literature on risk factors for heart disease, examined existing scales and measures for a wide range of risk and protective factors related to heart disease, and where no existing scales or items seemed appropriate, developed new items or adapted existing ones. Academic partners contributed knowledge of the peer-reviewed literature and existing measures to this process, and community members and health service providers offered valuable insights into community dynamics and conditions. Some discussions in the survey subcommittee centered on the intent or purpose of sections of the survey and on the use of particular language to ensure relevance and meaning for community respondents. For example, the subcommittee modified a question asking respondents whether they had ever been tested for "diabetes" to include lay language commonly used in Detroit, that is, had they had a test for "blood sugar." During this development period, the subcommittee reviewed drafts of the entire survey multiple times, as did the full SC at two of its monthly meetings.

The HEP Survey Subcommittee used established literature on risk factors for cardiovascular disease as well as themes identified by the focus groups as guidance on areas to be covered by the survey. For many focus group themes, existing scales could be used, sometimes with minor adjustments. Thus the results of the focus groups supported use of these existing instruments, as they independently raised issues and concerns that had been previously identified and for which measurement tools existed. Focus group participants also raised issues and concerns for which the survey subcommittee was unable to identify existing scales and items. In these cases new items or response categories were developed, pretested, and piloted. For example, some white focus group participants felt that they experienced employment discrimination as residents of Detroit, and some Latino respondents reported that limited English language skills and being born outside of the United States were sources of discrimination. The survey subcommittee used these focus group results to modify response options to questions developed by Williams, Yu, Jackson, and Anderson (1997) to assess perceived reasons for discrimination. Specifically, the subcommittee added "because you live in Detroit," "because of your English language skills," and "because you were not born in the U.S." to the response options offered in the original scale (such as "because of your race," "because of your age"). (See Appendix C.)

Getting Feedback and Fine-Tuning the Survey Questionnaire: Pretesting and Discussion with Community Residents

In October 2001 and again in January 2002, the steering committee helped recruit neighborhood residents and offered community sites to pretest the survey questionnaire. In each pretest the draft survey was administered to six to twelve community residents, followed by a group debriefing to discuss specific feedback on the survey instrument. Project staff recorded the start and end times for each section of the survey, and calculated the mean time for completion of each section of the survey. This information was used to aid committee members as they considered modifications or sections of the survey for trimming, along with interviewers' notes regarding particular difficulties that arose in the course of the pretest. The mean length of time for completion of the surveys at the second pretest was one hour and twenty minutes (which did not include time needed to complete the informed consent statement and the anthropometric measures (height, weight, hip, and waist measures) that were to be included in the survey). The goal was no more than one and one-half hours average completion time for the survey, inclusive of anthropomorphic measures and the informed consent process, so the subcommittee reviewed and discussed potential cuts to reduce the length.

The group debriefing with community members who had participated in each pretest involved discussion of the language used, meanings (what the respondents were thinking of when they gave their answers), the flow and comprehensiveness of survey sections, and survey clarity and interpretability. The debriefings resulted in a number of changes to specific survey items. For example, there was substantial discussion among community members of how to frame and interpret questions about police interactions with community residents and about groups of youths who were "hanging around" in neighborhoods. Community members' diverse experiences and interpretations of the questions were used to fine-tune question wording. Two subsequent pretests were conducted, with similar debriefings and modifications, before the survey was finalized and formal interviewing began. The final version of the survey included 342 psychosocial items plus 160 additional questions specific to frequency and quantity of food intake. Constructs assessed in the survey were categorized along six dimensions: stressors (for example, police stress, family stress); neighborhood indicators (for example, sense of community); health-related behaviors (for example, tobacco use, physical activity); social integration and social support (for example, perceived instrumental social support); responses to stressors (for example, hopelessness, anger); and health outcome indicators (for example, blood pressure) (see Appendix D).

Steering Committee: Oversight of Field Period

The HEP Survey Subcommittee held its final meeting in January 2002. Following that date, several critical discussions and decisions were made by the full steering committee. For example, the SC discussed survey items intended to identify community resources, focusing on the definition of neighborhood or community to be used. Initially, these items asked about resources (parks, recreation areas, stores) located within a fifteen-minute drive from the respondent's home. After substantial discussion about the proportion of residents in the survey areas without cars and about various definitions of neighborhood, the SC modified the question so that it referred to resources within a "half mile" of the respondent's home, and further described a "half mile" as "within a 10–15 minute walk or a 5-minute drive" of their home.

As HEP prepared to enter the field with the survey, the SC embarked on a series of conversations about subcontracting the administration of the survey to a professional survey group not affiliated with the partnership. The principal investigator felt that it was important to subcontract the administration of the survey to a group with expertise in this area. In exploring options the principal investigator held a number of conversations with survey organizations to explore the feasibility of contracting out for this service. By the time the results of these conversations were brought to the SC, it was very near the time that the survey was scheduled to go into the field: at this point the principal investigator had narrowed the pool to one survey administration group.

SC members raised a number of questions and concerns about this potential subcontractor. Although some members felt that this was an administrative decision and were less concerned with input into it, others felt strongly that opportunities for input and for discussion of this contract had been inadequate. Some members of the SC had prior relevant experiences and felt that the truncated timeline limited their opportunities to bring their insights to inform the partnership's decision.

In response to these concerns the principal investigator initiated a series of conversations with members of the research team, the SC (individually, in small groups, and with the full SC), and the potential subcontractor. A number of concerns were discussed in these conversations, and mechanisms put in place in an effort to address them. Steering committee members felt strongly that if HEP were to retain the services of the proposed subcontractor, HEP must maintain a visible presence and active influence in the administration of the survey. An agreement was reached with the subcontractor that addressed key concerns regarding ownership and attribution of the study. Specifically, the SC wanted assurance that the "face" of the survey as it was conducted in the community would be that of HEP and not the subcontracting organization.

Toward this end, the revised contract included language specifying that

- Detroit community residents would be hired as interviewers for the survey.

- Interviewers would wear name badges that identified them as interviewers for HEP (rather than as employees of the subcontracting organization).

- Study materials and phone lines would identify HEP (rather than the name of the subcontracting organization).

- Study materials and data gathered would be the sole property of HEP.

- HEP staff would be actively involved in the training of interviewers.

- The survey administrator would attend monthly SC meetings to provide updates on survey progress and discuss survey-related issues.

The subcontractor worked closely with HEP staff to assure that all decisions made related to the survey were carried out in close communication with the project.

Interviewers were recruited through a variety of mechanisms, including word of mouth, referrals, flyers distributed by SC members, and ads in local newspapers (such as *El Centrál,* a newspaper for the Hispanic community). Although the subcontractor had primary responsibility for conducting the interviewer training, HEP staff and SC members were actively involved. For example, the HEP project manager, research secretary, research assistants (including a community resident as well as doctoral and master's degree students working with HEP), and faculty researchers worked closely with the survey contractor to develop the training manual. In addition, HEP staff and students involved with the project were actively involved in training interviewers, covering topics such as the overall study goals, the backgrounds of the partnership and the partner organizations, the rationale behind specific survey items, and how to perform anthropomorphic measures. Finally, staff from the Detroit Department of Health and Wellness Promotion, one of the HEP partners, provided in-depth training for the interviewers in taking blood pressure readings, which were to be obtained from all survey participants as part of the interview.

As specified in the agreement, the subcontractor participated in monthly SC meetings for several months prior to the initiation of the survey and for the entire period that the survey was in the field (April 2002 to March 2003). The subcontractor provided regular updates on survey progress, including issues, questions, and concerns arising in the course of the field period. The SC was actively involved in problem solving related to survey issues. For example, the HEP study communities had been defined based on demographic information available from the 1990 census (the 2000 census results were not yet available when the sample was drawn). As the field period progressed, it became apparent that some areas of the city that had substantial white populations in 1990 had far fewer white residents in 2000. This had serious implications for the HEP sample, which had been designed to examine similarities and differences across white, African American, and Hispanic residents of the city. The project faced the prospect of having insufficient numbers of white respondents to provide the statistical power necessary for these analyses.

Over a two-month period the SC embarked on a series of discussions in regularly scheduled meetings and in separate meetings with subgroups of the SC and the sampling expert, who was a part of the HEP research team and the survey subcommittee. During this time the SC and affiliated researchers considered several potential alternatives for addressing this sampling issue, drawing on a number of strategies that had been employed previously by researchers facing similar sampling challenges. All members of the SC felt that whatever decision was reached should not compromise the scientific merit of the study, so that the findings would be credible to scientific and policy audiences as well as useful in informing local interventions. The SC also considered the technical challenges that would be involved with implementation of the decision reached, and the sensitivity of the communities involved in the study. Partner organizations were all located in and members of the study communities and they, as well as

HEP as a whole, expected to continue their relationships with the communities over long periods of time. Therefore it was a high priority that the solution to this problem be one that would be both scientifically sound and acceptable to the communities in which the study was conducted.

Ultimately, the SC decided on a strategy of oversampling blocks in areas with high proportions of white households that retained the random sample selection needed for generalizability of results. This approach substantially increased the number of white respondents in this area of the city, allowing for improved statistical power in the subsequent examination of the interplay of race and class as risk factors for cardiovascular disease.

Results of Survey Implementation

HEP completed 919 valid interviews with residents of the three Detroit communities selected for this study, 92 percent of the initial goal of 1,000 interviews. Overall, 56 percent of respondents reported their race as non-Hispanic black, 21 percent as non-Hispanic white, 20 percent as Hispanic, and 2 percent as "other." The proportion of respondents in each of the three racial or ethnic groups of interest in this study varied in each of the three communities, as was expected. On Detroit's east side, 97 percent of HEP survey respondents were African American, consistent with the proportion of African Americans found in that community by the 2000 census. As described earlier, the survey subcommittee had initially projected that 50 percent of respondents in northwest Detroit would be non-Hispanic white and 50 percent non-Hispanic black, but had then found that the proportion of whites had declined considerably between the 1990 and 2000 censuses. As a result of the strategies already described, HEP succeeded in completing 35 percent of the northwest interviews with non-Hispanic white respondents; the majority of the remaining interviews (61 percent) were conducted with non-Hispanic black residents. In southwest Detroit, the most racially diverse area of the city, 47 percent of the interviews were conducted with Hispanic residents, 26 percent with non-Hispanic white residents, and 20 percent with non-Hispanic black residents. The mean duration of the interviews was 1.57 hours (the range was from 1.15 to 3.45 hours). Participants received a $25 cash incentive for participation in the survey. In addition, all survey participants were invited to participate in a second component of the study that involved collection of biomarker samples (saliva and blood), with an additional $50 cash incentive.

Faculty, students, and the project's data manager are currently engaged in analyses of the survey data, including construction of scales, cleaning data, and merging survey data with data collected through other components of the HEP study (such as the biomarker component and the neighborhood observational checklist). As preliminary descriptive results are available, they are shared with the SC at regularly scheduled monthly meetings. As data preparation is completed, analysis turns to addressing specific study questions and developing papers that discuss those analyses. Members of the SC are involved in interpretation of the results and development of manuscripts. Because not all SC members participate in all manuscripts developed from the study, the SC devotes a section of each month's meeting to presentation and discussion of ongoing analyses. This helps ensure that each SC member has in-depth knowledge about some aspects of the study findings, through participation in interpretation and writing, and that all SC members have some familiarity with all analyses conducted through the project, building capacity for dissemination of findings.

Dissemination of Survey Results: Community Outreach and Education Program

Dissemination of results and feedback of study results to the community are important HEP priorities. Study participants received immediate feedback about their blood pressure readings at the time the survey was administered, along with recommendations based on American Heart Association guidelines for follow-up. In addition, members of the SC worked with project faculty and students to design personalized nutrition and biomarker feedback forms for respondents whose nutrition and biomarker data had been collected. The forms included recommendations for actions that might be taken to reduce the risk of heart disease. Personalized nutrition feedback forms were produced and mailed to each HEP study participant, and those who participated in the biomarker component of the study also received a personalized biomarker feedback form. (For a discussion of the community-based participatory process used to develop the template for these forms, see Kannan and colleagues, 2003.)

HEP's Community Outreach and Education Program specifies that findings be disseminated to the study communities through a variety of mechanisms, including presentations to community groups and publications in local media. In keeping with the dissemination principles adopted by the HEP SC, presentations are, whenever possible, conducted by a team consisting of members of the SC representing academic and community-based or health service–providing organizations. Working collaboratively to interpret study findings helps build capacity for collaboration in the dissemination of findings to the involved communities as well as in the peer-reviewed literature. (See Chapter Thirteen for further discussion of dissemination in a CBPR project.)

CHALLENGES ENCOUNTERED AND LESSONS LEARNED

As the Healthy Environments Partnership developed and implemented the community survey, we encountered a number of challenges and learned (or relearned) a few lessons about using a survey in the context of a community-based participatory research effort. We are not the first CBPR partnership to encounter many of these challenges (Green et al., 1995; Krieger et al., 2002) and will therefore focus our discussion on selected challenges and lessons learned in this process.

Specifically, HEP faced challenges in effectively eliciting and synthesizing input from multiple groups, including community residents, representatives from community-based organizations, health service providers, and academic researchers from multiple disciplines. These challenges might be briefly summarized as the question of *which* groups to ask for *what* input, *when,* and *how?* Effective participation in survey development and implementation takes time and commitment on the part of partners involved, community members, and staff whose role it is to facilitate and support that participation. Assuring that participation occurs in a manner that minimizes that burden while maximizing informed input and appropriate and shared influence in decision making is an ongoing challenge. A CBPR process that meets this first challenge of ensuring participation then faces a second: how to effectively manage and synthesize the diverse insights, perspectives, and agendas of these groups into a product—in this case a community survey. That integration requires synergy, willingness to compromise, and at times, the ability to make difficult decisions about priorities. Finally, like any other community-based participatory research process, the HEP survey highlighted challenges and offered lessons related to the importance of establishing mutually agreed upon objectives and processes for conducting the survey as well as interpreting and disseminating survey results. In the following paragraphs, we discuss lessons learned with regard to each of these challenges as they arose in the process of developing and conducting the HEP community survey.

Creating mechanisms for multiple forms of participation from diverse groups. Perhaps the most commonly mentioned challenge for community-based participatory research projects is time, and the HEP survey was no exception. Members of the HEP SC, as well as community members who participated in the development of the survey questionnaire, juggled multiple roles and responsibilities in their lives, and time for participation had to be set aside or negotiated in the context of these other commitments. For example, one member of the HEP Steering Committee was a nurse for a large hospital, and her participation in the survey subcommittee and the SC had to be fitted within her day-to-day responsibilities for management, training, and hospital floor work. Similarly, community residents have important insights into relationships between their environments and their health. Mechanisms that support opportunities for community residents to offer those insights may differ from those that facilitate participation by health care professionals or representatives from community-based organizations.

The four mechanisms and strategies described in the preceding sections—steering committee, focus groups, survey subcommittee, and pretest and discussion—reflect HEP's efforts to structure opportunities for different types of participation for people with varying degrees of involvement with the partnership. For example, focus group participants were involved for roughly one two-hour period, and influenced the content of the survey items through the insights they offered into community stressors and protective factors. Survey subcommittee members participated intensively for over a year, and shaped decisions about which items were included in the survey questionnaire and how they were presented. Community residents participating in pretesting were involved for about three hours and helped to identify problematic question wording. And SC members were involved on a monthly basis over a five-year period, influencing survey administration, key decisions about sampling procedures, and interpretation and dissemination of study findings.

Addressing geographical distance and difference. The Healthy Environments Partnership experienced particular challenges related to the geographical locations of the study communities and involved organizations. Community-based and health service organizations working with the project were dispersed widely throughout Detroit, and the University of Michigan's main campus is located an hour's drive from the city. Several strategies facilitated participation in HEP-related meetings. On the one hand, for example, all SC meetings were held at Detroit-based partner organizations and scheduled well in advance to ensure that SC members could plan their attendance. Survey subcommittee meetings, on the other hand, rotated between locations at the University of Michigan and in Detroit, often with several members present in a room together while other members participated via speakerphone. This process allowed participation without requiring extensive travel. However, these conference calls were not without their challenges. For example, telephone participants commented on their inability to observe interpersonal cues and interactions or to see illustrations or ideas that might be sketched out by a participant at another site. HEP sought to at least spread these challenges equitably among partners by rotating locations so that all members could participate in at least some meetings in person. This in turn led to some logistical problems in accessing appropriate speakerphone links, so even this solution had its challenges.

Providing flexible and organized support for participation. Engaging SC members and community residents in these processes required flexibility and organization to ensure that meetings were a productive use of all members' time. Strategies for maximizing the use of participants' time varied depending on the format. For example, preparation for SC meetings involved crafting agendas, preparing background materials necessary for informed participation, ensuring appropriate opportunities to influence decisions, and documenting and disseminating results. For focus groups, a well-organized schedule, trained facilitators, and mechanisms to reduce distractions (for example, child care and room arrangements) helped ensure that participants' time was well spent and that they came away from the experience knowing that their insights had been heard and valued.

Meetings with community residents were most often scheduled on weeknights or weekends: one series of focus groups was held in a church following Sunday services because many men in that community worked Saturdays. Finding times when all members of the HEP SC and Survey Subcommittee were available was an ongoing challenge, and sometimes required alternating meeting days and times to ensure that all members could participate in at least some meetings. Meeting minutes were circulated to all members to provide detailed information about decisions made, recognizing that not everyone could participate in all meetings. HEP made extensive use of phone calls, conference calls, e-mails, and debriefings with individual members who had been unable to attend scheduled meetings, to facilitate participation and influence in the face of the multiple commitments juggled by members of the SC and survey subcommittee.

Substantial time and energy were required from competent and committed project staff to organize the multiple schedules involved and to ensure that meetings were well planned and organized. A full-time project manager, research secretary, and several part-time student research assistants coordinated schedules; arranged meeting locations, speaker phones, and conference call lines (see below); developed agendas; followed up between meetings, and were responsible for the multiple behind-the-scenes tasks essential for progress between meetings and for effective use of time when working groups were together. A project manager with skills in communication, attention to detail, adeptness at planning ahead on multiple fronts, and a commitment to ensuring that all partners were engaged in major decisions was essential.

Recognizing when participation is needed and from whom. Recognizing that members of HEP have many obligations and responsibilities beyond their participation in HEP also involved judgments about which decisions needed participation from whom and at what point in the process. Too much participation or poorly coordinated participation can lead to frustration among all partners and an inability to move forward effectively. Conversely, assumptions about which decisions require input can lead to surprises and at times tensions.

We have described multiple mechanisms used to facilitate different forms of participation in the development of the HEP survey. Coordinating the roles of the different groups and the timing of their activities and clarifying which decisions would be made by which group and when were all challenges that HEP grappled with in constructing the community survey. For example, a first cut at content for the survey questionnaire was provided by academic partners experienced in cardiovascular health, suggesting the broad content areas to be included in the survey (for example, psychosocial stressors, dietary factors, and health indicators). Input from the focus groups helped to fine-tune specific questions and at times suggested additional content for inclusion in the survey questionnaire. The survey subcommittee reviewed and discussed specific content for the questionnaire, incorporating insights from the focus groups as well as insights from the pretesting process. Finally, the full SC reviewed the sections of the survey at several points in time, as well as the full questionnaire, contributing comments before it was finalized. Lessons learned in this process included the importance of clarifying the roles of various decision-making bodies and of having effective staff coordination between meetings.

A second, and related, challenge has to do with determining which decisions should be made by project staff, which should be brought to the SC, and when. Challenges related to the contract for administration of the community survey reflected a misjudgment on the part of the principal investigator in the timing of engaging the steering committee in this subcontracting process. As it turned out, the SC had a lot to say on this issue, and concerns were voiced about the lack of adequate participation in this decision. These concerns were addressed through several additional discussions with individuals and small groups and in full SC meetings, allowing SC members' insights to be brought into the decision-making process. This process led to several important modifications in the survey contract, and illustrated the degree to which the SC felt ownership of and shared responsibility for the study. More broadly, it served as a reminder of the importance of explicit conversations about which decisions must be brought to the SC for discussion, which require input or insights from outside sources, and which might be made by project staff (Israel et al., 2003).

Balancing multiple priorities. Success in eliciting multiple perspectives and insights goes hand in hand with the challenge of what to do with all the input and all those priorities. In an ideal world, with no limitations of time or funding, all perspectives and priorities might be accommodated. However, the first version of the HEP survey questionnaire would have taken several hours to administer to each respondent. Given the realities of fixed budgets, participant burden, project timelines, and complex issues, it was essential to prioritize, negotiate, and make difficult decisions about which content would remain and what would be eliminated. The survey subcommittee held lengthy conversations about how to contain the length of the survey without unduly compromising the scientific integrity of the data or the usefulness of the results for informing planned community change.

A particular challenge with which the survey subcommittee grappled was the tension between capturing issues that might help explain similarities and differences in CVD risk within and across the three Detroit communities involved in HEP and an interest in comparing local findings with those from regional and national studies. The SC and survey subcommittee recognized and discussed at length the relative advantages and disadvantages of using established and validated scales that would allow comparisons with other national studies but might be less sensitive to the specifics of Detroit communities. Mechanisms for coming to agreement on such decisions facilitated difficult decision-making processes and helped the group continue to work effectively together. The 70 percent consensus rule for decision making, described earlier in this chapter, was one such mechanism. Similarly, integration of existing literature on cardiovascular disease risk with results from focus groups and from pretests of survey questionnaires helped survey subcommittee members prioritize areas for inclusion. In many cases, academic researchers identified established scales that addressed issues raised by focus group participants, and discussion of items with community residents identified modifications in the language of those scales that would enhance their reliability and validity for this population (for example, adding the term "blood sugar" to an item assessing diabetes). Where new items or response categories were developed, pretested, and piloted as part of the HEP survey, HEP analyses examined the extent to which these new indicators contributed to our understanding of variations in cardiovascular disease risk.

Demonstrating that contributions are valued. It is essential to demonstrate actively that contributions to any community-based participatory research effort are valued, and contributions to a community survey are no exception. In keeping with the multiple forms of participation we have described, it is appropriate that such recognition takes many forms. Listening respectfully and honestly to feedback offered and providing concrete support for participation (for example, stipends for time) demonstrate that contributions are valued. Community residents participating in focus groups and pretesting were paid. Focus group participants also received a follow-up packet thanking them for their time and contributions and a summary of results and actions taken. Public recognition of contributions also demonstrates that contributions are valued. For example, we expressed appreciation to focus group participants in materials summarizing focus group results and listed all partner organizations in survey materials disseminated to community and academic audiences. SC members attended professional meetings and copresented on the study process and results at these meetings, a recognition of their ongoing contributions to HEP's efforts.

Sustaining mutual commitment. The Healthy Environments Partnership was the first project undertaken as part of the Detroit Community-Academic Urban Research Center that did not include a specific intervention component, due to specifications of the funding mechanism. As a result, community members and public health providers who participated in the project invested considerable time and energy in the design and implementation of a research effort with few direct and immediate benefits to the study communities. Contributions were made on faith and agreed-upon commitments that the results would contribute to improved understanding of determinants of heart health in Detroit and to the development of interventions and policies to address these determinants.

HEP established and agreed upon CBPR principles for the partners' working together, as well as for the dissemination of study results, early in that work. These principles specified the partnership's common goals and processes for sharing both responsibility and credit for the partnership's work. Discussion of and mutual agreement to these principles made explicit the commitment of all partners to contribute to the development and implementation of the community survey (as well as other data collection and analysis undertaken by HEP), and to the use of the study findings to address community health concerns. Thus, as discussions were carried out within the SC about the survey questionnaire, items were weighed in terms of their importance in understanding factors that contribute to CVD, and their potential importance in understanding opportunities for change.

CONCLUSION

Mounting a community survey is an enormous undertaking under any circumstances: doing so using a community-based participatory process requires both commitment and resources to ensure the active engagement of multiple, geographically dispersed partners with diverse perspectives, insights, and priorities. In the preceding pages, we described four different types of structures and processes that were put in place to provide opportunities for participation and influence from a wide range of partners in the design and implementation of the HEP community survey. The HEP Steering Committee provided input and oversight for the community survey, as well as for other aspects of the project prior to, during, and following completion of the community survey. This role allowed ongoing interaction with project staff and considerable input, influence, and insight into the conduct of the study, as well as long-term follow-up and assurance of accountability. Community focus groups provided detailed insights into aspects of the social and physical environments experienced by community residents, the interpretations and meanings of these environmental aspects, and their potential implications for cardiovascular disease. The survey subcommittee, made up of SC representatives along with a broad group of academically based researchers with particular expertise in survey design, sampling, and cardiovascular disease, provided a mechanism for detailed, ongoing, and intensive input during the period in which the survey questionnaire was designed. And finally, pretesting and debriefings or discussions with community residents offered opportunities to test the questionnaire and to gain essential insights into nuances of language, meaning, and experience relevant to finalizing and interpreting survey results.

A community-based participatory process may not always be the most appropriate method for conducting a community survey. However, each of the mechanisms described here provided opportunities for critical insights into aspects of the social and physical environments in the study communities, and each contributed to understanding environmental variations that might underlie disparities in risk of cardiovascular disease. Community-based and health service partners facilitated conversations with members of the study communities; contributed a depth of knowledge of community histories, resources, and dynamics; and helped build HEP's credibility in the community. Academic partners brought in-depth knowledge of specialized literatures in both content (for example, air quality monitoring) and process (for example, sampling design, survey administration, and community-based participatory research).

The challenges and lessons learned as the Healthy Environments Partnership developed and implemented its community survey are in many ways variations on themes or lessons that have been described by many other CBPR efforts. They include challenges associated with the time and energy that must be devoted to ensuring appropriate and effective participation, the importance of attention to partnership processes and their implications for outcomes, and the negotiation of multiple perspectives and priorities (Israel et al., 1998). Our experience reiterates the importance of flexibility and organization; a variety of opportunities for participation; adequate and competent staff support; respect for and recognition of the contributions of all partners; patience and a commitment to listen to, learn from, and respect each other; a commitment to equity; and mutually agreed upon guidelines and procedures for the collective work of the partnership. All contribute to opportunities for co-learning and capacity building that can build a basis for broad community movement toward the common goal of greater equity in health.

References

Fink, A., & Kosecoff, J. (1998). *How to conduct surveys: A step-by-step guide.* Thousand Oaks, CA: Sage.

Fowler, F. J. (2001). *Survey research methods* (3rd ed.). Thousand Oaks, CA: Sage.

Green, L. W., George, M. A., Daniel, M., Frankish, C. J., Herbert, C. J., Bowie, W. R., et al. (1995). *Study of participatory research in health promotion.* Ottawa: Royal Society of Canada.

Israel, B. A., Lichtenstein, R., Lantz, P. M., McGranaghan, R. J., Allen, A., Guzman, J. R., et al. (2001). The Detroit Community-Academic Urban Research Center: Development, implementation and evaluation. *Journal of Public Health Management and Practice, 7*(5), 1–19.

Israel, B. A., Schulz, A. J., Parker, E. A., & Becker, A. B. (1998). Review of community-based research: Assessing partnership approaches to improve public health. *Annual Review of Public Health, 19,* 173–202.

Israel, B. A., Schurman, S. J., & House, J. S. (1989). Action research on occupational stress: Involving workers as researchers. *International Journal of Health Services, 19*(1), 135–155.

Israel, B. A., Schulz, A. J., Parker, E. A., Becker, A. B., Allen, A. J., & Guzman, J. R. (2003). Critical issues in developing and following community-based participatory research principles. In M. Minkler & N. Wallerstein (Eds.), *Community-Based Participatory Research for Health* (pp. 56–73). San Francisco, CA: Jossey-Bass.

Kannan, S., Arya, I., Benjamin, A., Wyman, L., Roy, R., Schulz, A. J., et al. (2003, November 17). Designing personalized nutrition feedback for participants in the community-based Healthy Environments Partnership (HEP) study. Paper presented at the American Public Health Association meeting, San Francisco.

Krieger, J. W., Allen, C., Cheadle, A., Ciske, S., Schier, J. K., Senturia, K. D., et al. (2002). Using community-based participatory research to address social determinants of health: Lessons learned from Seattle Partners for Healthy Communities. *Health Education & Behavior, 29*(3), 361–382.

Nardi, P. M. (2002). *Doing survey research: A guide to quantitative research methods.* Boston: Pearson Allyn & Bacon.

Parker, E. A., Schulz, A. J., Israel, B. A., & Hollis, R. (1998). Detroit's East Side Village Health Worker Partnership: Community-based health advisor intervention in an urban area. *Health Education & Behavior, 25*(1), 24–45.

Schulz, A. J., Kannan, S., Dvonch, J. T., Israel, B. A., Allen, A., House, J. S., et al. (under review). *Social and physical environments and disparities in risk for cardiovascular disease: The Healthy Environments Partnership conceptual model.*

Schulz, A. J., Parker, E. A., Israel, B. A., Becker, A. B., Maciak, B. J., & Hollis, R. (1998). Conducting a participatory community-based survey: Collecting and interpreting data for a community intervention on Detroit's east side. *Journal of Public Health Management and Practice, 4*(2), 10–24.

Schulz, A. J., Parker, E. A., Israel, B. A., & Fisher, T. (2001). Social context, stressors and disparities in women's health. *Journal of the American Medical Women's Association, 56,* 143–149.

Williams, D. R., Yu, Y., Jackson, J., & Anderson, N. B. (1997). Racial differences in physical and mental health: Socioeconomic status, stress and discrimination. *Journal of Health Psychology, 2,* 335–351.

CHAPTER SIX

Using a CBPR Approach to Develop an Interviewer Training Manual with Members of the Apsáalooke Nation

Suzanne Christopher, Linda Burhansstipanov, and
Alma Knows His Gun-McCormick

This chapter will focus on how a community-based participatory research (CBPR) approach was used to develop and implement an interviewer training manual for a preintervention survey (see Chapter Five for a more detailed discussion of the development of a community survey using a CBPR process). The project Messengers for Health (MFH), conducted on the Apsáalooke Reservation, uses a lay health advisor approach to decrease cervical cancer screening barriers, increase knowledge regarding screening and prevention of cervical cancer, and increase Apsáalooke women's participation in cervical cancer screening. We describe the CBPR process used to modify interviewer training protocols, developed for use with non-Native groups, to increase the cultural acceptability of this approach and the accuracy of the data gathered from women on the Apsáalooke Reservation. Both the cultural acceptability and the accuracy and reliability of survey data are essential for the development of effective efforts to reduce the high rates of cancer of the cervix among Native American women of the Northern Plains.

Acknowledgments: Portions of this chapter were adapted from "Development of an Interviewer Training Manual for a Cervix Health Project on the Apsáalooke Reservation," by S. Christopher, A. Knows His Gun-McCormick, A. Smith, and J. C. Christopher, *Health Promotion Practice* (in press). Adapted with permission of the publisher. Reprinted with permission from Sage Publications.

The support of the American Cancer Society (Margaret Ann Wise Grant TURSG-01-193-01-PBP) is acknowledged with gratitude. We also want to thank community members and project staff who were involved in the development of the training manual, our advisory board, Little Big Horn College faculty and staff, and Eugenia Eng.

COMMUNITY SETTING

The Fort Laramie Treaty established the Apsáalooke Reservation in 1851. Originally 38 million acres, the reservation has been eroded by treaty changes, and now stands at approximately 2.25 million acres. Apsáalooke means "children of the large beaked bird," and this name was communicated in sign language by flapping one's hands to resemble a bird's wings in flight. White explorers and traders misinterpreted the sign as referring to the crow, and used that word in reference to the Apsáalooke. Apsáalooke community members asked the research team to use the term Apsáalooke during this project, although use of the term Crow is ubiquitous on the reservation.

Apsáalooke traditions remain very strong and are part of the Apsáalooke way of life today. Among women who completed the MFH survey, 80 percent reported speaking Apsáalooke at home. In the Apsáalooke culture, one's clan, immediate family, and extended family are very close and these ties are extremely important. For example, a cousin is tantamount to one's brother or sister, an aunt is analogous to one's mother, and an uncle to one's father. So, if one's mother were to pass away, other women in the family would take her place as one's mother. These strong clan and family ties form the basis for the information networks of communication and support that lie at the core of the MFH project (Lowie, 1935).

As shown in Table 6.1, Native Americans from the Northern Plains, where the Apsáalooke Reservation resides, have significantly higher rates of cervical cancer mortality than women in other regions of the United States. Native American women of the Northern Plains have the highest rate of cancer of the cervix across all regions and races of the United States (Espey, 2003).

Table 6.1. Indian Health Service (IHS) Age-Adjusted Cervical Cancer Mortality Rates, by Region, 1994–1998

U.S. all races	2.6
All IHS regions	3.7*
Alaska	1.5
East	4.3*
Northern Plains	4.7*
Pacific Coast	2.4
Southwest	3.9*

Note: Rates are mortality per 100,000 population per year, adjusted to the 2000 U.S. population.

*Denotes a rate significantly higher than the overall U.S. rate.

Source: Data are from Espey, 2003.

CBPR PARTNERSHIP BACKGROUND

Alma Knows His Gun-McCormick, Apsáalooke tribal member and project coordinator for MFH, and Suzanne Christopher, faculty member at Montana State University and principal investigator on this study, began meeting early in 1996 while working through the Montana Department of Public Health and Human Services on the CDC-funded Breast and Cervical Health Project. Alma informed Suzanne of her desire to provide cancer education and outreach on the Apsáalooke Reservation and Suzanne shared with Alma her interest in writing a proposal for a collaborative grant for a cancer project with the Apsáalooke Nation. MFH evolved as a result of more than five years of meetings among Alma, Suzanne, and selected members of the tribe (most of whom later became members of the project's advisory board).

Most CBPR projects include working with existing community-based organizations (CBOs). Reservations typically have few formalized CBOs. However, comparable organized bodies have decision-making and leadership capabilities in these tribal communities. On the Apsáalooke Reservation, these groups include the Crow Tribal Legislature, the Tobacco Society, and the Crow Tribal Health Board. In addition, tribal members also recognize many individuals as being in positions of leadership. Examples are leaders of traditional groups or organizations (such as sacred societies), those who have been given the right to lead traditional ceremonies (such as the sun dance, the sweat lodge, or Peyote meetings), leaders of tribal clans, individuals who do traditional healing, and elders. Hence Native American community partners involved in this project represented a variety of groups and individuals in a number of leadership positions. In addition, Native American Cancer Research (NACR), an American Indian CBO that works with tribal organizations throughout the North American continent and has conducted multiple studies on cancer prevention and control (Burhansstipanov, 1999; Burhansstipanov, Dignan, Wound, Tenney, & Vigil, 2000; Burhansstipanov, Gilbert, LaMarca, & Krebs, 2002; Orians et al., 2004) provided technical assistance to the project on an as-needed basis.

Partners for the project included the project coordinator, the principal investigator and staff from Montana State University-Bozeman (including students who were members of the Apsáalooke Nation and other Native American tribes), members of the advisory board, and individuals in leadership roles in the community. (All these partners are hereinafter referred to as the *research team* or, more simply, the *team*.) The advisory board included individuals who helped with planning the grant, cancer survivors, tribal elders and leaders, and women who worked with or were interested in women's health. (See Chapter Two for additional discussion of the development of community partnerships.)

DEVELOPMENT OF INTERVIEWER TRAINING MANUAL

Before an interviewer training manual could be developed, a survey instrument had to be designed that was culturally, geographically, and scientifically relevant to the Apsáalooke community. The goal of the survey interviews was to gather accurate and comprehensive information to guide the development of a culturally competent, community-driven educational intervention. The survey development process included, but was not limited to the advisory board's reviewing community-driven priorities and question phrasing, expert (scientific and cultural) panel reviews, and multiple meetings to discuss the phrasing and concepts behind the phrasing. This process required one year, and the final tool included 120 items. (See Chapter Five for a description of the development of a survey instrument within the context of a community-based participatory research partnership.)

Although the team was able to locate multiple survey instruments used with Native communities, it was able to procure only one detailed interviewer training manual developed for use with Native communities. The team determined that that manual was not culturally acceptable for the Apsáalooke community (because it was almost identical to other manuals developed for use with non-Indian populations). Thus the team used a manual developed for non-Indians as a template, revising this template line by line, discussing the appropriateness of the content, and making changes to increase the cultural acceptability of the manual to the local community.

Although every part of the manual had significant changes from the template, we will focus our discussion here on six areas:

- The goals of survey research
- Recruitment and enrollment
- The manner of the interviewer
- Beginning the interview
- Language use
- Dissemination and use of survey findings

Goals of Survey Research

The goals of most survey research are to "produce accurate statistics" (Fowler & Mangione, 1990, p. 12) and "to ensure as far as possible that 'bias' factors do not have an effect on the data collected" (Salazar, 1990, p. 569). Although collecting valid data was a key component of this study as well, when the team first discussed the survey, Apsáalooke team members suggested that having respect for the women interviewed and for the community was a primary goal.

As we demonstrate in the remainder of this section (and in discussing beginning the interview), these goals are in fact inseparable: the ability to collect accurate and valid data is dependent on demonstrating respect for the women interviewed.

The Apsáalooke members of the research team called attention to their long and repeated experiences with previous research and the ways in which it was disrespectful—by, for example, failing to invite Native Americans to be involved with research taking place in their community or by not giving community members access to data collected from them. Thus the team needed to implement procedures that would address earlier cultural affronts to the community and poor research ethics, such as community members' providing information to researchers who were never heard from again. It would be essential for all participants in this study to view their participation as voluntary and as contributing to their community rather than to the researcher's career, promotion, or salary. The team felt strongly that community members, regardless of their direct participation in the survey process, should be assured that the information shared in interviews would

- Remain confidential
- Be brought to the community (for example, findings would be made anonymous and then shared locally prior to release of information outside of the community)
- Be used to directly help improve Apsáalooke women's health

Apsáalooke women who worked with the training manual wanted these points spelled out in the manual to avoid problems of past research with Native Americans. These concerns and practices are not typical of those addressed in the interviewer training manuals that the team reviewed in this process. The research team believed that specifying and implementing such guidelines would increase the likelihood that the project would be perceived as trustworthy and would subsequently result in the women welcoming the interviewers into their homes and feeling comfortable sharing information.

Recruitment and Enrollment

Much of the interviewer training literature mentioned addressing the process of persuading potential participants to agree to the interview. For example, Suskie (1996) suggested that interviewers remain neutral at all times except during this interaction. He stated that "it is then and only then that we use our powers of persuasion to get a prospective respondent to agree to an interview" (p. 168).

When looking over the template manual, tribal members stated that such tactics would be detrimental to this study because it is neither appropriate nor acceptable in the Apsáalooke culture to coerce or push someone into doing something. In Apsáalooke, the term *iisáatchuche,* which translates as "bold face" or "hard face," is used to describe someone who is being blunt, not taking no for an answer, being bold, or not respecting others. Persons who act that way are being disrespectful and inconsiderate; thinking of themselves rather than thinking of others. Another term that describes someone like this is *baaiilutchichíhletuk.* The elders pass on to the younger generations that this is not an appropriate manner in which to behave. Hence the research team concluded that interviewers should not be trained to behave this way, and team members changed the original version of the interviewer training manual to a new version that stated "do not try to persuade her [the potential participant] to complete the interview."

The revised interviewer training manual discussed approaching a potential study participant through a respectful and open dialogue. The team concurred that women were more likely to want to participate in the study if they fully understood that the purpose of the interview and survey results were to provide information for subsequent interventions in the local community (that is, the team sought understanding rather than coercion). Elders emphasized that the words we speak are sacred. They said that people should speak to each other using kind words. There is an Apsáalooke term, *baaleéliaitchebaaluúsuuk,* that means it is easy to speak good words. Thus the team determined that a person would be more willing to respond to something said to them when kind and good words were used.

This method differs from the stronger methods suggested in some literature, such as prodding (Suskie, 1996, p. 168). Given the atmosphere of distrust already existing around research, the interviewers were coached not to do any type of prodding. With interviewers trained to use open and respectful dialogue when approaching women to participate in the study, only 2 of the 103 women approached declined, yielding a response rate of 98 percent.

Manner of the Interviewer

The usual advice in the interviewer training literature was to encourage the interviewer to be neutral, distant, and businesslike (Gillham, 2000; Sapsford, 1999; Suskie, 1996). For example, Salazar (1990) states that "one of the greatest challenges of interviewing is combining some important human qualities such as kindness, sensitivity, and concern with a general sense of detachment" (p. 569). This recommended manner assumes a cultural homogeneity that does not exist in the United States (Christopher, Christopher, & Dunnagan, 2000; Taylor, 1989). For instance, Voss and colleagues (1999) drew out distinctions between the white and the Lakota cultures and stated that "often, what is viewed as good, healthy, and confident behavior in the dominant [non-Native] culture is based on a high valuation of the individual. This is in direct contradiction to the traditional Lakota valuation of tribalism" (p. 293). In tribalism, the emphasis is on the extended family and kin over the individual. This more collectivistic view also fits with the Apsáalooke worldview and affects interactions between individuals, including interactions during survey interviewing.

When conducting focus groups to develop interview methods for a survey with Native Hawaiians, Banner and his colleagues (1995) found "negative reactions to the standard neutral voice tone and lack of interviewer responsiveness to respondent answers" (p. 450). They altered their methods to reflect Hawaiian cultural norms, and interviewers were encouraged to use their normal speech patterns and rhythms. Likewise, the MFH research team made changes from its template to encourage the interviewers to feel relaxed during the interview and to display a compassionate attitude and interest in the women that were consonant with the Apsáalooke culture. The team's manual stated that "sincerity and interest in the woman's feelings and family will help establish rapport."

Beginning the Interview

Another change that came about through the team's collaborative work on the manual affected beginning the interview. The team's training manual discussed proceeding with the interview at a pace that was comfortable to both the interviewer and the participant. This might mean taking time before the interview started to make sure that the participant was comfortable and familiar with the interview process and to describe what would happen with the information she shared. A common and important Apsáalooke custom is that when two people come together they introduce themselves by stating the family they belong to and where they come from geographically. Most interview guides however discourage the practice of disclosing personal information. As Fowler and Mangione (1990) state, "[a]lthough an interviewer may volunteer information or explanation, this behavior is only to prepare for the question asking event" (p. 9). However, team members stated that such disclosure is culturally expected and required for a trusting conversation or interview to follow.

The team's training manual said that interviews conducted with Native people on reservations and in tribal community settings (including urban Indian clinics) may be preceded with a visit, a snack, and a cup of coffee or tea. Although some non-Native procedures (Suskie, 1996) admonished against such practices, others acknowledged that they may be sometimes appropriate. However, the research team recognized that an interview is a social situation and in a social situation giving and accepting food is a traditional way of welcoming someone and revealing a family's generosity and is an important part of the Apsáalooke culture. The serving of a plate of food when a person comes to a home for a visit or to a gathering is common; to ask if someone is hungry before offering food is impolite. This giving of substance happens at clan meetings, after going into the sweat lodge, and at any time where people come together.

It is disrespectful to turn down a participant's offer of hospitality, and if an interviewer does refuse it, the subsequent interview is typically incomplete and includes misinformation. As one Native woman said, "If they don't trust me enough to visit with me and to eat my food, why should I trust them with my personal knowledge? I told them all kinds of wild stories. They didn't deserve the truth" (NACR, 1996).

Language Use

Crazy Bull (1997c) has stated that "language is the medium for the transmission of culture" (p. 21). Regarding language, the usual advice given is that "the research interview should be conducted in the respondent's preferred language" (Keats, 2000, p. 82). As stated previously, 80 percent of the women interviewed for this study stated that they spoke the Apsáalooke language at home. It is the preferred language for many Apsáalooke people. This language is mainly oral; most people who speak Apsáalooke are not able to read or write it with the same proficiency. Native American culture has often been carried on orally rather than through writing (Hodge, Fredericks, & Rodriguez, 1996). The team did not find any literature on training interviewers or conducting interviews in a language that is predominately oral. The usual advice given is that "[i]f the study population does not speak the primary language of the interviewer, which is usually English, then data collection instruments must be translated" (McGraw, McKinlay, Crawford, Costa, & Cohen, 1992, p. 283).

Because the Apsáalooke language is predominantly oral, the research team decided that it would not be practical or workable to translate the interview into Apsáalooke and have the interviewers read the script. It would also not be culturally acceptable to ask the participants to speak only in English. The team's training manual therefore noted that it might be necessary for the interviewers to translate the questions from English into Apsáalooke. It added that such interpreting would not only help the participants to better understand certain questions but would also allow them to feel more comfortable and would provide a means of more effective communication for both the interviewer and the participant. It asked the interviewers to conduct the interview in the language preferred by the participant, and this usually meant alternating between Apsáalooke and English. During the interviewer training, the interviewers practiced conducting the interview in this manner. It appeared to be comfortable and natural for the interviewers, as tribal members often speak in this manner in everyday conversation. The project coordinator, a fluent Apsáalooke speaker, observed the interviewers practicing, and the interviews were conducted without hesitation and with mutual understanding between those playing the roles of questioner and respondent. Some researchers are uncomfortable with real-time translation and clarification of items during survey administration and feel that the exact wording of a question and its various possible responses should be retained (Keats, 2000; Suskie, 1996). We understand that the direct translation may have subtle variations from interviewer to interviewer, but believe that the MFH method yielded the best results. After the interviews were completed the interviewers stated that using this method, they could go through the interview with the assurance that the participant was clear about what was being asked and that using the Apsáalooke language allowed the participants to feel at ease, feel free to answer personal questions, and feel that they were not being judged.

Another point about language concerns the words used to describe the interviewers, participants, and their work. This language is often mechanistic. For example, Groves and McGonagle (2001) discuss the "displayed behavior" of the participants, other authors discuss what participants say as "an utterance" (Schmidt & Conaway, 1999), and other literature refers to the interviewer as a "research instrument" instead of as a person (Gillham, 2000). Although those who use mainstream English language may be accustomed to the strategic, instrumental, and detached connotations of this discourse, it is crucial for those working cross-culturally to realize that such language is characteristic of a particular cultural outlook, namely that of "utilitarian individualism" (Bellah, Madsen, Sullivan, Swindler, & Tipton, 1985; Taylor, 1989). This technique was discarded by the team as culturally disrespectful to the Apsáalooke. Some survey research literature also suggested ways of dealing with "inadequate or irrelevant" responses. Schmidt and Conaway (1999) state that the "response may be incomplete, or an answer may be irrelevant to the question. Some responses are so poorly organized that they are difficult to follow. Sometimes inaccurate information is given" (p. 42). Weisburg, Krosnick, and Bowen (1996) mention replies that are unclear, vague, or "off the track." Fowler and Mangione (1990) discuss "probing inadequate answers" (p. 37) and what to do if what the respondent says is "not a complete and adequate answer" (p. 33). Seeing this advice in the template training manual, one Apsáalooke woman working on the training manual stated that there was no such thing as an inadequate or irrelevant response and that whatever the participants had to offer was valid and informative. Burhansstipanov (1999) encourages interviewers to listen carefully to the stories the respondent tells because they will frequently provide answers to subsequent interview questions and the stories usually help clarify the responses. The training manual developed by the team discussed how to probe to receive answers that fit the closed-ended question responses.

The team also added to the manual the point that if the woman is talking about other things, the interviewer needs to be patient and courteous. This is another example of looking at the women who were sharing information in a respectful manner and is consistent with Apsáalooke cultural practices. Long (1983) noted that among the Apsáalooke people, "[o]ne does not correct others or indicate that the other's perceptions are incorrect. Tolerance of others is highly valued, and is practiced through silence and nonintrusive behavior" (p. 124). The training manual included some neutral probes that interviewers could use without appearing to judge an offered response when that response did not fit the question. For example, the template training manual advised the interviewer to say, "What do you mean?" This was felt to be too negative a response, and alternatives were given such as, "Could you tell me a little more about . . . ?" or, "I'm not sure I understand what you mean." The team's manual also advised interviewers to write any additional information given in the interview on the side of the questionnaire form, in order to include all responses.

Dissemination and Use of Survey Findings

Most research projects consider dissemination and use of survey findings a task to be addressed during the latter portion of a study. The team did not see this issue addressed in any of the literature on interviewer training. However, dissemination and use of findings was an important component of the interviewer training manual for MFH. The team added this material because a common and valid complaint in Indian Country is that communities rarely receive survey findings, nor do they receive benefits from surveys done in their communities. Due to this history, there is resistance to taking part in contemporary surveys.

The interviewers received information on how previous research had been conducted and how this project would be different in the ways in which findings from this study would be used and shared with the community. The training manual specified how MFH planned to continuously update the community on the progress of the project. These plans included holding multiple community meetings to share results of the survey and developing easy-to-understand handouts on the survey results that would be widely distributed. The manual also stated that the survey information would be used to help all Apsáalooke women to be healthier and specifically that survey findings were going to be used to determine

- The focus of training of the lay health advisors
- The information that would be emphasized by the lay health advisors in educating women in the community
- The nature and focus of the educational materials provided to the community

Use and dissemination of survey findings was part of the information given by interviewers to potential participants.

THE INTERVIEWERS

As has been true for other successful surveys conducted with Native populations, hiring and training local community members to conduct the survey demonstrated respect for the community and increased the accuracy of the data. Some researchers (Singleton & Straits, 2002) suggest that race matching is of limited utility and that few studies have found any association between interviewer demographics and the answers obtained from participants. Other survey experts recommend cultural awareness of the acceptability of matching or not matching on race (Keats, 2000) as well as on gender.

Apsáalooke team members contended that the only way to receive honest and accurate information would be to hire Apsáalooke interviewers. The trust essential for Apsáalooke women to discuss personal health issues would not exist with nontribal interviewers. Further, they considered it important that the interviewers be female and speak Apsáalooke. Cross-gender taboos would prohibit male interviewers from being successful in this situation, and those working on the manual stated that many community members felt more comfortable talking in Apsáalooke than in English. Likewise, there are subtleties of nonverbal communication (such as individuals' proximity to one another and eye contact) that required the interviewers to be intimately familiar with the culture. Thus the team decided that Apsáalooke women living in and known by the community, who practiced typical Apsáalooke cultural behaviors and norms, would be selected as interviewers.

The interviewers were recruited by a professor at Little Big Horn College (LBHC), a tribal college on the reservation. The interviewers came from all areas of the reservation and ranged in age from the late twenties through the late fifties. The interviewer training took place over the course of one day at LBHC, with a follow-up meeting one week later to discuss progress, questions, and concerns. The training covered the following topics: the purpose and focus of the study, confidentiality and privacy protocols, cervical health and cervical cancer, roles and responsibilities of the interviewer, and interviewing procedures and techniques. Interviewers were trained to conduct interviews in a standardized manner, for example, not varying the order of the questions. The interviewers also practiced role playing the interview. Interviewers were paid with project funds at rates agreed to by the study team, and support and supervision were provided by the project coordinator. To ensure confidentiality interviewers signed a confidentiality statement. The statement read:

> I (insert name) agree to keep the identity of all persons in the study and any information on these persons that I gain access to as a result of this study completely confidential. I will maintain confidentiality in order to protect the rights and well-being of the women participating in this study. By doing so, I agree to

never discuss any information on the women participating in this study with anyone but this research team (including significant others, family, friends, other interviewers, or other women being interviewed), nor will I allow anyone who is not a member of this research team to view interviews, study files, or data.

LESSONS LEARNED AND IMPLICATIONS FOR PRACTICE

In this chapter we have discussed various lessons learned in the process of using a CBPR approach to develop an Apsáalooke-specific interviewer training manual. Specifically, we have described a history of inequality, manifest in disrespectful interactions and in the community's inability to access, influence, or make use of information generated through research to improve health in the community. We have described several specific ways that this history of disrespect and inequality shapes current perspectives and responses to research, and the implications for training survey interviewers to collect information to improve the cervical health of women on the Apsáalooke Reservation. In this section we summarize the lessons learned and their implications for public health research and interventions.

Both historical events and the cultural values of the specific population need to be taken into account in determining the content of the interviewer training manual and in the process of creating the manual. To be successful at integrating these implications researchers must be prepared to spend a considerable amount of time and energy with and in the community of concern. In this process a broad range of historical events should be taken into consideration, including those that have involved research, researchers, governmental agencies and employees, and health care institutions. For example, community members shared with the MFH team stories of researchers who gathered personal and sensitive information from them never to be heard from again. They did not know what happened to the information or how it was used, and they doubted that the information was used to directly help the community.

Others have described additional research indiscretions that potential researchers need to be aware of as they conduct research with Native Americans. These include (Alfred, 1999; Ambler, 1997; Christopher, in press; Deloria, Foehner, & Scinta, 1999; Deloria, 1969, 1980, 1991; Dixon & Roubideaux, 2001; Freeman, 1993; Red Horse, Johnson, & Weiner, 1989; Smith, 1999; Trafzer & Weiner, 2001; Trimble, 1977)

- Grouping all tribes together
- Failure to invite Native American individuals and communities to be involved with research taking part in their own communities

- Failure to inform Native communities of study findings or to allow access to data collected from them

- Research that does not benefit Native American communities

- Research that reinforces stereotypes and emphasizes negative behaviors

- Research that blames individuals or communities as the cause of problems rather than identifying historical events and inequalities that shape these challenges

- Researchers who place their own interests ahead of those of the people they are working with

Because of this history, many Native communities, including the Apsáalooke community, are wary about participating in studies of a community's health. The research team took this history into account when developing the interviewer training manual. The team's manual addressed these issues up front and discussed how team members were aware of this history and were actively working to establish a different precedent. The interviewers were instructed to discuss these issues with potential respondents. If this had not been a part of the interviewer training manual, women might not have been interested in taking part in the interview, might have shared information just to get the interview completed, might have participated but not in a manner of open disclosure, might have provided inaccurate information, or might have felt uncomfortable or disturbed by the interaction and subsequently less open to future interviews (Ambler, 1997; Trimble, 1977). Other important recommendations for working successfully with Native American individuals and communities have been spelled out and include working honestly and cooperatively with communities, working from a standpoint of respect, spending time with communities, working with tribal colleges, and ensuring that Native communities are involved in all stages of the research endeavor (Banner et al., 1995; Crazy Bull, 1997a; Davis & Reid, 1999; Harrison, 2001; Kritek et al., 2002; Macaulay, 1994; Marín et al.,1995; Mihesuah, 1993; Nason, 1996; Stubben, 2001; Swisher, 1993; Weaver, 1997, 1999).

It is also necessary to gain an understanding of cultural values, including appropriate and inappropriate ways of behaving during interactions, with particular attention to behaviors that signal disrespect. For example, a part of the Apsáalooke culture is that a person will not always look another person in the eye during a conversation. It would have been inappropriate to put in the manual that the interviewer should look the respondent in the eye during the interview as is typically recommended in the literature. It is also important to understand how cultural values around the survey topic area may affect survey interactions. For example, the team's manual included a discussion of how the words *cancer, breast,* and *cervical* or *cervix* may bring about feelings of discomfort among some women. Traditionally, the use of certain words has been taboo, and the word *cancer* has had negative associations. For example, there is no specific word in the Apsáalooke language for cancer. The phrase used to describe it translates as "dreadful, awful disease." These topics were dealt with directly in the manual. It stated: "Because of outreach education that has been done in this area of health, women are responding better to the use of these words and people are understanding that not all people who are diagnosed with cancer will die. Now we have Crow cancer survivors. We want women to feel comfortable to use these words because it's important for women's health and we hope that this interview will help to overcome some barriers to using these words."

Without the CBPR approach, the manual would have been unlikely to have addressed the cultural nuances referred to throughout this chapter. Because thousands of surveys have been implemented in Indian Country, the team was surprised to learn that no culturally appropriate interviewer manuals were available to use as a template (the one that had been used with Native communities had few cultural modifications). The manual described here is available from the first author upon request.

Like other CBPR projects and products, the development of this manual required several years for the researchers to become acquainted with the community, learn how to work within the community, and gain trust from community members. This was accomplished through frequent team meetings in community settings for more than five years before funding was received. Additionally, the principal investigator read many books about the Apsáalooke Nation, attended cultural and community events, and talked with tribal members to learn about the culture. This demonstrated to the community that the university members were committed to helping and were not just interested in furthering their own careers.

Time was also required for the tribal leaders and key members of the community to become members of the research team. The team collaboratively developed drafts of the manual that were reviewed and revised by tribal leaders and lay members of the community. These meetings and discussions revealed patterns of tribal communication among the Apsáalooke that were incorporated into the manual. As a result, this knowledge about tribal communication was used in a way that could potentially facilitate trust and respect between the interviewer and the study participant. Such information required considerable time to uncover, not because of deliberate attempts to hide information but because for the local community, as for all of us, this type of information is typically implicit and not immediately accessible to conscious awareness and reporting.

CONCLUSION

The historical legacy of interactions between Native communities and government officials, health researchers, and health workers has impeded the success of research intended to improve health. Individuals working with Native communities "are likely to be confronted with some of the grief and anger over losses and injustices of the past. They will be better able to deal with these confrontations if they have gained some insight into the events that caused the pain" (Harrison, 2001, p. 9).

We close by quoting from Cheryl Crazy Bull's (1997b) eloquent explanation of a culturally respectful research process. This process is in line with a CBPR approach and was an inspiration for us in developing a training manual respectful of the Apsáalooke community and culture.

> As we seek our own understanding of tribal research and scholarship, we must remember the people of the community are the source of our profound understanding of tribal life, values, and rituals. We must hear their voices and participate in their stories and ritual in order to attain the wisdom we seek. As we explore the world of scholarship, the everyday people and everyday rituals must form the foundation for the lodges we build [p. 16].

References

Alfred, T. (1999). *Peace, power, righteousness: An indigenous manifesto.* Oxford: Oxford University Press.

Ambler, M. (1997, Summer). Native scholarship: Explorations in the new frontier. *Tribal College: Journal of American Indian Higher Education, 8,* 8–10.

Banner, R., DeCambra, H. O., Enos, R., Gotay, C., Hammond, O., Hedlund, N., et al. (1995). A breast and cervical cancer project in a Native Hawaiian community: Wai'anae cancer research project. *Preventive Medicine, 24,* 447–453.

Bellah, R., Madsen, R., Sullivan, W., Swindler, A., & Tipton, S. (1985). *Habits of the heart: Individualism and commitment in American life.* New York: HarperCollins.

Burhansstipanov, L. (1999). Native American community-based cancer projects: Theory versus reality. *Cancer Control: Journal of the Moffitt Cancer Center, 6*(6), 620–626.

Burhansstipanov, L., Dignan, M. B., Wound, D. B., Tenney, M., & Vigil, G. (2000). Native American recruitment into breast cancer screening: The NAWWA project. *Journal of Cancer Education, 15*(1), 28–32.

Burhansstipanov, L., Gilbert, A., LaMarca, K., & Krebs, L. (2002). An innovative path to improving cancer care in Indian Country. *Public Health Reports, 116*(5), 424–433.

Christopher, S. (in press). Recommendations for conducting successful research with Native Americans. *Journal of Cancer Education.*

Christopher, S., Christopher, J. C., & Dunnagan, T. (2000). Culture's impact on health risk appraisal psychological well-being questions. *American Journal of Health Behavior, 24*(5), 338–348.

Crazy Bull, C. (1997a, Summer). Advice for the non-Native researcher. *Tribal College: Journal of American Indian Higher Education, 8,* 24.

Crazy Bull, C. (1997b, Summer). in the center of the earth i am standing and i am praying as i stand. *Tribal College: Journal of American Indian Higher Education, 8,* 16.

Crazy Bull, C. (1997c, Summer). A Native conversation about research and scholarship. *Tribal College: Journal of American Indian Higher Education, 8,* 17–23.

Davis, S. M., & Reid, R. (1999). Practicing participatory research in American Indian communities. *American Journal of Clinical Nutrition, 69,* 755–759S.

Deloria, B., Foehner, K., & Scinta, S. (Eds.). (1999). *Spirit & reason: The Vine Deloria, Jr. reader.* Golden, CO: Fulcrum.

Deloria, V., Jr. (1969). *Custer died for your sins.* Norman: University of Oklahoma Press.

Deloria, V., Jr. (1980). Our new research society: Some warnings for social scientists. *Social Problems, 27*(3), 265–271.

Deloria, V., Jr. (1991). Commentary: Research, redskins, and reality. *American Indian Quarterly, 15*(4), 457–468.

Dixon, M., & Roubideaux, Y. (Eds.). (2001). *Promises to keep: Public health policy for American Indians & Alaska Natives in the 21st century.* Washington, DC: American Public Health Association.

Espey, D. (2003). *Regional patterns of cancer mortality in American Indians and Alaska Natives in the U.S., 1994–98.* Paper presented at the meeting of the American Public Health Association, San Francisco.

Fowler, F. J., & Mangione, T. W. (1990). *Standardized survey interviewing: Vol. 18. Minimizing interviewer-related error.* Thousand Oaks, CA: Sage.

Freeman, W. L. (1993). Research in rural Native communities. In M. J. Bass, E. V. Dunn, P. G. Norton, M. Stewart, & T. Fred (Eds.), *Conducting research in the practice setting* (Vol. 5, pp. 179–196). Thousand Oaks, CA: Sage.

Gillham, B. (2000). *The research interview.* London: Continuum.

Groves, R. M., & McGonagle, K. A. (2001). A theory-guided interviewer training protocol regarding survey participation. *Journal of Official Statistics, 17*(2), 249–265.

Harrison, B. (2001). *Collaborative programs in indigenous communities: From fieldwork to practice.* Walnut Creek, CA: Altamira Press.

Hodge, F. S., Fredericks, L., & Rodriguez, B. (1996). American Indian women's talking circle: A cervical cancer screening and prevention project. *American Cancer Society, 78*(Suppl.), 1592–1597.

Keats, D. M. (2000). *Interviewing: A practical guide for students and professionals.* Buckingham, UK: Open University Press.

Kritek, P. B., Hargraves, M., Cuellar, E. H., Dallo, F., Gauthier, D. M., Holland, C. A., et al. (2002). Eliminating health disparities among minority women: A report on conference workshop process and outcomes. *American Journal of Public Health, 92*(4), 580–587.

Long, K. A. (1983). The experience of repeated and traumatic loss among Crow Indian children: Response patterns and intervention strategies. *American Journal of Orthopsychiatry, 53*(1), 116–126.

Lowie, R. H. (1935). *The Crow Indians.* Lincoln: University of Nebraska Press.

Macaulay, A. C. (1994). Ethics of research in Native communities. *Canadian Family Physician, 40,* 1888–1890.

Marín, G., Burhansstipanov, L., Connell, C. M., Gielen, A. C., Helitzer-Allen, D., Lorig, K., et al. (1995). A research agenda for health education among underserved populations. *Health Education Quarterly, 22*(3), 346–363.

McGraw, S. A., McKinlay, J. B., Crawford, S. A., Costa, L. A., & Cohen, D. L. (1992, Summer). Health survey methods with minority populations: Some lessons from recent experience. *Ethnicity & Disease, 2,* 273–287.

Mihesuah, D. A. (1993). Suggested guidelines for institutions with scholars who conduct research on American Indians. *American Indian Culture and Research Journal, 17*(3), 131–139.

Native American Cancer Research. (1996). *Interview transcripts.* Pine, CO: Author.

Nason, J. D. (1996, Fall). Tribal models for controlling research. *Tribal College: Journal of American Indian Higher Education, 7,* 17–20.

Orians, C., Erb, J., Kenyon, K., Lantz, P., Liebow, E., Joe, J., et al. (2004). Public education strategies for delivering breast and cervical cancer screening in American Indian and Alaska Native populations. *Journal of Public Health Management and Practice, 10*(1), 46–53.

Red Horse, J., Johnson, T., & Weiner, D. (1989). Commentary: Cultural perspectives on research among American Indians. *American Indian Culture and Research Journal, 13*(3–4), 267–271.

Salazar, M. K. (1990). Interviewer bias: How it affects survey research. *AAOHN Journal, 38*(12), 567–572.

Sapsford, R. (1999). *Survey research.* Thousand Oaks, CA: Sage.

Schmidt, W. V., & Conaway, R. N. (1999). *Results-oriented interviewing: Principles, practices, and procedures.* Needham Heights: Allyn & Bacon.

Singleton, R. A., & Straits, B. C. (2002). Survey interviewing. In J. F. Gubrium & J. A. Holstein (Eds.), *Handbook of interview research: Context and methods* (pp. 59–82). Thousand Oaks, CA: Sage.

Smith, L. T. (1999). *Decolonizing methodologies: Research and indigenous peoples.* London: Zed Books.

Stubben, J. D. (2001). Working with and conducting research among American Indian families. *American Behavioral Scientist, 44*(9), 1466–1481.

Suskie, L. A. (1996). *Questionnaire survey research: What works* (2nd ed.). Tallahassee, FL: Association for Institutional Research.

Swisher, K. G. (1993). From passive to active: Research in Indian Country. *Tribal College: Journal of American Indian Higher Education, 4*(3), 4–5.

Taylor, C. (1989). *Sources of the self: The making of the modern identity.* Cambridge, MA: Harvard University Press.

Trafzer, C. E., & Weiner, D. (Eds.). (2001). *Medicine ways: Disease, health, and survival among Native Americans.* Walnut Creek, CA: AltaMira Press.

Trimble, J. E. (1977). The sojourner in the American Indian community: Methodological issues and concerns. *Journal of Social Issues, 33*(4), 159–174.

Voss, R. W., Douville, V., Soldier, A. L., & Twiss, G. (1999). Tribal and shamanic-based social work practice: A Lakota perspective. *Social Work, 44*(3), 228–241.

Weaver, H. N. (1997). The challenges of research in Native American communities: Incorporating principles of cultural competence. *Journal of Social Service Research, 23*(2), 1–15.

Weaver, H. N. (1999). Assessing the needs of Native American communities: A Northeastern example. *Evaluation and Program Planning, 22,* 155–161.

Weisberg, H. F., Krosnick, J. A., & Bowen, B. D. (1996). *An introduction to survey research, polling, and data analysis* (3rd ed.). Thousand Oaks, CA: Sage.

CHAPTER SEVEN

The Application of Focus Group Methodologies to Community-Based Participatory Research

Edith C. Kieffer, Yamir Salabarría-Peña, Angela M. Odoms-Young, Sharla K. Willis, Kelly E. Baber, and J. Ricardo Guzman

The *focus group* is a qualitative research method in which a trained moderator facilitates a guided discussion with a small group of people (often six to eight) who have personal or professional experience of the topic being studied (Brown, 1999, Morgan, 1998a). They may be the sole data collection method, or they may be used in combination with other qualitative methods (such as in-depth interviews, observation, and case studies) or quantitative methods (such as close-ended structured questionnaires).

Acknowledgments: The project described in this chapter was conducted in collaboration with the Detroit Community-Academic Urban Research Center, whose members provide unfailing guidance in conducting community-based participatory research. The authors thank the Promoting Healthy Lifestyles Among Women Steering Committee, whose continual efforts and dedication to the well-being of Detroit residents made this work possible. Committee members included the Butzel Family Center, Community Health and Social Services Center (CHASS), the Detroit Department of Health and Wellness Promotion, Friends of Parkside, Henry Ford Health System, Kettering/Butzel Health Initiative, Latino Family Services, the Michigan Department of Community Health, the REACH Detroit Partnership, and University of Michigan Schools of Public Health and Nursing. The authors also thank the community focus group moderators, the host sites, and the project staff and students for their contributions and commitment to the project and the focus group participants for sharing their time and ideas. This project was supported by the Centers for Disease Control and Prevention, Division of Nutrition and Physical Activity (grant U48/CCU515775-/SIP 10), with additional support from the REACH Detroit Partnership (grant U50/CCU522189) and the W. K. Kellogg Foundation–funded Community Health Scholars Program.
    This chapter was coauthored by Yamir Salabarría-Peña in her private capacity. No official support or endorsement by the CDC is intended or should be inferred.

Focus groups can help researchers understand social experience by answering such questions as: What is going on here? Why and how do things happen the way they seem to? and, Why and how do people think and behave the way they do? (Brown, 1999; Denzin & Lincoln, 2000; Morgan, 1998b). Through focus groups, community members have explored a wide array of public health issues: formulating research questions and hypotheses (O'Neill, Small, & Strachan, 1997); building knowledge and capacity (Parsons & Warner-Robbins, 2002); analyzing systems of care and barriers to service utilization (Loevy & O'Brien, 1994; Walters, Simoni, & Horwath, 2001); and planning, developing, and evaluating programs (Kieffer, Willis, Arellano, & Guzman 2002; Kieffer et al., 2004; Piran, 2001). Focus groups may be used to identify problems and to plan and implement projects and assess their processes and outcomes (Morgan, 1998b).

Focus groups offer participants the opportunity to exchange ideas, express opinions, and assert differences and commonalties. Many researchers consider focus groups to be a culturally sensitive method, reaching those who may feel intimidated by one-on-one encounters and fitting well with cultures and groups that value collectivity (Denzin & Lincoln, 2000; Madriz, 2000). Ideally, the questions and interactions elicited during focus groups generate rich and diverse stories as participants share experiences in their own words and language. This group dynamic may help balance the power between researchers, moderators, and participants because the flow of interactions and opinions empowers participants' voices. The multiple voices, dialogues, and debates among participants may decrease their interaction with the moderator, giving more validation and importance to participants' thoughts and ideas (Madriz, 2000). Holding focus groups in settings familiar to participants (such as community centers and churches) may further enhance the participants' influence in the interview process.

In this chapter we concentrate on the use of focus groups in the context of community-based participatory research (CBPR) and related approaches, such as participatory action research, that share an emphasis on participation and action linked with research (Israel, Schulz, Parker, & Becker, 1998). Groups and community members become agents of change by telling their stories, articulating their perspectives on the health and social issues affecting them, and recommending strategies for addressing these issues that are grounded in the realities of their environment and experience. We will present a brief description of focus groups conducted in two CBPR projects, and an in-depth discussion of a third project that developed from these earlier experiences. (For a full description of how to plan and implement focus groups, see Morgan & Krueger, 1998; Crabtree & Miller, 1999a. See Chapter Fourteen in this volume for an examination of the use of in-depth group interviews.)

CBPR AND THE PROJECT BACKGROUND

The ongoing community-based participatory research partnership projects that are described in this chapter take place in the southwest and eastside communities of Detroit, Michigan. The eastside community is 89 percent African American, and at least 35 percent of the ethnically diverse southwest community is Latino (U.S. Census Bureau, 2000). These communities experience the effects of fifty years of economic decline, including an outmigration of employment opportunities and middle-class residents and businesses and an increased concentration of poverty and ethnic segregation, high crime rates, and a decaying and inadequate public infrastructure (Sugrue, 1996). Nonetheless, community-based organizations provide a range of social, health, and advocacy services and have long-standing ties to neighborhoods and residents. Several of these organizations are members of the Detroit Community-Academic Urban Research Center (URC), a partnership of community-based organizations, service providers, and academic institutions. Initiated with funding from the Centers for Disease Control and Prevention (CDC) in 1995, the URC supports interdisciplinary, community-based participatory research that strengthens the ability of its partners to develop, implement, and evaluate health interventions aimed at improving the health and quality of life of families and communities (Israel et al., 2001).

Several URC-affiliated CBPR projects, using community surveys and focus groups, identified diabetes and its risk factors, including obesity, physical inactivity, and poor diet, as major concerns to community residents and used these results to plan appropriate interventions (Kieffer et al., 2001, 2002, 2004; Schulz et al., 2002). In one of these projects, Latino women from southwest Detroit participated in a series of three focus groups, two during pregnancy and one postpartum, which engaged the same participants in an active process that moved from issue identification to data analysis and interpretation to program planning (Kieffer et al., 2002). During the first focus group these women discussed their beliefs about diabetes and factors affecting their risk, including physical activity and eating. In their second focus group they discussed and extended the major ideas that had emerged during their first meeting, and identified strategies for reducing barriers to physical activity. During their third focus group they developed detailed recommendations for a culturally appropriate program to provide group social support and safe opportunities for exercise. This process resulted in increasingly open discussion and interaction among participants that built toward problem solving (Kieffer et al., 2002). It also captured changes in the women's perceptions of themselves and of the barriers in their environment as they moved through pregnancy and the postpartum period.

To support the recommended program and other potential diabetes-related interventions, URC partners formed the REACH Detroit Partnership, which responded to the CDC's Racial and Ethnic Approaches to Community Health (REACH) 2010 initiative to reduce health disparities. During its planning year the REACH Detroit Partnership Steering Committee invited eastside and southwest Detroit families to participate in focus groups to plan interventions aimed at reducing the prevalence and impact of diabetes (Kieffer et al., 2004). The committee held six gender- and age-specific focus groups in each community that brought people ages eight to eighty together to share their perspectives and suggest strategies for reducing barriers to healthy eating, regular physical activity, and diabetes prevention and management. Recommendations from the REACH focus groups resulted in a CDC-funded multilevel (community, social support group, health system, and family) intervention that began in eastside and southwest Detroit in 2000. Community resident *family health advocates* work with families and health care providers to improve diabetes self-management and health care. *Community facilitators* and *community health advocates* work with community organizations and residents to increase awareness of diabetes and its risk factors and to develop resources needed to reduce those risks.

The URC board and the REACH Detroit Partnership Steering Committee also supported the development of Promoting Healthy Lifestyles Among Women/ Promoviendo Estilos de Vida Saludables entre Mujeres, a CBPR project designed to plan interventions to reduce risk factors for excessive weight gain during and after pregnancy and for subsequent obesity and diabetes among Latino and African American women. The CDC's Division of Nutrition and Physical Activity funded the project from October 2000 to September 2001, with an unfunded extension of activity through September 2002.

The project steering committee (SC) was made up of representatives of URC-affiliated community, service provider, and academic organizations, including the Butzel Family Center, Community Health and Social Services Center (CHASS), the Detroit Health Department, Friends of Parkside, Kettering Butzel Health Initiative, Latino Family Services, and University of Michigan School of Public Health. The SC invited Michigan Department of Community Health representatives and Detroit community resident women of childbearing age, including a pregnant woman, to join. The SC was the research team, participating in all phases of the project. SC members built on their experience in conducting CBPR with URC-affiliated projects and in working with African American and Latino women of childbearing age. Team members from those ethnic groups brought essential cultural and linguistic backgrounds and skills needed to plan and conduct the proposed methodology. Academic team members had backgrounds and experience in conducting qualitative research related to nutrition, physical activity, and maternal and child health. The W. K. Kellogg Foundation–funded

Community Health Scholars Program supported the work of several academic team members. Between monthly meetings of the full committee, members worked individually and in small groups on project activities.

RESEARCH DESIGN

Promoting Healthy Lifestyles Among Women/Promoviendo Estilos de Vida Saludables entre Mujeres used a multimethod qualitative approach that included in-depth individual interviews and focus groups. The project steering committee planned a three-phase data collection sequence to engage an increasing number and range of community residents and organizations in developing and analyzing the information needed to plan useful, acceptable, and accessible community interventions. The first phase of data collection, which lasted four months, involved conducting forty-three semistructured, in-depth individual interviews with pregnant and postpartum African American and Latino women from eastside and southwest Detroit, respectively. A person designated by each woman as most likely to influence her beliefs and practices was interviewed separately. The interviews focused on beliefs related to weight, diet, and physical activity and on practices, barriers, and facilitators during and after pregnancy. (See Chapters Four, Ten, and Twelve for discussion of the use of in-depth interviews.)

During the three-month second phase, the SC conducted separate focus groups with pregnant and postpartum women in each community to discuss, confirm, and expand on the key results of the individual interviews and to identify potential intervention strategies. During the two-month third phase, the SC summarized and shared the results of the individual interviews and women's focus groups with two community-specific focus groups made up of policy, program, and organization leaders with community-, local-, or state-level responsibilities for health, social, or community development services. These focus groups sought to ascertain these leaders' perspectives on community-identified issues and potential solutions and to obtain their ideas and investment in identifying the best possible intervention approaches.

The SC recommended that the project facilitate the design of interventions culturally and linguistically tailored to the needs of English-speaking African American women in eastside Detroit and Spanish-speaking Latino women in southwest Detroit, because these groups represented the majority of pregnant women in their communities. The SC recommended that recruitment be limited to women who were pregnant or six to twelve weeks postpartum and who were at least eighteen years of age, due to prior experience with barriers to obtaining consent from parents or guardians and due to the belief that interventions should vary between younger teenagers and adults.

FOCUS GROUP INTERVIEWS WITH PREGNANT AND POSTPARTUM WOMEN

All the partners were involved in the steps required to develop and implement the focus group interviews. These steps, described in the following sections, were developing focus group guides, recruiting and training staff, recruiting participants, and implementing the focus groups.

Development of the Pregnant and Postpartum Women Focus Group Guides

The focus group guides provided a structure to ensure that moderators asked questions that confirmed and extended the results of the individual interviews in a clear, consistent fashion. After reviewing and discussing the individual interview results, the SC designed four guides that used a common structure (for example, topics related to weight, physical activity, and eating were addressed in each) but were tailored to probe issues specific to each community and to pregnant and postpartum women. Within each topic, the guides explored major themes that had arisen from the individual interviews, followed by questions and suggested probes. For example, the guides reviewed women's views about pregnancy-related weight gain. The eastside postpartum women's guide said: "Some women told us that they worried about gaining too much weight during pregnancy, or not losing weight after pregnancy. Others were less concerned about these things." This statement was followed by the question: "How important is it for women to return to the weight, size or shape that they had before becoming pregnant?" A probe explored advantages and disadvantages of weight change. The southwest women's guide was similar in structure and many areas of content, but also explored the influence of acculturation to the United States, for example. This Spanish-language guide was translated into English for use by non-Spanish speaking SC members. The final section in each of the guides focused on women's intervention recommendations, including issues and resources needed to make participation feasible for community women.

Recruitment and Training of Recruiters, Moderators, and Note Takers

The SC discussed position roles, responsibilities, and selection criteria and then interviewed and selected focus group recruiters, moderators, and note takers. SC members suggested that the most important position that required a trained community resident was the moderator. Criteria for this role sought women who had experienced pregnancy and the postpartum period, had the same ethnic background as participants, and had some experience facilitating group discussions. SC members nominated several women who met the criteria. One moderator was a pregnant woman who had joined the SC after participating in an individual interview. Moderators received $250 to compensate for their time and effort given to the project. The SC decided that the project's graduate student research assistants and a community resident staff member would serve as recruiters and note takers. These women were familiar with the project's purpose and CBPR principles and had demonstrated skills in these roles. Academic SC members trained the recruiters on the recruitment protocol and materials, participant selection criteria, and confidentiality.

Academic SC members conducted two community-specific training workshops for moderators and note takers to prepare them for their challenging roles (see Chapter Six for a discussion of interviewer training). Both workshops were held two weeks before the planned date of the focus groups and were hosted by the eastside and southwest community organizations that also hosted the focus groups. The aim was to build individual and team skills, a shared sense of the focus group purpose, and familiarity with procedures and the host setting.

The moderators and note takers received a training manual one week prior to the workshop date. The workshop for southwest trainees was conducted in Spanish to prepare them to work in the language spoken by the focus group participants. Because written Spanish language material on focus group methodology was scarce, research assistants translated training materials into Spanish under the guidance of one of the academic SC members.

The training workshop curriculum covered introductions; the project background; a focus group definition; moderator and note-taker roles before, during, and after focus groups; the importance of and procedures for protecting confidentiality; the purpose, content, and administration of the focus group guide; a demographic sheet (to collect information on participant characteristics for use during data analysis); informed consent (including descriptions of procedures for audiotaping and for protecting confidentiality); summary report procedures; and role-playing exercises using the focus group guides. The workshops concluded with the administration of a process evaluation questionnaire. Strengths of the workshop noted by participants included both the inherent capacity building and the practicality of concepts learned. During the period between the workshop and the focus groups, academic research team members were available to discuss any concerns or questions with the moderators and note takers. All participants in both workshops received certificates of completion.

Recruitment of Pregnant and Postpartum Women

Project SC partner organizations and recruiters distributed flyers advertising the project at prenatal, postpartum, and Women, Infants, and Children (WIC) program clinics and Baby Fairs (health education events for pregnant and postpartum women) held by SC partners in each community. Recruiters approached women in clinic waiting rooms and Baby Fair information tables and described the purpose of the study. The recruiters administered a brief eligibility questionnaire to women who wanted to learn more about participating. Interested and eligible women provided contact information so that recruiters could confirm participation, transportation needs, and the focus group date, time, and place. Women who requested child care also provided the ages and names of their children. Recruiters left a project information sheet with women who were unsure about their interest and with those who were interested and eligible. The sheet described project activities and potential benefits, incentives, risks, and protections for participants. To assist with project planning, women who declined to participate were asked to provide their reasons.

A week before the focus group, project staff mailed a letter to each woman that thanked her for accepting the invitation, reviewed logistics and the incentive, and provided a contact number for questions and attendance changes. Project staff called each woman to confirm arrangements two to three days prior to the focus group meetings, to help plan for and address participants' needs. For instance, some women who had not previously expressed a need for child care or transportation requested these services during the call. Others told the caller they could not participate due to illness or other daily life commitments. Although, ideally, the same person who had recruited a woman made the call to her, other recruiters whose schedules better matched the women's schedules sometimes made these calls. Multiple follow-up calls were needed to reach some women; others had disconnected telephones. Of the women who initially agreed to participate, approximately two-thirds confirmed their appointments, and one-half ($n = 12$) of southwest and one-third ($n = 10$) of eastside women ultimately participated in the focus groups.

IMPLEMENTATION AND DATA COLLECTION

The focus groups were conducted in meeting rooms of SC community partner organizations. On the morning of the focus group, a note taker greeted each participant and explained and administered the demographic information and informed consent forms. She addressed questions or concerns and collected the signed forms. She provided the participant with a name tag, introduced mothers and children to the child-care provider, escorted women to the focus group meeting room, and introduced them to the focus group moderator. During this informal period before all of the women had assembled, the focus group moderator welcomed the women and offered them fresh fruit and beverages.

The meetings began with a welcome and an icebreaker exercise, during which the moderator, note taker, and participants introduced themselves. The moderator discussed the ground rules, which included guaranteeing confidentiality by identifying participants only by their first names, destroying the audiotapes at the conclusion of the study, and not using identifiers in any of the reports. Then, using the focus group guide as previously described, the moderator read brief summaries of the key themes from the individual interviews for each major topic. The moderator asked women to reflect on, react to, and expand on the themes developed from the individual interview results and to generate and discuss program recommendations. The note taker assigned each participant a position number at the table and used that number as she took detailed field notes, including notes on speaker order and observations of nonverbal cues that added meaning to the discussion (Denzin & Lincoln, 2000). The note taker operated two tape recorders with external microphones as a safeguard against equipment failure.

The focus groups lasted approximately ninety minutes. At the conclusion the note taker presented a brief (three-minute) summary of the key themes, based on her notes, and invited participants to offer additions or corrections (Krueger, 1998b; Kreuger and King, 1998b). The moderator thanked participants for sharing their time, energy, and ideas and told them that the SC would mail them a summary report of the focus group results, including recommendations for action. Each participant received $20.

FOCUS GROUP INTERVIEWS WITH POLICY, PROGRAM, AND ORGANIZATION LEADERS

The organization leader focus groups were designed to engage in the process of intervention planning with a variety of individuals and organizations whose interests, responsibilities, and resources could contribute to planning and implementing the intervention ideas and recommendations that emerged from the individual interviews and women's focus groups.

Development of the Organization Leader Focus Group Interview Guide

The SC reviewed and discussed summary analyses of key themes and illustrative quotations from the women's focus groups (see the section on data analysis later in this chapter). In a process that lasted approximately one month, the project steering committee created two interview guides with a common structure, tailored to include community-specific themes, illustrative quotations from the indepth interviews and women's focus groups, and questions with probes. The SC recommended that focus group participants read each quotation aloud, to facilitate their engagement with the women's experiences.

Recruitment and Training of Moderators

The SC nominated potential moderators who had lived or worked extensively in one of the two communities. The two selected moderators were women from the same ethnic group as the potential population for the planned interventions, and included one SC member. Both had extensive experience moderating focus group discussions in similar communities and had played leadership roles in nonprofit organizations similar to the roles of most of the invited participants. During this phase the women's focus group note takers again filled the note-taking roles.

The SC recommended that the REACH Detroit Partnership eastside and southwest community facilitators serve as hosts, greeters, and observers to make explicit and visible the central role of community organizations in planning and implementing the focus groups. The SC also thought the community facilitators' strong relationships with local and community organizations and REACH Detroit's objective of promoting diabetes prevention programs for pregnant and postpartum women would provide continuity with organization leader participants during subsequent phases of grant writing and program development. Two academic SC members were also observers.

Moderators, note takers, and observers participated in a training workshop similar to those conducted for the women's focus groups and conducted by the same academic SC members. Because the moderators and note takers had focus group experience, the primary objective was to develop a shared vision of the focus group goals, roles, procedures, and materials used before, during, and after the focus group sessions. An additional objective was to increase the capacity of all participants to use focus groups for future CBPR activities and to extend their skills to others through similar workshops (Krueger & King, 1998b). Trainees also reviewed the content of the focus group guides and participated in practice sessions using the guide.

Recruitment of Organization Leaders

The SC and the REACH Detroit community facilitators compiled the names and contact information of policy, program, and community organization leaders from programs that directly or indirectly provided services or leadership related to pregnancy, health, social services, community development, safety, food and nutrition, or recreation and physical activity. The SC gave priority to leaders whose organizations' service mandate included eastside or southwest Detroit.

Each SC member personally contacted one or more of the leaders to inform them about the purpose of the focus group interview and the importance of their participation and to determine their availability. SC members used a telephone script drafted by project staff. The project principal investigator and the REACH Detroit community facilitators signed and mailed formal invitation letters to the leaders or representatives designated during the phone calls. Each SC member, supplemented by staff as needed, made follow-up contacts by telephone or e-mail to confirm participation. A follow-up letter thanked confirmed participants and provided detailed focus group logistics information.

IMPLEMENTATION AND DATA COLLECTION

The SC conducted two community-specific focus groups simultaneously in separate meeting rooms belonging to a SC partner whose building was centrally located between, but not within either of, the two communities. Participants were assigned to the eastside or southwest Detroit group based on their organization's primary service area, and those with broader service areas (for example, the state or the city of Detroit) were distributed between the two groups. An ice storm that closed most public facilities in southeast Michigan the day of the focus groups reduced participation to half of those who had confirmed (six for the eastside group; seven for the southwest).

The REACH Detroit community facilitators greeted participants in the building lobby and checked them off the list of invited participants. A note taker escorted them to their designated meeting room and administered the demographic information sheet. The SC planned to use the demographic information to assess the potential influence of participant age, gender, ethnicity, type of organization, or geographical area of responsibility on the results. Because this phase of data collection involved people in the public sector, whose identity would be difficult to disguise, the University of Michigan Institutional Review Board suggested that participation in the day's activities demonstrated informed consent, so no written consent forms were administered. Moderators invited participants to chat and share fresh fruit and beverages while waiting for their group to assemble. During this period the moderator approached several participants to invite them to read one of the selected quotations. She gave a sheet of paper with a quotation typed in bold text to those who agreed.

The ninety-minute focus group interviews began with the introduction of the moderator, note taker, and observers. The moderator reviewed the project background, focus group objective, and ground rules. She asked participants to introduce themselves during a brief icebreaker and then presented a review of major themes, during which participants read the selected quotations aloud to the group. The discussion included participants' reactions to what they had heard and their own perspectives about barriers and facilitators to healthy eating and exercise. The moderator asked participants to comment on the feasibility of the women's recommendations, identify factors that might impede or facilitate implementation, and add their own recommendations for planning, implementing, and maintaining interventions, including necessary resources and training, environment, program, and policy components. She encouraged participants to discuss their potential roles in such activities.

Moderating, note-taking, audiotaping, summarizing, thanking, and reporting procedures were similar to those described in the previous section. The moderator told participants that the project steering committee would review the ideas generated in both groups and recommend the next steps in the planning process. She invited participants to continue their involvement in planning by contacting the REACH Detroit community facilitator who had attended their focus group. Participants also could complete a form with their name, organization, contact information, and area of interest in follow-up planning. Within two weeks, the SC mailed thank-you letters to participants, and to people who had confirmed but not attended, that described the next steps in the planning process to those who had expressed interest in participating. The SC mailed a summary report to all participants. Several became involved in subsequent activities.

DATA ANALYSIS

Community members were involved in each phase of data analysis (Kemmis & McTaggart, 2000). This involvement was inherent in the study design, as first women and then organization leader focus group participants reviewed, gave meaning to, and confirmed, revised, and extended the findings from the previous phase. The SC used summary analysis processes adapted from several used previously in community-based research to facilitate rapid feedback of results to the SC for each phase of planning (Kieffer et al., 2002, 2004; Kreuger, 1998a; Scrimshaw & Hurtado, 1987).

Following each focus group meeting, moderator and note-taker pairs met for ten minutes to discuss their overall impressions and key ideas and insights from the interview. Then the moderators, note takers, and observers held a thirty-minute debriefing meeting facilitated by an academic SC member. The group members exchanged impressions of the major themes from each focus group and discussed process issues such as interpersonal and environmental factors that may have affected the quality of the data. Academic SC members took notes during this meeting.

Within a week following the focus group meetings, the note takers typed detailed field notes, using the audiotapes to ensure accuracy. Community moderators, note takers, and observers also completed a summary analysis form. This form was an expanded version of the focus group guide, with space for noting new topics that focus group participants had introduced and observations of nonverbal dynamics. The SC encouraged those completing this form to include quotations that allowed the words of participants to illustrate the major themes that they listed.

The SC held summary analysis meetings with community moderators, note takers, and observers one week following the focus groups. Each person used her or his summary analysis form to report key themes for each topic until those present agreed that the resulting lists for each focus group represented that group's outcomes. Those attending these meetings identified overarching themes and the relative importance of items within each theme, and noted themes related to specific populations and communities. The meetings were audiotaped to provide backup confirmation of written themes, to allow SC members who were not present to listen if they desired, and to produce a tool for future training in the summary analysis process. The SC used oral and typed reports of the results of the summary analysis meetings at its meetings.

Each focus group audiotape was transcribed verbatim in English or Spanish, as appropriate, and Spanish language transcripts were also translated into English. Each session note taker reviewed the relevant transcript for accuracy in its original language and made corrections as needed, integrating the field notes into the transcription to give a more complete picture of the environment and the nonverbal aspects of the focus groups and identifying speakers by seating number to protect participant confidentiality.

Procedures described by Krueger (1998a) guided in-depth analysis of the focus group transcripts. This phase confirmed that the summary analysis process had retrieved accurate results and allowed the extraction of illustrative quotations for SC use. The results of this analysis provided in-depth data needed for development of grant proposals and intervention materials. At least two academic SC members read each of the final transcripts to confirm themes that emerged during the summary analysis and extract additional themes related to target issues. Community SC members' time constraints limited their involvement in these readings. After the initial reading, SC members and several community moderators discussed, confirmed, and refined themes. They expanded a codebook developed for analysis of the individual interview data to include new themes derived from the focus groups, so that the widest range of relevant ideas would be available to the SC for intervention planning. The codebook included code definitions, inclusion and exclusion criteria, and examples (Crabtree & Miller, 1999b; Miles, 1994). Two research assistants coded the final transcripts, using Atlas.ti qualitative software, Version 4.1 (Muhr, 2000). Academic SC members reviewed and recoded any text that received less than 80 percent agreement during intercoder reliability assessment (Carey, Morgan, & Oxtoby, 1996). The SC selected direct quotations to illustrate major themes.

DATA FEEDBACK, USE OF DATA AND PRODUCTS, AND RESULTING CBPR INTERVENTIONS

Following each data collection phase, the SC used community (eastside, southwest) and population-specific (pregnant, postpartum) summaries to generate recommendations for the next phase of data collection. Project staff mailed final summary reports to focus group participants, SC members, and other interested URC-affiliated projects and community partners. The SC members and staff of other URC-affiliated projects in both communities have adapted many of the focus group-related methods and materials developed for this project, such as participant consent forms, focus group training manuals, and summary analysis forms.

Finally, the SC used the focus group recommendations to develop two large CBPR projects, tailored to the characteristics, cultural contexts, and needs of the eastside and southwest communities. Promoting Healthy Lifestyles Among Women (now renamed Healthy Mothers on the Move) is a five-year National Institutes of Health–funded project that aims to reduce risk factors for type 2 diabetes. Community resident women's health advocates facilitate a social support group intervention designed to improve pregnant and postpartum women's ability to increase their healthy eating and physical activity practices and to limit excessive weight gain and retention during and after pregnancy. Promoting Healthy Eating in Detroit is a three-year CDC-funded policy and organization-level intervention designed to increase demand for and use of healthy foods. The Michigan Department of Community Health, an SC partner, funded pilot phases of both projects. Funds for the Promoting Healthy Lifestyles Among Women pilot went to CHASS, as lead agency for the REACH Detroit Partnership, to ensure continuity. Both projects involve full collaboration among community, health, and academic partners, guided by project steering committees.

CHALLENGES AND LIMITATIONS

The success of any CBPR project rests on maintaining the delicate balance between the need for the active involvement of community organizations and residents and the effects of this participation on their time and resources. Many organizations and individuals who most represented community interests and needs also faced the greatest challenges to participation. Leaders of small, grassroots community organizations sometimes could not participate to the extent either they or other SC members had anticipated because of competing obligations and staff and budget constraints that involved their survival.

Some women identified as either prospective SC members or focus group moderators could not assume these roles because of life barriers, for example, competing schedules and responsibilities, language, transportation, and legal status.

Identifying individuals with adequate competencies to serve as moderators, note takers, transcribers, and translators was difficult, even with extensive training available for these roles. A Spanish surname or African American ethnicity did not automatically credential a person as linguistically or culturally competent to interact with focus group participants or to understand the language they used. The SC faced a major challenge in identifying fully bilingual and bicultural individuals and focus group training materials. The SC members and staff of other CBPR projects recommended people with whom they had worked successfully. Nonetheless, it took more time and resources to develop materials and to recruit and train moderators and note takers than had been anticipated in the original grant budget and timeline.

We did not intend the focus groups to generate data for use across broad populations, even those with characteristics, such as ethnicity, language, and life stage, similar to participants' characteristics. Seen in the context of CBPR, this potential limitation is a strength. The data are most useful for their immediate purpose and context, that is, for generating the perspectives of those whose voices should be heard, for improving understanding about issues and concerns, and for planning programs and policies. Triangulation, or use of multiple data sources, methods, or theoretical perspectives, to address similar questions was one way to increase the credibility of the focus group results, whether in the immediate or a broader context (Gilchrist & Williams, 1999). The SC used a relatively unstructured first data collection phase to explore a broad range of issues that might have affected the beliefs and behaviors of concern. These ideas were discussed with separate groups of individuals with similar backgrounds (women's focus groups) and with groups of others with at least some different characteristics (organization leaders). The SC confirmed most themes and found additional insights during each new phase of data collection.

LESSONS LEARNED AND IMPLICATIONS FOR PRACTICE

The steering committee's experience with this project led to a number of lessons learned and implications for the use of focus groups. Some of these are discussed here.

Involvement of community experts in conducting focus groups was essential. Focus group moderators were either native Detroiters or Latino immigrants living in the city, were of the same ethnic background as the participants, and had participated either in the in-depth interviews or in facilitating group discussions in their respective communities. They had recent experiences as pregnant or postpartum women that helped them relate to the issues raised by the focus group participants, they were acquainted with the key themes of the in-depth interviews (which formed the basis for the focus groups), and they were thoroughly familiar with the questions discussed because they were engaged in the entire process. These experiences and skills served as groundwork for the focus group workshop and contributed to these individuals' success as moderators.

Adequate resources and logistical support for community experts is essential. Scheduling focus group training and some SC meetings on weekends in Detroit and providing stipends or honoraria enhanced participation by community SC members and resident moderators. The project eventually provided child care, transportation, and translation services to facilitate participation. Including support for such services in the project budget would have reduced barriers to participation for some potential community partners from the start.

CBPR provides the opportunity for community capacity building. Including women from the community of identity (Israel et al., 1998) in leadership positions as moderators was a powerful form of capacity building, as they developed or enhanced professional and personal skills and abilities and served as role models for other women in the community. Some trainees planned to use their facilitation and observation skills at their jobs, in church-related activities, when communicating with their families, or in other research projects.

Anticipating the need to provide child care, refreshments, and transportation maximized attendance and minimized inconveniences to focus group participants. These services facilitated participation by a broader cross-section of community women than would otherwise have participated, including those who were the most isolated, underserved, and often unheard. Offering on-site child care was essential for many women with newborns and young children. Some women were reluctant at first to use the child-care services due to concerns about safety or trust. Allowing participants to tour the child-care facility and interact with the providers helped them to relax and decide to use the services. Because many residents of Detroit and similar cities lack cars or reliable public transportation, the project offered or supported transportation to enhance recruitment and retention of focus group participants. Drivers who knew the communities and could communicate well with participants enhanced participants' trust in the service. Refreshments served as people arrived provided an opportunity for participants to chat with each other and feel at ease, which set a welcoming tone for the focus groups.

Having reputable connections in the community was a positive force. The SC included representatives of respected and committed organizations based in the communities in which the project took place. These organizations hosted and actively participated in meetings and were strong believers in the project benefits and results for the communities they served. This connection facilitated the selection of data collection locations and recruitment of focus group moderators and participants. Conducting focus groups in these reputable places provided credibility and removed some barriers to attendance. Links to trustworthy organizations within the community helped to dissipate mistrust.

Adequate budgets for transcription and translation services were also essential. Transcription of focus group tapes required special care to distinguish adequately among participants. Translation of all project materials and meetings was expensive but essential to the success of the project. Although the budget supported translation services, the needs far exceeded available resources, and the search for appropriate materials and service providers was a challenge. CBPR projects that use focus groups must adequately budget for such services.

Participatory processes can affect the timeline for focus groups. Although the SC helped to recruit moderators and note takers, it was very difficult to identify nonacademic individuals with the time to receive training and conduct the focus groups. This process took approximately four months, resulting in timeline delays. Using a participatory data analysis process was also time consuming. The SC was made up of very committed but busy people who contributed their time and insights during and between meetings and whose tasks included reviewing, discussing, and revising materials. It might have been faster if academic SC members and research assistants had planned and implemented the data collection and analysis. However, this would have sacrificed the richness of participation and would not have fully allowed the voice and understanding of community members to manifest.

Ensuring immediate benefits to the community from focus group interviews. All phases of the research involved a trust-building process among participants. Staying connected and committed to those project aims that extended beyond data collection and analysis, and that included returning results to the community, were essential to maintaining this trust and the success of subsequent activities. Summary reports and presentations were provided to community residents and organizations. Maintaining the SC and extending membership to interested community residents who participated in data collection were also important steps. Collaborative development and implementation of successful grant proposals that addressed community issues and recommendations, and participation by community and academic SC members in other forms of community capacity building are examples of continuing mutual commitments that strengthen and maintain relationships that arise from CBPR.

CONCLUSIONS AND FUTURE DIRECTIONS

The use of focus groups has become increasingly popular in the last decade in public health projects. The growing emphasis on social inequalities and racial or ethnic disparities in health has encouraged researchers to acknowledge the importance of community members' knowledge, experiences, and perspectives when developing effective strategies to address risk and protective factors associated with health and disease. The focus group method is ideal for community-based participatory research, where community members are equal partners in the research process and knowledge translates into action and social change (Wallerstein & Duran, 2003). In this context, focus groups are a vehicle to capture the *voice* (Stewart, 2000) of community members, particularly marginalized populations whose cultural norms and realities may not "fit" with the norms of dominant mainstream society. Although focus group methodologies have specific features at their core, community partnerships can vary their design sufficiently to target the needs and specific aims of the community, population, and type of intervention under consideration.

In CBPR, focus group processes provide opportunities for community members to engage actively and equally in planning and implementing the primary means of data collection, interpreting its results, and developing intervention strategies. Community moderators and focus group participants often develop a common bond based on shared perceptions of health and social issues as well as an investment in solutions that they themselves suggest (Kieffer et al., 2002, 2004; Whitehorse, Manzano, Baezconde-Garbanati, & Hahn 1999). Focus groups, as used in the three projects described in this chapter, captured the voice of two communities and translated words into actions. The project members forged an expanded and lasting partnership that obtained the resources needed to build and sustain ongoing CBPR projects.

Nevertheless, the lessons learned during this project suggest that CBPR partnerships need to consider the roles that all partners play in the research process and to address the barriers that may limit participation by community residents and partner organizations. CBPR projects that use focus groups must carefully plan adequate timelines, budgets, and other resources needed to ensure truly equal community participation.

References

Brown, J. B. (1999). The use of focus groups in clinical research. In B. F. Crabtree & W. L. Miller (Eds.), *Doing qualitative research* (2nd ed., pp. 109–124). Thousand Oaks, CA: Sage.

Carey, J., Morgan, M., & Oxtoby, M. (1996). Intercoder agreement in analysis of responses to open-ended interview questions: Examples from tuberculosis research. *Cultural Anthropology Methods, 8,* 1–5.

Crabtree, B. F., & Miller, W. L. (Eds.). (1999a). *Doing qualitative research* (2nd ed.). Thousand Oaks, CA: Sage.

Crabtree, B. F., & Miller, W. L. (1999b). Using code manuals: A template organizing style of interpretation. In B. F. Crabtree & W. L. Miller (Eds.), *Doing qualitative research* (2nd ed., pp. 163–177). Thousand Oaks, CA: Sage.

Denzin, N. K., & Lincoln, Y. S. (2000). The discipline and practice of qualitative research. In N. K. Denzin & Y. S. Lincoln (Eds.), *The handbook of qualitative research* (2nd ed., pp. 1–28). Thousand Oaks, CA: Sage.

Gilchrist, V. J., & Williams, R. L. (1999). Key informant interviews. In B. F. Crabtree & W. L. Miller. (Eds.), *Doing qualitative research* (2nd ed., pp. 71–78). Thousand Oaks, CA: Sage.

Israel, B. A., Lichtenstein, R., Lantz, P., McGranaghan, R., Allen, A., Guzman, R., et al. (2001). The Detroit Community-Academic Urban Research Center: Development, implementation and evaluation. *Journal of Public Health Management and Practice, 7*(5), 1–19.

Israel, B. A., Schulz, A. J., Parker, E. A., & Becker, A. B. (1998). Review of community-based research: Assessing partnership approaches to improve public health. *Annual Review of Public Health, 19,* 173–202.

Kemmis, S., & McTaggart, R. (2000). Participatory action research. In N. K. Denzin & Y. S. Lincoln (Eds.), *Handbook of qualitative research* (2nd ed., pp. 567–605). Thousand Oaks, CA: Sage.

Kieffer, E. C., Carman, W. J., Gillespie, B., Nolan, G., Worley, S., & Guzman, J. R. (2001). Obesity and gestational diabetes among African-American and Latino Women: Implications for disparities in women's health. *Journal of the American Medical Women's Association, 1*(56), 181–187.

Kieffer, E. C., Willis, S., Arellano, N., & Guzman, R. (2002). Perspectives of pregnant and postpartum Latino women on diabetes, physical activity and health. *Health Education and Behavior, 29*(5), 542–556.

Kieffer, E. C., Willis, S., Odoms, A., Guzman, R., Allen, A., Two Feathers, J., et al. (2004). Reducing disparities in diabetes among African American and Latino residents of Detroit: The essential role of community planning focus groups. *Ethnicity and Disease, 14*(Suppl. 1), S1-27–S1-37.

Krueger, R. A. (1998a). The Analysis Process. Chapter 5 in D. L. Morgan & R. A. Krueger (Eds.), *Focus group kit* (Vol. 6 Analyzing and reporting focus group results (pp. 41–59). Thousand Oaks, CA: Sage.

Krueger, R. A. (1998b). What do you need to do during the focus group. Chapter Four in D. L. Morgan & R. A. Krueger (Eds.), *Focus group kit* (Vol. 4, Moderating focus groups, pp. 15–35). Thousand Oaks, CA: Sage.

Krueger, R. A., & King, J. A. (1998a). How to involve volunteers. Chapter Two in D. L. Morgan & R. A. Krueger (Eds.), *Focus group kit* (Vol. 5, Involving community members in focus groups, pp. 15–49). Thousand Oaks, CA: Sage.

Krueger, R., & King, J. A. (1998b). Learning exercises. Chapter Three in D. L. Morgan & R. A. Krueger (Eds.), *Focus group kit* (Vol. 5, Involving community members in focus groups, pp. 51–84). Thousand Oaks, CA: Sage.

Loevy, S. S., & O'Brien, M. U. (1994). Community-based research: The case for focus groups. In A. J. Dan (Ed.), *Reframing women's health: Multidisciplinary research and practice* (pp. 102–110). Thousand Oaks, CA: Sage.

Madriz, E. (2000). Focus groups in feminist research. In N. K. Denzin & Y. S. Lincoln (Eds.), *The handbook of qualitative research* (2nd ed., pp. 835–850). Thousand Oaks, CA: Sage.

Miles, M. (1994). *Qualitative data analysis: An expanded sourcebook* (2nd ed.). Thousand Oaks, CA: Sage.

Morgan, D. L. (1998a). What focus groups are (and are not). Chapter Four in D. L. Morgan & R. A. Krueger (Eds.), *Focus group kit* (Vol. 1, The focus group guidebook, pp. 29–35). Thousand Oaks, CA: Sage.

Morgan, D. L. (1998b). Why should you use focus groups? Chapter Two in D. L. Morgan & R. A. Krueger (Eds.), *Focus group kit* (Vol. 1, The focus group guidebook, pp. 9–15.). Thousand Oaks, CA: Sage.

Morgan, D. L., & Krueger, R. A. (1998). *The focus group kit.* Thousand Oaks, CA: Sage.

Muhr, T. (2000). Atlas.ti, Version 4.1. Berlin: Scientific Software Development.

O'Neill, J., Small, B. B., & Strachan, J. (1997). The use of focus groups within a participatory action research environment. In M. Kopala & L. A. Suzuki (Eds.), *Using qualitative methods in psychology* (pp. 199–209). Thousand Oaks, CA: Sage.

Parsons, M. L., & Warner-Robbins, C. (2002). Formerly incarcerated women create healthy lives through participatory action research. *Holistic Nursing Practice, 16*(2), 40–49.

Piran, N. (2001). Reinhabiting the body. *Feminism & Psychology, 11*(2), 172–176.

Schulz, A. J., Parker, E. A., Israel, B. A., Allen, A., Decarlo, M., & Robinson M. (2002). Addressing social determinants of health through community-based participatory research: The East Side Village Health Worker Partnership. *Health Education & Behavior, 29*(3), 326–341.

Scrimshaw, S.C.M., & Hurtado, E. (1987). *Rapid assessment procedures for nutrition and primary health care: Anthropological approaches to improving programme effectiveness.* Los Angeles: UCLA Latin American Center.

Stewart, E. (2000). Thinking through others: Qualitative research and community psychology. In J. Rappaport & E. Seidman (Eds.), *Handbook of community psychology* (pp. 725–739). New York: Kluwer Academic/Plenum.

Sugrue, T. J. (1996). *The origins of the urban crisis: Race and inequality in postwar Detroit.* Princeton, NJ: Princeton University Press.

U.S. Census Bureau. (2000, June). *Census of population and housing.* Data generated by the Michigan Metropolitan Information Center, Wayne State University.

Wallerstein, N., & Duran, B. (2003). The conceptual, historical, and practice roots of community-based participatory research and related participatory traditions. In M. Minkler & N. Wallerstein (Eds.), *Community-based participatory research for health* (pp. 27–52). San Francisco: Jossey-Bass.

Walters, K. L., Simoni, J. M., & Horwath, P. F. (2001). Sexual orientation bias experiences and service needs of gay, lesbian, bisexual, transgendered, and two-spirited American Indians. *Journal of Gay and Lesbian Social Services, 13*(1–2), 133–149.

Whitehorse, L. E., Manzano, R., Baezconde-Garbanati, L. A., & Hahn, G. (1999). Culturally tailoring a physical activity program for Hispanic women: Recruitment successes of La Vida Buena's Salsa Aerobics. *Journal of Health Education, 30*(2), S18–S24.

CHAPTER EIGHT

Application of CBPR in the Design of an Observational Tool

The Neighborhood Observational Checklist

Shannon N. Zenk, Amy J. Schulz, James S. House,
Alison Benjamin, and Srimathi Kannan

A large body of research demonstrates that living in economically disadvantaged neighborhoods is associated with poorer health, independent of individual socioeconomic position (Ellen, Mijanovich, & Dillman, 2001; Pickett & Pearl, 2000). Research also suggests that neighborhood socioeconomic position helps to explain racial disparities in health (Browning, Cagney, & Wen, 2003; Haan, Kaplan, & Camacho, 1987). The mechanisms by which neighborhood environments affect health and contribute to racial disparities in health are less clear (Diez-Roux, 2001; Macintyre, Ellaway, & Cummins, 2002). Identifying the characteristics of neighborhoods that affect the health of residents and

Acknowledgments: The Neighborhood Observational Checklist (NOC) was developed by the Healthy Environments Partnership (HEP), a project of the Detroit Community-Academic Urban Research Center (www.sph.umich.edu/urc). HEP (www.sph.umich.edu/hep) is funded by the National Institute of Environmental Health Sciences, grant RO1 ES10936–0. The HEP Steering Committee includes representatives from the Brightmoor Community Center, Detroit Department of Health and Wellness Promotion, Friends of Parkside, Henry Ford Health System, Southwest Detroit Environmental Vision, Southwest Solutions, University of Detroit Mercy, University of Michigan Schools of Public Health, Nursing, and Social Work, and the Survey Research Center. We thank other members of the NOC Subcommittee: Pat Miller, William Ridella, and Zachary Rowe. We appreciate the contributions of Sachiko Woods (field coordinator) and Clarence Gravlee (W. K. Kellogg Foundation–funded community health scholar) to the development of the NOC and training of observers. HEP is grateful to the researchers involved in the Chicago Community Adult Health Study (CCAHS) for sharing their Systematic Social Observation instrument, experiences with its use, and sampling advice.

contribute to health disparities is important so that interventions can be directed at transforming neighborhood environments to promote health and eliminate socioeconomic and racial disparities in health (House & Williams, 2000).

Understanding how the social and physical environments of neighborhoods affect health requires a comprehensive assessment of neighborhoods (Caughy, O'Campo, & Patterson, 2001). At the most basic level, a variety of information is available from the decennial census, including several indicators of socioeconomic position (for example, median household income, median home value, and percentage employed). Administrative sources provide data on numerous economic, social, and environmental subjects, such as crime, toxic emissions, housing code violations, day-care licenses, and student school performance (Kingsley, Coulton, Barndt, Sawicki, & Tatian, 1997). Still some types of data, such as normative beliefs and community social dynamics, can be gathered only by talking with the residents themselves through focus groups (see Chapter Seven), in-depth interviews (see Chapters Ten and Twelve), group interviews (see Chapter Fourteen), or surveys (see Chapter Five) to gain their perceptions and insights (Caughy et al., 2001; Macintyre et al., 2002). Other neighborhood characteristics—for example, the nature and quality of public space and of residential, commercial, and other properties—may be difficult for survey respondents and interview participants to accurately describe and quantify (Raudenbush & Sampson, 1999). Therefore direct assessment of physical and social conditions can make valuable contributions to understanding how neighborhoods affect health (Caughy et al., 2001). Direct observation of neighborhoods, whereby trained observers systematically document preselected, well-defined aspects of neighborhoods, is a method of measuring neighborhood conditions that allows comparisons across neighborhoods. It is also referred to as *systematic observation* or *systematic social observation* (Reiss, 1971; Sampson & Raudenbush, 1999). Direct observation can also address same source bias, which may result when the same informant provides information on both health determinants, such as neighborhood conditions and health outcomes (Raudenbush & Sampson, 1999).

In this chapter we begin by reviewing how direct neighborhood observation has been used in research, including community-based participatory research (CBPR). We then describe how community and academic partners of the Healthy Environments Partnership (HEP), a CBPR project in Detroit, Michigan, worked together to design an observational instrument, the Neighborhood Observational Checklist (NOC). As part of this discussion, we highlight how HEP sought input from and engaged other community residents in this process. Then we share selected outcomes of HEP's participatory process. Finally, we discuss challenges encountered and lessons learned in applying a CBPR approach to the design of a neighborhood observational tool, with particular attention to implications for the use of neighborhood observation in future CBPR efforts.

REVIEW OF EXISTING NEIGHBORHOOD
OBSERVATIONAL INSTRUMENTS

Arguably, two of the most influential neighborhood observational instruments, both in terms of shaping the content of subsequent observational instruments and crafting innovative methodology for data collection and analysis, are the Block Environment Inventory, developed by Taylor and his colleagues (Perkins, Meeks, & Taylor, 1992; Taylor, Gottfredson, & Brower, 1984), and the Systematic Social Observation instrument from the Project on Human Development in Chicago Neighborhoods (PHDCN) (Sampson & Raudenbush, 1999). Investigators have used both tools primarily to examine neighborhood-level determinants of crime and delinquency. Taylor and colleagues' Block Environment Inventory includes measures of constructs such as physical incivilities (for example, vandalism or graffiti), defensible space (for example, public street lights), and territorial functioning (for example, private plantings) and has been used to collect data at the level of the block face (block segment on one side of a street) (Taylor, Shumaker, & Gottfredson, 1985; Perkins et al., 1992). The PHDCN Systematic Social Observation provides perhaps the most comprehensive assessment of neighborhoods within an urban area (Sampson & Raudenbush, 1999). The PHDCN collected data in 196 Chicago census tracts by observing and videotaping streets from a sport utility vehicle moving at five miles per hour. From the videotapes and observer logs, 126 variables were coded. The reliability and validity of measures of physical disorder (for example, cigarettes or cigars in the street or gutter) and social disorder (for example, drinking alcohol in public) have been documented (Raudenbush & Sampson, 1999).

Several neighborhood observational instruments have been developed for health research from Taylor and colleagues' Block Environment Inventory and the PHDCN's Systematic Social Observation instrument. Adapting these tools for use in a project in Baltimore, with a particular focus on the well-being of children and families, Caughy and colleagues (2001) developed an observational instrument consisting of forty-five items. In addition to creating measures of physical incivilities and territoriality, they developed a neighborhood indicator of available play resources (for example, the proportion of homes with yards, a public playground in good condition). To help test the impact of neighborhood environments on the health of residents, the Chicago Community Adult Health Study (CCAHS) collaborated with the PHDCN to create an observational instrument (Morenoff, House, & Raudenbush, n.d.). The CCAHS instrument and PHDCN instrument include many of the same variables. However, instead of driving through and videotaping neighborhoods, the data collectors (survey interviewers) in the CCAHS walked through neighborhoods and recorded data on standardized coding sheets.

Community Action Against Asthma (CAAA), a project of the Detroit Community-Academic Urban Research Center, developed the thirty-one-item CAAA Environmental Checklist for use in the context of its CBPR project to address childhood asthma (Farquhar, 2000). Adapted in part from Taylor and colleagues' Block Environment Inventory, the CAAA Environmental Checklist was designed to evaluate the presence of neighborhood deterioration and blight (for example, abandoned factories, vacant industrial lots), annoyances (for example, heavy traffic, stray animals), industry and technological stressors (for example, chemical plants, landfills), and neighborhood assets (for example, parks, playgrounds, gardens, block club lamps) in neighborhoods located in eastside and southwest Detroit. Members of the CAAA Steering Committee, representing each partner organization (for example, a university, community-based organizations, health service agencies), had the opportunity to delete from, add to, and otherwise modify the draft list of environmental stressors generated by academic partners and were also involved in identifying and selecting the checklist raters. In addition to these instruments, the number of audit tools to evaluate observable neighborhood conditions that may affect residents' physical activity is growing rapidly (Emery, Crump, & Bors, 2003; Moudon & Lee, 2003; Pikora et al., 2002).

Investigators have begun to test relationships between neighborhood conditions, as assessed through observation, and health. In one study in New Orleans, secondary data on public high schools were combined with observational data to create a "broken windows" index: the percentage of homes with cosmetic, minor, or major structural damage; the percentage of streets with trash, abandoned cars, or graffiti; and the number of physical problems and building code violations in public high schools (Cohen et al., 2000). Among high-poverty neighborhoods, those with high scores on the broken windows index had significantly higher gonorrhea rates than those with low scores. In another study, Weich and colleagues (2002) collected data in two electoral wards in north London with a twenty-seven-item observational checklist designed to assess aspects of the built environment. They found that people who were identified as being depressed, based on a dichotomous split on the Centers for Epidemiologic Studies Depression Scale (CES-D), were more likely to live in areas characterized by residential properties that had predominately deck access for entering the dwellings and were of recent (post-1969) construction (adjusting for individual socioeconomic status, floor of residence, and structural housing problems) (Weich et al., 2002). In a Canadian study a latent neighborhood environment score based on eighteen observations, such as variety of destinations and traffic, was positively associated with walking to work (Craig, Brownson, Cragg, & Dunn, 2002).

Direct observation as a data collection method has tremendous potential to illuminate the pathways by which neighborhood environments influence health. Still, relatively few studies to date have used observational data to test relationships between neighborhood conditions and health. In addition, community involvement in the process of developing neighborhood observational instruments (for example, deciding what to measure and how to measure it) has been limited. As a result it is not clear to what extent existing observational instruments reflect residents' experiences in and insights about their neighborhoods. The ability to identify unique characteristics of neighborhoods and to understand their meaning and relevance for health can be critically enhanced by engaging community residents in the process of designing neighborhood observational instruments.

OVERVIEW OF THE HEALTHY ENVIRONMENTS PARTNERSHIP

The Healthy Environments Partnership (HEP) is a CBPR project designed to identify and address aspects of the social and physical environments that contribute to racial and socioeconomic disparities in risk and protective factors for cardiovascular disease in three large communities of Detroit, Michigan: eastside, southwest, and northwest (Schulz, Kannan, et al., under review). Established in October 2000 as a part of the National Institute of Environmental Health Sciences' Health Disparities Initiative, HEP is part of the Detroit Community-Academic Urban Research Center. HEP comprises a number of community partners (including community-based and health service organizations) and academic partners: the Brightmoor Community Center, Detroit Department of Health and Wellness Promotion, Friends of Parkside, Henry Ford Health System, Southwest Detroit Environmental Vision, Southwest Solutions, University of Detroit Mercy, University of Michigan Schools of Public Health, Nursing, and Social Work, and the Survey Research Center. Representatives of these partner organizations make up the HEP Steering Committee, which meets monthly and is involved to varying extents in all aspects of the research process, consistent with the principles of CBPR (Israel, Schulz, Parker, & Becker, 1998).

The HEP Steering Committee developed a conceptual model in which the physical and social environments of neighborhoods were conceptualized as intermediaries in the pathway through which race-based residential segregation and concentrated poverty influence more proximate factors that ultimately influence physiological responses (for example, body mass index, cortisol as an indicator of allostatic load, and hypertension) and cardiovascular health (Schulz, Kannan, et al., under review). The proximate factors fall into the following categories: social (for example, stress, social networks), behavioral (for example, physical activity), psychological (for example, hopelessness), community (for example, community capacity), and biological (for example, micronutrient status). To achieve as complete a picture as possible of the social and physical environments of the three Detroit study communities, HEP conducted the following data collection activities: compiled data from the 2000 U.S. Census; obtained air quality data collected by a sister Urban Research Center project in two study communities over a three-year period (Keeler et al., 2002) and amassed additional air quality data in the third community; held six focus groups with African American, Latino, and white residents of the study communities on neighborhood stressors and resources; and conducted a survey of Detroit residents ($n = 919$) that included questions about their perceptions of neighborhood resources, social dynamics, and stressors (see Chapter Five). In addition, following a decision made by community and academic partners who participated in writing the initial grant proposal, HEP designed and systematically recorded observations of neighborhood environments using the Neighborhood Observational Checklist (NOC).

DESIGN OF THE NEIGHBORHOOD OBSERVATIONAL CHECKLIST

The HEP Steering Committee developed the Neighborhood Observational Checklist (NOC) by refining and extending available observational instruments according to the project's goals and for use in the three Detroit study communities. This involved adding some items and omitting others, modifying response options and rating scales, and especially, revising operational definitions. The extensive participatory process HEP employed to design the NOC is the focus of this chapter. This process involved the following steps:

1. Review of previous data collection efforts
2. Formation of the NOC Subcommittee
3. Content discussions among the NOC Subcommittee members and HEP Steering Committee members
4. Pilot testing

The community and academic partners who made up the HEP Steering Committee and the community residents who were involved in the focus groups and NOC pilot testing contributed to the design of the NOC. The NOC development took place over an eleven-month period in 2002 and 2003, followed by approximately fifteen weeks of data collection (Table 8.1).

Review of Previous Data Collection Efforts

From August to November 2002, two HEP academic partners (the principal investigator and a graduate student research assistant) conducted preliminary work

Table 8.1. Design and Implementation of the Neighborhood Observational Checklist:
Major Tasks, Participants, and Timeline

Major Tasks	Participants	Timeline
Decision to use neighborhood observation in grant proposal	Community and academic partners	Spring 2000
Review of literature and existing instruments, review of focus group results, and construction of first draft of NOC	Academic partners	August–November 2002
HEP Steering Committee discussion of NOC implementation and formation of NOC Subcommittee	Community and academic partners	October 2002
One-on-one discussions of NOC first draft between NOC Subcommittee members	Community and academic partners	December 2002
NOC Subcommittee meeting to discuss revised version of NOC	Community and academic partners	January 2003
HEP Steering Committee discussion of further refined version of NOC	Community and academic partners	February 2003
Refinement and extension of NOC based on feedback from NOC Subcommittee and HEP Steering Committee	Community and academic partners	January–February 2003
Pilot-testing and revision of NOC	Academic partners and HEP staff	March 2003
Training of observers and additional pilot-testing and revision of NOC	Academic partners, community residents, and HEP staff	April–June 2003
Data collection with NOC	Community residents with HEP staff supervision	June–October 2003

on the NOC design. These academic partners first identified neighborhood observational instruments available in the literature, including some of those reviewed earlier in this chapter. They also met with investigators from the Chicago Community Adult Health Study (CCAHS) to discuss that study's

Systematic Social Observation instrument. Given that the CCAHS Systematic Social Observation was among the most comprehensive neighborhood observational instruments, its framework was used as the basis of the NOC.

The academic partners systematically compared the Systematic Social Observation items to community survey content areas and themes of the focus groups conducted with African American, Latino, and white residents of the three Detroit study communities two years previously (see Chapter Five in this volume and Schulz, Israel, et al., 2004). Topics discussed in the focus groups included challenges and major changes in the participants' neighborhoods that contribute to stress and how neighborhood residents respond to these challenges and changes. (See Chapter Five for additional information on the content areas and the process of developing the HEP survey.)

To assist with these comparisons, the academic partners constructed a grid that showed

- Neighborhood stressors, resources, and responses to stress identified by community residents during the focus groups

- Items in the HEP community survey to assess these stressors, resources, and responses

- Items on these topics from the CCAHS Systematic Social Observation instrument

This comparison allowed the identification of gaps where the NOC could complement and extend the other data collected by HEP and improve the assessment of neighborhood conditions. For example, focus group participants identified alcohol use as a response to stress for some people in their neighborhoods. The community survey included items on the frequency and amount of respondents' alcohol consumption. The NOC offered an opportunity to look for environmental cues that might encourage alcohol use, such as the presence of bars, liquor stores, and advertisements for alcohol.

When topics found in the focus group results or the community survey were not addressed in the CCAHS Systematic Social Observation instrument, the academic partners either identified relevant items from other observational tools (Caughy et al., 2001; Farquhar, 2000; Perkins et al., 1992) or created new items. For example, focus group participants identified truck traffic as a significant stressor in their neighborhoods. Truck traffic not only may be a source of psychosocial stress but may also have implications for air quality. As a result, an item on the volume of truck traffic was added to the draft of the NOC, adapting an item from the Community Action Against Asthma Environmental Checklist (Farquhar, 2000). (Later, in a discussion with the NOC Subcommittee, this item was revised to measure the presence of semis [tractor-trailer trucks], a source of noxious diesel exhaust and particulate matter—one of the main physical environmental variables of interest to HEP.) In other cases, new items were developed for the NOC based on focus group themes. For example, focus group participants described crumbling and broken sidewalks as a problem in their neighborhoods. Because poorly maintained sidewalks may impede physical activity, an item was drafted for the NOC on the condition of sidewalks. Table 8.2 displays a sampling of comparisons among focus group themes, community survey items, and final NOC items.

Table 8.2. Examples of Neighborhood Stressors Identified by Residents in Focus Groups, Included in the HEP Survey, and Included in the HEP Neighborhood Observational Checklist

Stressor Identified in Focus Groups	Item(s) in the HEP Survey	Items in the HEP Neighborhood Observational Checklist
Dumping, including on sidewalks	Streets, sidewalks, and vacant lots in my neighborhood are kept clean of litter and dumping. (Rated on a 5-point agree-disagree scale.)	Are there any piles of garbage or dumped materials on the block face? Is there strewn garbage, litter, broken glass, clothes, or papers on the block face?[a] Is a "No Dumping" sign visible on the block face?[b]
Roads and sidewalks in disrepair	Quality of street maintenance in your neighborhood, for example, filling potholes or replacing burned-out street lights. (Rated on a 4-point scale, from excellent to poor.)	Condition of the street.[a] Condition of the sidewalk.
Deteriorated and abandoned homes	Houses in my neighborhood are generally well-maintained. (Rated on a 5-point agree-disagree scale.) My neighborhood has a lot of vacant lots or vacant homes. (Rated on a 5-point agree-disagree scale.)	Based on street-level frontage, is there a vacant home on this block face?[a] How would you rate the condition of *most* of the houses/ residential buildings on the block face?[a]

[a]Adapted from the Systematic Social Observation instrument (Morenoff et al., n.d.).

[b]Adapted from Brief Neighborhood Observational measure (Caughy et al., 2001).

Formation of the Neighborhood Observational Checklist Subcommittee

In October 2002, the HEP Steering Committee began concrete discussions about how to conduct neighborhood observation in the study neighborhoods. Academic and community partners reviewed a first draft of the NOC, HEP's conceptual model, and the grid linking focus group themes, community survey items, and possible NOC items. Several important issues were raised during the discussion among the steering committee members. First, some members brought up the uniqueness of Detroit, noting that issues that are relevant elsewhere may not be in Detroit and vice versa. They noted the importance of making comparisons with communities outside the city and gathering data that accurately capture the context of the study communities. Second, steering committee members raised concerns about the limited assessment of neighborhood assets and resources in existing instruments. The steering committee was particularly interested in achieving a balance in the NOC between neighborhood resources and stressors. In addition, some members expressed their hopes that the NOC would be comprehensive enough to meet future research needs of other Detroit Community-Academic Urban Research Center projects and thus would minimize duplication of efforts in creating observational instruments in the future.

Given the importance of these issues, the HEP Steering Committee decided to form a subcommittee with responsibility for reviewing the NOC in further detail and making additions, modifications, and deletions. The NOC Subcommittee consisted of two academic partners (the principal investigator and graduate student research assistant) and four community partners—two from community-based organizations and two from health service organizations. A postdoctoral fellow working with HEP and the NOC field coordinator who was a Detroit resident participated in several of these discussions as well.

The work of the NOC Subcommittee unfolded as follows. First, in December 2002, the graduate student research assistant met with each other member of the subcommittee to discuss the current content of the NOC and to identify possible revisions. The research assistant compiled the suggestions and revised the NOC accordingly. The entire subcommittee met in January 2003 to discuss the revised version of the NOC and recommend further modifications to items and operational definitions, which the research assistant then made. Finally, in February 2003, the subcommittee presented a further refined version of the NOC to the entire HEP Steering Committee and facilitated discussion among the broader membership.

Content Discussions Among the NOC Subcommittee and HEP Steering Committee Members

The content discussions among the NOC Subcommittee and HEP Steering Committee members proved invaluable and served to clarify the purpose of the Neighborhood Observational Checklist, probe the meaning of proposed NOC items, examine the appropriateness of items for Detroit and the study communities, and add items to capture more community assets. Each of these functions is described in the following sections.

Clarifying the Purpose of the NOC. One of the first issues that became apparent in discussions of the NOC was a desire for the NOC to be comprehensive. One strength of HEP is its diversity of community and academic partners. The academic partners represent, for example, health behavior and health education, environmental health sciences, and sociology. The community partners include health service organizations and community-based organizations that represent three different Detroit communities (eastside, southwest, and northwest). Although sharing commonalities, these communities also have unique histories, populations (see www.hepdetroit.com for further information on the neighborhoods involved), health concerns, and assets.

Thus the NOC Subcommittee members identified a wide range of topics they deemed important for cardiovascular health. The length of the initial list made it clear that the subcommittee and the partnership as a whole would need to establish priorities to guide decisions about which items would be included in the final instrument. After discussion, the subcommittee agreed that the purpose of the NOC was to measure neighborhood conditions that create or protect against stress, influence social relationships, and affect health behaviors (that is, diet, physical activity, alcohol consumption, and tobacco use); thus, the NOC would capture both neighborhood stressors and neighborhood assets. Though still ambitious in scope, these mutually agreed-upon purposes served as a basis for making decisions about items to include, and partners took responsibility for asking how various topics and items fit these purposes.

Probing the Meaning of NOC Items. Probing the meaning of proposed NOC items was another function of conversations among subcommittee and steering committee members. One example of this probing relates to "This Building Is Being Watched" signs. These signs are placed on abandoned houses and buildings in Detroit as part of a citywide effort to prevent vandalism and arson. Two subcommittee members independently suggested assessing the presence of these signs because they thought the signs reflected community mobilization. Other members of the subcommittee noted that because the signs are placed on every abandoned house or building, they reflect very little about community mobilization. After discussion the subcommittee decided to omit this item from the NOC because of the lack of clarity regarding the meaning of these signs.

There was considerable discussion of whether to include an item on the presence of block club lamps. Block club lamps are matching lights in residential yards, historically used by Detroit block clubs as visual symbols of neighborhood collective action to protect against crime. Some subcommittee members thought that block club lamps had little current meaning in terms of collective action, that in some neighborhoods where collective action no longer exists these lamps were present simply because they had been left by previous home-owners, whereas in neighborhoods that did have extensive mobilization efforts lamps might not be present because residents lacked resources to install them. Other members pointed out that one of the three study neighborhoods had never made use of these lamps and noted that previous collective action can serve as a basis for future mobilization. Ultimately, the subcommittee decided to include an item assessing the presence of block club lamps, even though rec-ognizing the challenges that would be involved in interpreting this item in terms of contemporary collective mobilization. (This item was later refined based on community residents' feedback during pilot testing.)

In yet another example of how the subcommittee probed the meaning of NOC items, its members discussed the interpretation of a proposed NOC item assessing the presence of dumping and piles of trash as indicators of physical disorder. Members noted if blocks were observed around the time of the monthly bulk pickup day, their score on this item would not provide an accu-rate indicator of disorder. To address this issue, community partners on the sub-committee obtained maps showing the monthly bulk pickup schedules so that the field coordinator could avoid assigning blocks for data collection within a week of their monthly bulk pickup.

Examining the Appropriateness of NOC Items for Detroit. As part of NOC Subcommittee and HEP Steering Committee discussions, members also examined the appropriateness of proposed NOC items for Detroit. For example, items in existing observational tools assessed the overall condition of residen-tial buildings and grounds. Focus group participants had identified deteriorated housing as a problem in their neighborhoods, suggesting the importance of eval-uating this aspect of the neighborhood environment with the NOC. In discus-sions, however, subcommittee members noted that the conditions of buildings and grounds in Detroit neighborhoods are often mixed. By assessing only the condition of most, HEP might miss neighborhoods where some residents invest considerable energy to maintain their properties and grounds, even though gen-eral conditions are poor. Conversely, HEP might fail to capture the effects of a few badly deteriorated homes in neighborhoods where overall conditions are fairly good. Several strategies were discussed for capturing these situations, and the subcommittee ultimately decided to assess the condition of the *best, worst,* and *most* residential buildings and residential grounds on each block face.

Adding Items to Capture More Community Assets. As mentioned earlier the HEP Steering Committee was particularly interested in achieving a balance between neighborhood stressors and resources in the NOC items. The NOC

Subcommittee members struggled with how to capture and operationalize the neighborhood resources and assets they identified. Ultimately, they settled on the addition of several items intended to capture positive social relationships and community capacity. For example, the Systematic Social Observation instrument includes an item assessing the presence of vacant lots, which can be conceptualized as a community stressor or as an indicator of deterioration. Subcommittee members pointed out that some vacant lots are kept up and cared for by neighbors, some have been turned into informal playgrounds, and some are places for neighborhood socialization (set up with chairs and furniture, for example). Items were added to document signs that vacant lots were being transformed for positive purposes, as indicators of community investment and community social ties.

Subcommittee members representing southwest Detroit, a community in which 60 percent of residents are Latinos, noted that a considerable strength of the community was the vibrancy of the ethnic enclave. They felt that the community reflected and seemingly reinforced a sense of ethnic identity and connectedness among the residents and provided services tailored to the needs of the large number of recent immigrants (for example, passport services, money-wiring services, foods imported from Mexico, Spanish-speaking service providers and employees). The question of how to capture these dimensions of southwest Detroit neighborhoods initially sparked considerable discussion among subcommittee members and project staff. For example, is a display of green, red, and white colors a symbol of ethnic identity? Is a Mexican restaurant always an ethnic business? Are businesses with names or signs that include the words "Mexican" or "Latino" or a Spanish name or surname always ethnic businesses? Does it matter whether a business is owned and operated by Latinos or is targeting Latinos as a clientele, and is it possible to discern this fact about the business by observation?

The discussions moved from operational to larger conceptual issues around the following questions: What underlying structures or processes do ethnic symbols and businesses ultimately reflect? What benefits or restrictions do these structures or processes confer? and, How might these be important for health? Ultimately, the subcommittee added an item to the NOC assessing the presence on the block face of sayings, symbols, or murals that reflected Latino identity or pride, and it also added several items intended to capture the presence of businesses and institutions with services or products oriented toward Latinos. Analogous items were also developed to capture symbols of African and African American identity and businesses tailored to African American preferences. (African Americans composed 70 to 90 percent of the populations of the other two study communities.) The discussions leading up to this decision raised issues related to the diverse histories and circumstances of Latinos, African Americans, and whites in Detroit and questions about the meanings of ethnic symbols and businesses for African Americans compared to those for Latinos. These discussions provided an opportunity to talk directly about race and ethnicity in Detroit and reinforced the steering committee's common goals of understanding and intervening to address factors that produce racial and ethnic disparities in health.

Pilot Testing and Implementing of the Neighborhood Observational Checklist

Following the steering committee's approval of a draft of the Neighborhood Observational Checklist in February 2003, the instrument was pilot-tested in two contexts over a four-month period (Table 8.1). First, in March 2003, academic members of the NOC Subcommittee (the principal investigator and graduate student research assistant) and HEP project staff (three additional research assistants, a postdoctoral fellow, the project manager, and the field coordinator), two of whom lived in Detroit, pilot-tested the NOC on several blocks in each of the three study communities and then met to discuss what had been learned. The graduate student research assistant compiled the feedback from each pilot test and modified the NOC.

The NOC was also pilot-tested as part of the observer training process. As we discuss in more detail later in the chapter, the hired observers, all of whom lived in Detroit, completed practice blocks as part of their training to collect data using the NOC. The practice blocks served as additional opportunities to pilot-test the NOC, and the subcommittee continued to revise NOC items and especially operational definitions based on the observers' feedback.

The feedback of HEP project staff and community residents on practice blocks was critical in further refining NOC items and operational definitions. For example, it became clear that distinguishing gang graffiti from other graffiti would require training that was beyond the scope of the project. As a result, the NOC included an item on the presence of any graffiti, but it did not ask observers to attempt to distinguish gang from other types of graffiti. Also, the NOC initially included "boarded windows" in the operational definition for residential and nonresidential buildings in "poor" condition. Pilot testing, however, revealed that some buildings were in otherwise good condition with the exception of a single boarded window, which observers pointed out might have been put up for security. Thus boarded windows were ultimately excluded from the operational definition for buildings in poor condition and other criteria were used instead.

The training and pilot testing were both rapid and time consuming and this limited the opportunities to convene the entire NOC Subcommittee to discuss modifications in the operational definitions. During this period, decisions were made by academic members of the subcommittee in close collaboration with the Detroit residents who were hired as observers and the NOC field coordinator (a Detroit resident). Updates were provided at monthly HEP Steering Committee meetings and revised versions of the NOC were periodically sent to all steering committee members to ensure that they were apprised of these changes.

Pilot testing informed two key implementation decisions. When planning the community survey, the steering committee had defined the precise boundaries of the three study communities. Initial interest in observing all the blocks in these defined study communities, and possibly even larger geographical areas, was quickly tempered as the amount of time required to make systematic observations became apparent. The time per block ranged from forty-five minutes to about two hours during pilot testing, and HEP did not have the resources to conduct neighborhood observation on this scale. After discussions between the academic partners on the subcommittee and sampling experts about several options for sampling blocks, a recommendation was made to collect data on the 147 blocks where community survey respondents lived and the blocks sharing a common border with these blocks (so-called rook neighbors) (Lee & Wong, 2001). The HEP Steering Committee agreed with this approach.

Another major decision involved the data collection method. Initially the NOC was planned as a paper-and-pencil observational tool. However, a postdoctoral fellow working with HEP had experience in collecting survey data with handheld computers and proposed using this method for the NOC. Use of handheld computers for data collection offered the potential advantages of improved data quality, faster turnaround time, and with a separate data entry step eliminated, reduced or equivalent costs (Gravlee, 2002), as well as the possibility of building capacity for the partnership and for observers. HEP community partners were enthusiastic about the opportunity to use this technology for NOC data collection. Handheld computer and paper-and-pencil approaches were compared during the initial NOC pilot testing. The vast majority of participants thought that the handheld computers facilitated data collection, and on the basis of this feedback, a decision was reached to computerize the data collection.

SELECT OUTCOMES OF THE NOC DESIGN PROCESS

The development of the 140-item Neighborhood Observational Checklist was the first outcome of the process we have described. The NOC covers a range of topics including land use; physical conditions of residential and nonresidential buildings and grounds, sidewalks, and streets; types of businesses and institutions; alcohol, tobacco, and fast-food advertisements; social and physical disorder; territoriality; residential stability; physical environmental exposures; activities of observed adults and teenagers; and symbols of ethnic identification. Items were measured at one of three spatial scales, or levels: block face (one side of a street extending from the middle of the street into the middle of the block), street, or block. The HEP Steering Committee and project staff are currently constructing scales and testing scale reliability and validity for theoretical constructs of interest. (The items included in the NOC are presented in Appendix E of this book.)

A second outcome was the recruitment of community residents as observers. The NOC field coordinator recruited community residents who had previously worked with HEP as interviewers for the community survey or with other research projects affiliated with the Detroit Community-Academic Urban Research Center. The NOC field coordinator also posted job announcement flyers at the Detroit Department of Health and Wellness Promotion, one of HEP's partner organizations, and distributed flyers to representatives of the other community-based and health service organizations in the HEP Steering Committee. Job qualifications included a high-school diploma or equivalent, ability to follow written and verbal instructions, excellent organizational skills and attention to detail, ability to read a map, access to a car, and a valid Michigan driver's license. The NOC field coordinator conducted interviews and hired sixteen qualified community residents to participate in the training.

The thirty-four hours of observer training included detailed instruction on and discussion of data collection procedures, operational definitions, and use of handheld computers for data collection; group and individual practice sessions; and feedback to observers of interrater reliability statistics based on observers' performance on practice blocks, including individualized feedback (Zenk et al., 2004). The training took place over a seven-week period from April to June 2003 and was structured to include all-day group sessions on weekends, evening group sessions on weekdays, and individual practice opportunities completed at the observers' discretion during designated time frames. The two academic partners from the NOC Subcommittee, the NOC field coordinator, a postdoctoral fellow working with HEP, and an additional research assistant prepared materials for and conducted the trainings. The training sessions were scheduled to accommodate the hired observers' employment schedules and to allow time for observers to complete practice blocks and for project staff to run interrater reliability statistics and prepare feedback between group training sessions. Community residents were paid for the training.

Of the fifteen community residents who completed the initial training sequence, eleven were eventually certified as observers to collect NOC data. Certification involved achieving at least 75 percent overall agreement (based on a kappa statistic) with a HEP staff member's "gold standard" ratings for a practice block. Observers were paid for the first two certification attempts and had an opportunity to review feedback on their performance with the field coordinator. The eleven certified observers collected data on 551 blocks across the three study neighborhoods over a fifteen-week period during the summer and early fall of 2003.

CHALLENGES ENCOUNTERED AND LESSONS LEARNED

A number of challenges were encountered and lessons learned in the design and implementation of a neighborhood observational checklist. Some of these are discussed in the following sections.

Community reservations about neighborhood observation and data sensitivity. The decision to collect data on neighborhood conditions was made by academic and community partners who participated in writing the initial grant proposal for HEP. When the HEP Steering Committee initiated discussions on designing and implementing an observational instrument a couple of years later, partners were still in agreement that an examination of the ways in which neighborhood environments contribute to racial and socioeconomic disparities in health required measuring both neighborhood resources and stressors. However, community partners also expressed concerns that the findings might contribute to negative representations of the study communities. Later, community residents who participated in the NOC training shared these concerns. Data collected with the NOC, like most social science data, are sensitive and subject to multiple interpretations.

Several factors allowed these important concerns to be discussed and addressed openly. There was a history of collaboration among partners in HEP and trust had been established through that collaboration. Several of the community residents hired as observers had previously worked on Urban Research Center projects, and they were comfortable raising concerns and asking direct questions about how the data would be used and also comfortable contributing their own perspectives on interpretation of NOC items. These concerns included, for example, that neighborhood deterioration and blight might be attributed to residents themselves, without recognition of the broader social and economic processes, such as institutional racism and economic restructuring, that contribute to those conditions. Discussions of these concerns were essential and produced opportunities to talk about the meaning and potential utility of the data in terms of a conceptual model that explicitly recognized relationships between fundamental social and economic processes and the neighborhood conditions assessed through the NOC (Schulz, Kannan, et al., under review). Those conversations led to modifications of items and data collection processes, opened opportunities for considering how results might most effectively be presented, and helped academic members of the team build trust in the insights offered by community members and, similarly, helped community partners build trust in the research being conducted in their communities.

A broad range of interests among partners. The diversity of the involved community and academic partners is a significant asset of HEP in that it is a source of multiple areas of expertise and perspectives on neighborhood environments and health. Exchanges drawing on these varied perspectives contributed to holistic thinking about social determinants of health and enhanced the content of the NOC. Yet the broad range of interests also created challenges in designing the NOC. Not only did partners agree that a number of indicators and scales from the literature were relevant (though often with some modification) for HEP goals and study communities but partners also offered numerous other suggestions for NOC items. Some of the identified topics reflected individual organization priorities and assessment needs, but almost all could be linked to cardiovascular health, the overall focus of HEP.

Thus decisions needed to be made about which items reflecting the multiple interests and priorities of partners would be included in the final NOC. Coming to consensus on the core purpose of the NOC was essential in this process. Even so, very real limitations of time and funding meant that at times the NOC traded breadth for depth and vice versa in the assessment of neighborhood conditions. Future efforts to design a neighborhood observational instrument using a participatory approach might benefit from explicit discussion of these trade-offs.

Community participation in all phases of NOC development. Another challenge was that designing and implementing the NOC was time intensive. As described in this chapter, the members of HEP were actively involved throughout the early stages of this process. HEP Steering Committee members were less involved in the day-to-day activities of pilot testing and training of observers and in the refinement of items and operational definitions that took place at these later stages.

Given the time required to design and implement a neighborhood observational instrument, it is important to consider which activities must involve the participation and influence of all members of a partnership and which may be moved forward by paid staff using a variety of means to keep all partners informed of significant modifications that may continue to develop at later stages. In this instance the NOC was one of several activities being carried out simultaneously by HEP and in which HEP Steering Committee members were participating. The intensive work carried out by the NOC Subcommittee established the content for the NOC and the subsequent refinements during pilot testing were made with a clear sense of the concerns and priorities of steering committee members. This experience suggests that frequent and cyclical changes to observational tools, and especially their operational definitions, can be expected during pilot testing and that the input of community members is critical to that process. Adequate planning and conversations about who needs to be involved in what decisions are important to ensure that all partners are involved appropriately throughout this process, recognizing that the level of participation may vary at different stages of the process.

CONCLUSION

Interest in direct observation of neighborhoods as a research method is growing. This may be attributable to the emergence of a large body of research that links neighborhood socioeconomic context to health, including cardiovascular disease risk and mortality (see, for example, Cubbin, Hadden, & Winkleby, 2001; Davey Smith, Hart, Watt, Hole, & Hawthorne, 1998; Diez-Roux et al., 2001; Sundquist, Malmstrom, & Johansson, 1999), yet provides less information about the pathways through which neighborhoods affect health. The data collected with the NOC will add to an understanding of the ways in which neighborhood conditions contribute to racial and socioeconomic disparities in cardiovascular disease risk and protective factors in Detroit. This understanding, in turn, will prove useful in designing interventions and making policy recommendations. The participatory process described here drew upon the expertise and understandings of community and academic partners of the HEP Steering Committee and also obtained community residents' perspectives (through focus groups and pilot testing) in order to develop a context-sensitive observational instrument, the results from which will inform future community change efforts. Such a community-based participatory research approach could greatly enhance future research efforts involving neighborhood observation.

References

Browning, C. R., Cagney, K. A., & Wen, M. (2003). Explaining variation in health status across space and time: Implications for racial and ethnic disparities in self-rated health. *Social Science & Medicine, 57,* 1221–1235.

Caughy, M. O., O'Campo, P. J., & Patterson, J. (2001). A brief observational measure for urban neighborhoods. *Health & Place, 7,* 225–236.

Cohen, D., Spear, S., Scribner, R., Kissinger, P., Mason, K., & Wildgen, J. (2000). Broken windows and the risk of gonorrhea. *American Journal of Public Health, 90,* 230–236.

Craig, C. L., Brownson, R. C., Cragg, S. E., & Dunn, A. L. (2002). Exploring the effect of the environment on physical activity: A study examining walking to work. *American Journal of Preventive Medicine, 23*(2), 36–43.

Cubbin, C., Hadden, W. C., & Winkleby, M. A. (2001). Neighborhood context and cardiovascular disease risk factors: The contribution of material deprivation. *Ethnicity & Disease, 11,* 687–700.

Davey Smith, G., Hart, C., Watt, G., Hole, D., & Hawthorne, V. (1998). Individual social class, area-based deprivation, cardiovascular disease risk factors, and mortality: The Renfrew and Paisley study. *Journal of Epidemiology and Community Health, 52,* 399–405.

Diez-Roux, A. V. (2001). Investigating neighborhood and area effects on health. *American Journal of Public Health, 91,* 1783–1789.

Diez-Roux, A. V., Merkin, S. S., Arnett, D., Chambless, L., Massing, M., Nieto, J., et al. (2001). Neighborhood of residence and incidence of coronary heart disease. *New England Journal of Medicine, 345,* 99–106.

Ellen, I. G., Mijanovich, T., & Dillman, K. (2001). Neighborhood effects on health: Exploring the links and assessing the evidence. *Journal of Urban Affairs, 23,* 391–408.

Emery, J., Crump, C., & Bors, P. (2003). Reliability and validity of two instruments designed to assess the walking and bicycling suitability of sidewalks and roads. *American Journal of Health Promotion, 18,* 38–46.

Farquhar, S. A. (2000). *Effects of the perceptions and observations of environmental stressors on health and well-being in residents of eastside and southwest Detroit, Michigan.* Unpublished doctoral dissertation, University of Michigan-Ann Arbor.

Gravlee, C. C. (2002). Mobile computer-assisted personal interviewing with handheld computers: The entryware system 3.0. *Field Methods, 14,* 322–336.

Haan, M., Kaplan, G. A., & Camacho, T. (1987). Poverty and health: Prospective evidence from the Alameda County study. *American Journal of Epidemiology, 125,* 989–998.

House, J. S., & Williams, D. R. (2000). Understanding and reducing socioeconomic and racial/ethnic disparities in health. In B. D. Smedley & S. L. Syme (Eds.), *Promoting health: Intervention strategies from social and behavioral science* (pp. 81–124). Washington, DC: National Academies Press.

Israel, B. A., Schulz, A. J., Parker, E. A., & Becker, A. B. (1998). Review of community-based research: Assessing partnership approaches to improve public health. *Annual Review of Public Health, 19,* 173–202.

Keeler, G. J., Dvonch, J. T., Yip, F., Parker, E. A., Israel, B. A., Marsik, F. J., et al. (2002). Assessment of personal and community-level exposures to particulate matter among children with asthma in Detroit, Michigan, as part of Community Action Against Asthma (CAAA). *Environmental Health Perspectives, 110*(Suppl. 2), 173–181.

Kingsley, G. T., Coulton, C. J., Barndt, M., Sawicki, D. S., & Tatian, P. (1997). *Mapping your community: Using geographic information to strengthen community initiatives.* Washington, DC: U.S. Department of Housing and Urban Development.

Lee, J., & Wong, D. W. (2001). *Statistical analysis with ArcView GIS.* New York: Wiley.

Macintyre, S., Ellaway, A., & Cummins, S. (2002). Place effects on health: How can we conceptualize, operationalize, and measure them? *Social Science & Medicine, 55,* 125–139.

Morenoff, J., House, J. S., & Raudenbush, S. W. (n.d.). Systematic social observation by survey interviewers: A methodological evaluation. Unpublished manuscript.

Moudon, A. V., & Lee, C. (2003). Walking and bicycling: An evaluation of environmental audit instruments. *American Journal of Health Promotion, 18,* 21–37.

Perkins, D. D., Meeks, J. W., & Taylor, R. B. (1992). The physical environment of street blocks and resident perceptions of crime and disorder: Implications for theory and measurement. *Journal of Environmental Psychology, 12,* 21–34.

Pickett, K. E., & Pearl, M. (2000). Multilevel analyses of neighborhood socioeconomic context and health outcomes: A critical review. *Journal of Epidemiology and Community Health, 55,* 111–122.

Pikora, T. J., Bull, F.C.L., Jamrozik, K., Knuiman, M., Giles-Corti, B., & Donovan, R. J. (2002). Developing a reliable audit instrument to measure the physical environment for physical activity. *American Journal of Preventive Medicine, 23,* 187–194.

Raudenbush, S. W., & Sampson, R. J. (1999). Econometrics: Toward a science of assessing ecological settings, with application to the systematic social observation of neighborhoods. *Sociological Methodology, 29,* 1–41.

Reiss, A. J. (1971). Systematic observations of natural social phenomena. In H. Costner (Ed.), *Sociological Methodology* (pp. 3–33). San Francisco: Jossey-Bass.

Sampson, R. J., & Raudenbush, S. W. (1999). Systematic social observation of public spaces: A new look at disorder in urban neighborhoods. *American Journal of Sociology, 105,* 603–651.

Schulz, A. J., Israel, B. A., Estrada, L., Zenk, S. N., Viruell-Fuentes, E. A., Villarruel, A., et al. (2004, November 6–10). *Engaging community residents in assessing their social and physical environments and their implications for health.* Paper presented at the annual meeting of the American Public Health Association, Washington, DC.

Schulz, A. J., Kannan, S., Dvonch, T., Israel, B. A., Allen, A., James, S. A., et al. (under review). Social and physical environments and disparities in risk for cardiovascular disease: The Healthy Environments Partnership conceptual model. *Environmental Health Perspectives.*

Sundquist, J., Malmstrom, M., & Johansson, S. (1999). Cardiovascular risk factors and the neighborhood environment: A multilevel analysis. *International Journal of Epidemiology, 28,* 841–845.

Taylor, R. B., Gottfredson, S., & Brower, S. (1984). Block crime and fear: Defensible space, local social ties, and territorial functioning. *Journal of Research in Crime and Delinquency, 21,* 303–331.

Taylor, R. B., Shumaker, S., & Gottfredson, S. (1985). Neighborhood-level links between physical features and local sentiments: Deterioration, fear of crime, and confidence. *Journal of Architectural and Planning Research, 21,* 261–275.

Weich, S., Blanchard, M., Prince, M., Burton, E., Erens, B., & Sproston, K. (2002). Mental health and the built environment: A cross-sectional survey of individual and contextual risk factors for depression. *British Journal of Psychiatry, 180,* 428–433.

Zenk, S. N., Schulz, A. J., Mentz, G., House, J. S., Miranda, P., Gravlee, C., et al. (2004, November 6–10). *Observer training strategies and interrater and test-retest reliability: The Neighborhood Observational Checklist.* Paper presented at the annual meeting of the American Public Health Association, Washington, DC.

CHAPTER NINE

Mapping Social and Environmental Influences on Health

A Community Perspective

Guadalupe X. Ayala, Siobhan C. Maty, Altha J. Cravey, and Lucille H. Webb

One of the earliest documented uses of maps to represent health risk factors was in the mid-1800s. Using colored maps, Cowan linked the prevalence of fever with overcrowding and economic disadvantage (Cowan, 1840, cited in Gordon & Womersley, 1997). Over the ensuing 150 years, researchers have continued to use maps to illustrate risk (Barry & Britt, 2002), prioritize resource allocation (Johnson, Ved, Lyall, & Agarwal, 2003; Taylor & Chavez, 2002), and better understand how behaviors fit within a given context (Morland, Wing, Roux, & Poole, 2002). Despite advances in the field, and in particular the use of geographical mapping software to facilitate the mapping process (Gordon & Womersley, 1997), there is scant evidence about how and why one should incorporate mapping techniques in a community-based participatory research project. Our objectives in this chapter are to illustrate ways of using mapping techniques in collaboration with community members to define

Acknowledgments: The authors would like to thank the funding agencies for their support of the research studies Hispanos Unidos en la Prevención de Obesidad, funded by the Program on Ethnicity, Culture and Health Outcomes at the University of North Carolina at Chapel Hill, and Your Crib, Your Grub, and Your Moves, funded by the W. K. Kellogg Foundation. Guadalupe Ayala would like to thank Kelley DeLeeuw, MPH, in the Department of Health Behavior and Health Education, University of North Carolina at Chapel Hill, for her significant contributions to the Familias Sanas, Comunidades Saludables research team. A final though no less important thanks goes to the many individuals and community groups who were involved in these studies.

community problems and ultimately refine research questions and subsequent action steps. We provide two case examples to illustrate these objectives.

Whether a project is mapping risk factors (Cowell & Cowell, 1999; Morrow, 1999) or prioritizing resource allocation (Bickes, 2000; Phillips, Kinman, Schnitzer, Lindbloom, & Ewigman, 2000; Taylor & Chavez, 2002), engaging community members in the process of mapping community concerns can contribute to understanding and ameliorating social, political, and structural influences on health. Although this chapter does not provide information on using geographical mapping computer software to achieve these goals, the use of such software may be an important next step, empowering community members to harness computer resources to document and address environmental influences on health (Gordon & Womersley, 1997).

THEORETICAL UNDERPINNINGS

A discussion of methods of mapping is incomplete without some reference to the theoretical underpinnings of the mapping approach. The studies presented in the following literature review acknowledge that social change requires a multidimensional understanding of the problem to be changed. Like photovoice methods that "enable people to identify, represent, and enhance their community through a specific photographic technique" (Wang, 1999, p. 188), mapping techniques provide a forum for graphically depicting external influences on health. The importance of using methods that enhance our understanding of environmental influences is supported by several well-known theoretical frameworks.

Social ecological frameworks recognize that behavior is often a function of the larger context of the individual's life (Breslow, 1996; Emmons, 2000). A person's desire to modify her or his own behavior may be impeded or facilitated by economic, social, and cultural contexts (Stokols, 1996). Social ecological approaches to health promotion suggest combining individually focused efforts at change with modifications of the physical and social surroundings.

Social cognitive theory also emphasizes the interactions between people's cognitions, behaviors, and the environment, through processes such as self-efficacy, outcome expectancies, reciprocal determinism, and vicarious or observational learning (Bandura, 1986). Bronfenbrenner (1979) identified five nested environmental systems whose interplay influences human development and human behavior, ranging from the microsystem (the immediate environment) to the macrosystem (societal norms and attitudes). Similarly, Emmons (2000) identified five levels for the development of interventions, as well as corresponding targets of change, ranging from the intrapersonal (individual skill development) to community-level change (social advocacy). Working in the context of ecological theory, Cohen, Scribner, and Farley (2000) proposed a structural model for health behavior change, with four specific factors (similar to those detailed by Moos, 1987): availability (for example, lean meat in the grocery store), physical structures (for example, bicycle lanes), social structures (laws and informal social controls such as household rule setting), and cultural and media messages (including interpersonal channels of communication). Together these theories and frameworks highlight the importance of considering the context of people's lived experiences in order to understand health-related change efforts. Mapping techniques provide a basis for understanding how individual behaviors fit into the context of the individual's environment. Working with community partners to identify environmental influences on health can be a first step in defining community problems and changing aspects of people's physical and social surroundings.

DESCRIPTION OF THE METHOD

Mapping of social and environmental influences has been applied in a variety of fields, such as medicine, public health, geography, urban planning, and anthropology. Before presenting our two case studies of the application of mapping in the context of community-based participatory research, we summarize the ways mapping techniques have been used in other research projects. Our goal in this section is to highlight differences in the types and amounts of resources required to implement mapping techniques (depending on whether participants drew maps or used printed maps) and to show how community members may be involved in the process of designing the mapping protocol. Where possible, we present the strategies used to engage and work with community members in using various mapping techniques. We include international studies because much of the research in this area has been done in countries other than the United States.

Drawing Maps

Emmel and O'Keefe (1996) involved community health workers (CHWs) in identifying clusters of tuberculosis and alcoholism in impoverished neighborhoods in India. Over the course of six participatory meetings, the CHWs used paper and pencil to

- Map the boundaries of their neighborhood
- Draw a detailed map of the households in their neighborhood, including the number of household members and their ages, the household members' occupations, and whether household members accessed services at a maternal and child health facility

- Identify households infected with tuberculosis and those in which they perceived alcohol use to be a problem
- Graphically examine the distribution of disease in their neighborhoods

Emmel and O'Keefe noted that the incorporation of mapping activities into discussions with CHWs was interactive, engaged the workers, and provided details about the distribution of disease at the household level without anyone's having to interview individual household members. The process of engaging CHWs in mapping disease within neighborhoods strengthened their capacity to see the problem at multiple levels and to visually see complex interactions of risk factors.

Mapping environmental risk factors is more difficult with highly mobile communities, such as seasonal migrant workers. In spite of these challenges, a project in North Carolina demonstrated that such transnational populations can use mapping techniques to gather important problem-defining information on pesticide exposure (Cravey, Arcury, & Quandt, 2000; Cravey, Washburn, Gesler, Arcury, & Skelly, 2001). There is great variety in exposure to pesticides among North Carolina farms and also extreme variation at the personal level in who is exposed, as some farm workers travel with young children whereas others, especially those on seasonal H2A visas, travel only with other adult males. To better understand the sources of these variations, at weekend workshops, teams of four to six Latino farm worker volunteers from several sites were asked to create a large map of the layout of the farm where they were working, including fields, housing, barns, machinery, eating areas, portable toilets, and other objects they deemed relevant. They then identified the different places where agricultural chemicals were stored or prepared for use, and marked these places with a red marker.

Through discussion of these maps, farm worker participants identified four principal avenues for further exploration: examining the locations of certain items within households; discussing the membership of the household; examining the relative locations of things such as household and field; and discussing the possible vectors of risk, exposure, and transmission. Although the mapping exercises in themselves did not change the difficult conditions encountered in North Carolina farms, they provided an initial means for dialogue about pesticide safety. Mapping can be a tool for personal transformation as well as means of strengthening social networks for subsequent collective efforts. In addition, the visual element of this mapping exercise helped to bridge varying levels of literacy and language ability (some of these Latino participants spoke an indigenous first language and Spanish as a second language). The maps helped students (and facilitators) identify constraints on safe work practices. Naming and discussing such difficulties is a first step toward identifying the potential for change.

Using Preprinted Maps

Siar (2003) and Walters (1997) worked with community members to identify the spatial relationships between the locations of fishery habitats and resources in a coastal zone of the Philippines populated by small-scale fisheries. Community members (adult men and women and children) participated in interviews and then in a pile-sorting task to identify and categorize types of fishing habitats and resources. Then, using printed maps drawn on a scale of 1:40,000, the groups color-coded the locations of these various habitats and resource sites. This mapping technique revealed that community residents had committed to memory much information about the locations of both habitats and resources that were not documented on nautical charts or maps (Siar, 2003). A key finding of this mapping technique was that approaches to space and resources were gendered. It illustrated that although both men and women accessed resources at common sites, they accessed different types of resources in these locations. Siar (2003) noted that "the characteristics and features of the environment are not only physically and biologically determined but socially constructed as well, in that users' perception and knowledge of that environment affect the way people respond to it" (p. 578). This mapping activity provided a depth of understanding about gender, space, and resources that was not gained from the interviews or the pile-sorting task. Thus the process of defining the problem should include consideration of possible methods for obtaining information about how gender and other social constructs (for example, race, social class) may influence perceptions and knowledge.

Steegmann and Hewner (2000) worked with community residents in Niagara County, New York, to identify environmental toxin exposure by asking adults about where they had played as children and the locations of active and inactive dump sites on maps. Retrospective reports covered a period of over sixty years. A detailed 40-by-40 cm map was created using a U.S. Geographic Survey topographic map and extensive ground observations using ethnographic techniques. The map depicted neighborhood streets, neighborhood dump sites, and other well-known dump sites. From among a sample of 209 residents who completed a brief survey, 40 men and women participated in the mapping activity. The map was shown to participants, and they were oriented to its features. They were then instructed to use a pencil and tracing paper to indicate the locations where they had played as children and the types of activities engaged in at these locations. Information from all participant maps was integrated into one comprehensive map to depict the most common places and activities. Despite the limitations associated with recall bias, evidence on the comprehensive map indicated that all participants had been directly exposed to toxins while playing in active and inactive dump sites. These findings were unexpected and highlighted the value of using maps to represent the relationship between play areas and exposure to toxins as a child. As a result of this mapping activity, the problem was refined by graphically depicting historical data held by community members.

In a third study using preprinted maps, 140 African American and European American residents in seven census-defined block groups (twenty residents per block group) marked the location of their homes and the boundaries of their neighborhoods using a printed map. The map showed their census block group in the middle surrounded by an eight-mile perimeter (Coulton, Korbin, Chan, & Su, 2001). The maps provided sufficient detail to orient the residents to their homes on the map, including street names and landmarks. The residents' maps were then entered into MapInfo, a geographical information system software, and analyzed on a number of different dimensions. For example, when compared with census-defined block groups, the area represented on the residents' maps was larger than their block group and typically included at least two census tracts and at least three block groups. This research highlighted the importance of understanding how residents perceive the boundaries of their neighborhoods, particularly because differences did emerge between residents' and researchers' perceptions of neighborhood boundaries.

Discussion

In this section we described the methods used in mapping activities in as much detail as was available. Other researchers have written about mapping influences but have provided insufficient detail to present the techniques used (Ghys, Jenkins, & Pisani, 2001; Johnson et al., 2003; Nemoto, Operario, Takenaka, Iwamoto, & Le, 2003; Sterk, 2002; Veale & Dona, 2003).

The use of mapping is consistent with the renewed focus on understanding environmental influences on the public's health. For example, a growing body of evidence links family and neighborhood environmental factors with risk for obesity (Dowda, Ainsworth, Addy, Saunders, & Riner, 2001; French, Story, & Jeffrey, 2001; Morland et al., 2002; Romero et al., 2001). This research suggests that the availability of fast food, media that promotes inactivity, large restaurant food portions, sedentary environments and the unavailability of fresh fruits and vegetables and recreational areas for physical activity all contribute to the growing obesity epidemic (French et al., 2001). Simultaneously, poorer neighborhoods house disproportionately fewer supermarkets with healthy food options (Morland et al., 2002; Dowda et al., 2001). Efforts to organize communities to reduce detrimental factors in their environments while increasing healthier aspects have been deemed a potential strategy for consideration in future research (Dowda et al., 2001).

Mapping is a method for gathering visual information that is not entirely dependent on answers to survey or interview questions. Completed maps can graphically depict factors in the immediate and extended environments that influence health and other characteristics. As evidenced in the examples presented, mapping can be accomplished with minimal resources (paper and pencil) or with more expensive resources such as preprinted maps or GPS units and GIS programs. The decision about what resources to use should be made in partnership with community members and researchers, and should recognize the influence on the mapping process and outcomes that may arise from community members' using unfamiliar resources. The two case studies that follow describe mapping techniques used in community-based participatory research projects.

WORKING WITH COMMUNITIES TO MAP SOCIAL AND ENVIRONMENTAL INFLUENCES

In this section we describe two community-based participatory research (CBPR) projects that incorporated mapping techniques into the study design. First, we discuss a study involving African American youths and their parents that examined environmental influences on eating and exercise behaviors. Second, we look at a study that examined environmental influences on eating and exercise behaviors among Latino families. The studies differ in the length of time the community and academic partners had been working together and in the mapping techniques that were used. We use these case studies to illustrate relationships between the research questions asked, available resources, community members and researchers, and the selection of appropriate mapping techniques.

Your Crib, Your Grub, and Your Moves

In the following case study, we describe the partnership background, the mapping technique used, and the role of the partners in each stage of the research process.

CBPR Partnership Background. The Your Crib, Your Grub, and Your Moves ("Your Crib") project was a collaborative endeavor involving Strengthening the Black Family, Inc. (STBF), a coalition dedicated to improving the quality of life of black families in Wake County, North Carolina; Project DIRECT, a community-based diabetes prevention intervention program in the African American community in southeast (SE) Raleigh, North Carolina; researchers and students from the University of North Carolina at Chapel Hill (UNC-CH); and members of the SE Raleigh community.

STBF was founded in 1980 and received 501(c)(3) status in 1987. It currently represents more than forty organizations in Wake County. The principal community partner in Your Crib, and a coauthor of this chapter, is Lucille Webb, president of the STBF board of directors and long-time collaborator with UNC-CH. Project DIRECT is a partnership established in 1993 between the Centers for Disease Control and Prevention (CDC), the North Carolina Department of Health and Human Services, Wake County Human Services, and the community of SE Raleigh. The Your Crib principal investigator, and a coauthor of this chapter, is Siobhan Maty, at the time a postdoctoral scholar in the W. K. Kellogg Foundation–funded Community Health Scholars Program at UNC-CH, who worked with two faculty mentors at the School of Public Health. The project was funded through the Scholars' Program for the 2002–2003 academic year.

The overarching goal of this partnership has been to work together to improve the health and well-being of families in the SE Raleigh community. Community partners have noted the reciprocal influence that family members have on each other as well as the influence that the community has on the individual and the family unit. Therefore the primary objective of the partnership has been to strengthen families and improve their daily living environments.

The Your Crib project represents one of many collaborative efforts between STBF and UNC-CH. This partnership was initiated in 1991 through the W. K. Kellogg Foundation–funded Community-Based Public Health Initiative. It has evolved through association with Project DIRECT (1994 to the present) and with several collaborative programs, such as Operation Health 27610, which focused on women's health issues in the Raleigh community defined by the zip code 27610 (1998 to 2001), and Brotha How's Your Health, an assessment of male gender socialization and men's health among African American men in SE Raleigh (2000 to 2002). This partnership has matured and strengthened over time and has reached a stage of successful, ongoing collaboration. Projects are designed and implemented, and decisions are made with the full participation of all partners, each of whom brings its respective expertise to the table.

CBPR Research Project Background. The primary purpose of Your Crib is to identify social and environmental influences on the eating and exercise behaviors of African American adolescents and their parents in SE Raleigh. Study participants chose the project name Your Crib, Your Grub, and Your Moves from a list created by community members and the project research advisory team; they found that this name reflected the key components of the study, which looked at environmental influences (*crib*) on eating (*grub*) and physical activity (*moves*). Community members noted the importance of these influences on weight control and diabetes and also noted the need to consider influences external to the home environment and not necessarily under the perceived control of the individual or family. A secondary project objective is to determine how to involve families in an intervention targeting, among other things, environmental change to prevent obesity and chronic illnesses.

Your Crib is a cross-sectional study using well-established formative research methods (for example, focus groups) in combination with the mapping activity. Families involved in Your Crib were convened at the STBF program facility in SE Raleigh. Data collection activities specific to this project were begun in December 2002 and are currently ongoing.

Research Process Stages and the Role of Partners. The Your Crib project was informed by Project DIRECT, a diabetes demonstration project funded by the CDC and modified by community members. In December 2001, members of Project DIRECT convened and expressed concerns about the health status of youths in the SE Raleigh community. In particular, community members noted that too many children were obese, their eating and exercise behaviors were unhealthy, and families needed to be empowered to improve their children's eating and exercise environments. In December 2002 and again in January 2003, Maty and Webb reconvened community members (thirty members in December 2002 and ten in January 2003) to assess whether these youth-related health topics were still of concern to the community and to identify possible steps to address key issues in the community. At these meetings it was decided that the project would focus on the social and environmental factors that influence healthy eating and exercise behaviors of community adolescents and their parents. Working together, Maty and Webb, along with Janice Dodds and Eugenia Eng, the faculty mentors involved from UNC-CH, decided that focus group interviews with parents and separate focus group interviews with youths were an appropriate methodology for retrieving information from study participants. Eng and Maty also suggested a mapping activity with youth participants as an additional data collection method that would provide spatial data, such as where youths congregate in the local community, and that would inform the development of tailored interventions by STBF and Project DIRECT. Community members were supportive of the suggested data collection methods.

A research advisory team was created that consisted of representatives from UNC-CH, STBF, Project DIRECT, and the SE Raleigh community. Throughout the ensuing months, and until data collection commenced, members of the Your Crib research advisory team met to design focus group interview guides, design recruitment materials, identify appropriate recruitment methods, create the mapping activity, and generate a list of possible project names. Institutional review board (IRB) approval was obtained from the IRB committee at UNC-CH. The final versions of the three youth focus group interview guides (discussed later in this chapter) were pilot-tested with youths involved in Teens Against AIDS, an AIDS-awareness, peer-educator program created and administered by STBF. Guided by the teen reviewers involved in the pilot test, modifications were made to the focus group interview guides in order to make the discussion issues and wording more relevant to the adolescent study population. (See Chapter Seven for a discussion of the development and implementation of focus group interviews.) For example, some phrasing in the original guides was not commonly used among the youth study participants and so it was changed to reflect cultural norms (for instance, "where do you live" became "where do you stay").

Development of Mapping Protocol. The Your Crib research team conceived the idea of the mapping activity, which was shared with the community partners and accepted as a data collection method for the project. The instrument used in the mapping activity drew on the activity space and place inventories methods used by Cravey and colleagues to locate social networks in rural North Carolina for the purpose of preventing diabetes. In this study (Cravey et al., 2001) the activity space method asked participants to recall the location, length, and frequency of their activities over the preceding seven-day period. The place inventory was a list of places in the community identified from windshield tours, public records, and the activity space data. Interviewers then asked study participants a series of questions about each place listed on the inventory, such as the type of information they received at each site and their evaluation of the location.

The Your Crib mapping activity combined and modified the activity space and place inventories methods. The activity required youth study participants to keep a log of all activities on three different days (two weekdays and one weekend day) over a two-week period. This log listed information about the location, time, duration, and purpose of each activity, as well as how the participant got to each location and with whom he or she visited the location. In addition, each participant had to describe what was observed going to and from each location that related to eating or exercise behaviors, such as advertisements for fast food or people on bicycles. Participants were also asked to identify the location of each of their activities on an individual map of Raleigh. Finally, all participants marked their activity locations on one large map.

Selection and Recruitment of Participants. Recruitment of participants for Your Crib occurred at two community forums. Community partners suggested recruitment forums as a way to share the project specifics and to answer questions with a group of potential study participants. Two forums were held at the YWCA in SE Raleigh, one on a weekday evening and another on a Saturday morning to increase the likelihood of participation. Food and child care were available at each meeting. Printed flyers announcing the forums were distributed throughout the local community, and community partners spread the word among their social networks. Members of the project research team and the local community assisted with the logistics for each forum, such as setting up and cleaning up the meeting space, distributing food, checking in attendees, answering questions, and taking notes. In addition, flyers were distributed advertising the focus group interviews, discussions were held with adult administrators of several youth organizations (such as Boys and Girls Club), and research team members, community members, and project participants were asked to recommend friends, family members, or coworkers to participate in the program (Babbie, 1979).

Criteria for participant inclusion were established during the initial community forums. Youths and their parents were eligible to participate if they resided or spent significant time in SE Raleigh and if the youths were between 14 and 17 years of age. The final sample in the Your Crib project consisted of thirty youths between 14 and 17 years of age (60 percent female and with a mean age of 15.4) and ten mothers. Having a child participate in the project was a requirement for adult participation; however, a youth could participate whether or not her or his parent participated.

Data Collection.   Focus groups were the primary data collection method, followed by the mapping activity. Parents participated in one focus group that collected data paralleling the data collected by the youth focus groups on the barriers and facilitators to healthy eating and physical activity encountered at home, work, school, or in their neighborhood.

The youth component comprised three consecutive focus group discussions followed by a mapping activity and a final wrap-up focus group discussion. The first two focus group discussions gathered information on youths' eating and exercise patterns at home, at school, and in their neighborhoods and environmental influences on these behaviors. The third focus group discussion checked on themes from the prior two focus groups; youths drew a picture of where and how they engaged in key activities, there was a discussion about using maps to better understand environmental influences, and instructions were given on how to conduct the mapping activity over the ensuing weeks.

The Your Crib mapping component collected information on the youths' activity spaces and environmental influences on their behavior. The mapping activity involved five steps. First, youths recorded their daily activities, especially activities related to eating and exercise behaviors in their lived environments. In the daily activity record exercise, they documented each major activity (for example, going to school, playing basketball) for a full three days (including one weekend day) over a two-week period. They answered several questions about each activity: where the activity was located, why they went to this location (for a specific activity, for example), how they were transported to this location, the time of day of the activity, how long they stayed in this location, and what they were exposed to at each location that related to eating and exercise behaviors. This activity provided information on typical activities for youths in SE Raleigh: key locales, frequency of visiting these locales, and the length of time spent at each locale.

Next, the youths graphically depicted their three days of activities on a city map. Each youth was given a map of Raleigh and asked to use colored markers to identify the locations visited, routes taken to get to each location, and key elements observed at each location. Key activity locations were indicated in red marker, and items of interest observed en route to that location were indicated in green marker. These maps provided information for each individual on the size of her or his activity space and what behaviors occurred in each location. As a group, they synthesized the information on one large community map.

The mapping activity was followed by a final focus group discussion about the mapping activities. It was at this meeting that all study participants' mapping data were combined on one larger map. This synthesis of mapping data helped illustrate overlap in activity spaces and patterns of environmental influences on adolescent behavior. Participants evaluated the mapping project for its usefulness in helping them identify patterns in their activities and activity locations that influence their eating and exercise behaviors. The final meeting also provided an opportunity to merge information gathered in the mapping activity with information from prior focus group interviews, to discuss possible intervention steps within the SE Raleigh community, and to evaluate the impact of involvement in the project on the eating and exercise behaviors of youth participants. All focus groups interviews were held after school at the STBF facility or a local community center in SE Raleigh. All focus group discussions were audiotaped and transcribed for data analysis purposes. Youths in the Your Crib project received $15 for each focus group interview they attended and $25 for completing the mapping activity. Parents who took part in the adult focus group interview received $20. Healthy food (fruit, water, vegetables, granola bars, and the like) was provided at all data collection events.

Data Analysis. The Your Crib research team analyzed the data. The principal investigator (PI) was responsible for getting the focus group discussions transcribed and distributed to all team members. All transcriptions were analyzed using a focused coding technique (Miles & Huberman, 1994). The PI created the initial coding scheme, using the interview guides to focus the codes, and used these codes to sort through large amounts of data. She then modified the original codes and added subcodes after several iterations of reading the data. The research team read each transcription and, using the preliminary coding scheme, analyzed a subset of the data. The research team then met via conference call and, drawing on each member's experience in analyzing the text, collectively modified the list of codes to be used for the final analysis.

Once the coding scheme was determined, the PI used Atlas.ti, Version 4.2 (2000), to recode all transcriptions using the final scheme. The text was then clustered by major and minor codes across all relevant transcriptions, and the PI began creating themes based on the code categories. Copies of the themes were distributed to the research team, who met several times via conference call to discuss and modify the themes. This stage of focus group data analysis concluded when the research team members agreed on the themes and the preliminary conclusions drawn from the data.

The location data from the mapping activity was geocoded and a computerized map was created that visually depicted the location and frequency of the multiple activities in which this adolescent cohort engaged during the summer of 2003. This map will be used by STBF and Project DIRECT to assist each organization in creating targeted interventions for youths in SE Raleigh.

Data Feedback. A findings forum is planned in which the Your Crib research team will share findings with youths and parents who participated in the study. They will be invited to interpret the results, finalize conclusions, and assist in drafting intervention plans based upon the results. A final project summary will be disseminated to the larger community either during Strengthening the Black Family's annual conference or at a separately convened community meeting. Study participants will be invited to play an active role in all dissemination efforts, such as assisting the research team in presenting study results at the STBF conference and to the larger community through other venues. We expect to submit study findings for publication in peer-reviewed journals, with each member of the research team being involved as a coauthor.

This community-based participatory research project integrated a mapping activity into a traditional focus group methodology in order to allow African American youths and their parents to develop a personal understanding of the environmental influences on their eating and exercise behaviors. The project discussed in the following section has similar goals but focuses on Latino families as the unit of analysis.

Hispanos Unidos en la Prevención de Obesidad

As we did for Your Crib, we will describe the partnership background, the mapping technique used, and the role of the partners in each stage of the research process for the project Hispanos Unidos en la Prevención de Obesidad (Hispanics United in the Prevention of Obesity).

CBPR Partnership Background. Hispanos Unidos en la Prevención de Obesidad is a collaborative effort between a university researcher, Guadalupe X. Ayala, an assistant professor at UNC-CH School of Public Health and a coauthor of this chapter, and members of Hispanos Unidos, a grassroots group of Latino families interested in improving the well-being of Latino families in North Carolina. The principal community partner is a woman from Costa Rica who lives in the community and who is dedicated to serving the Latino community through her church, work, and social activities. The Hispanos Unidos group is made up of approximately eight men and women (primarily husbands and wives) whose children participate in the youth soccer league. The Latino population in this county is relatively young (47 percent are between twenty-two and forty-four years old) and of low socioeconomic status, as indicated by the prevalence of poverty (23 percent) and low educational attainment (74 percent did not graduate from high school) (U.S. Census Bureau, 2000). The Hispanos Unidos en la Prevención de Obesidad project was originally funded by the Program on Ethnicity, Culture, and Health Outcomes at the University of North Carolina at Chapel Hill.

The Hispanos Unidos en la Prevención de Obesidad project represents the first collaborative effort between Latino families in North Carolina and the university researcher. The university researcher, new to the North Carolina area, was interested in building a partnership with a community group for several reasons:

- To better understand facilitators and barriers associated with leading a healthy lifestyle

- To better understand what it was like to be a Latino and a new immigrant in North Carolina

- To begin the process of designing a community-based intervention to prevent obesity

Through a colleague, the university researcher was introduced to a group of families interested in addressing the lack of healthy resources for Latinos in their community. The researcher met several community members at an exercise class and began attending these exercise classes weekly. Although most of the community members spoke only Spanish, language was not a barrier as the university researcher is bilingual (Spanish-English) and bicultural (Latina).

The group invited the researcher to attend its twice monthly Hispanos Unidos evening meetings. The group had been meeting for several months to discuss strategies for involving their youths in organized sports and to identify ways of involving more adults in the exercise classes. The group requested the researcher's participation to provide instruction on community organizing and empowerment skills. What unfolded from these meetings was recognition that both parties have something to offer that can be used to benefit the community. The researcher is perceived as a source of information about how to create change and has been relied upon for information about eating and exercise change, the factors to consider in program development, and potential funding sources. The community members are perceived by the university researcher as a source of information about context-specific risk factors for obesity and the acculturation process among new Latino immigrants to the southeastern region of the United States. However, despite the recognition that each partner has valuable information to share, during meetings the community members often seek a final decision from the university researcher. This is consistent with the literature on Latino cultural norms of respect (Marín & Marín, 1991). In addition, due to the relatively recent migration of Latino families into North Carolina, resources and services are primarily available in English. Thus being Latino (that is, knowing what it means to be Latino in the United States) and having English language skills are equated with power. This imbalance of power associated with the university researcher's having both English language skills and greater access to resources made the process of shared decision making more difficult than it might have been if the researcher and community partners had not shared a common ethnic background.

CBPR Research Project Background. The primary purpose of this project is to identify social and environmental influences on the eating and exercise habits of Latino families. The community members noted the importance of these behaviors for preventing diabetes and other chronic illnesses in their children. A secondary objective is to determine how to involve families in the design and implementation of an intervention: for example, training parents and their children to serve as peer health advisers.

The Hispanos Unidos en la Prevención de Obesidad project is a cross-sectional analysis of social and environmental influences on eating and exercise behaviors. The mapping activity is one of several methods used to gain information for intervention development purposes. Other methods are Hispanos Unidos meetings, community member focus groups, and in-depth interviews. Activities to date have taken place in the families' homes, in the PI's home, and at a community center. Data collection activities specific to this project were begun in March 2003 and are currently ongoing.

Research Process Stages and the Role of Partners. As will be illustrated below, the project began with development of a mapping protocol using various qualitative methods, recruitment of families to participate in the project, and implementation of research activities.

Development of Mapping Protocol. The mapping activity was informed by the university researcher's participation in the twice monthly Hispanos Unidos meetings and discussions with the principal community partner beginning in the early fall of 2002. Families involved in Hispanos Unidos had no experience in conducting research but were interested in understanding how to do this to obtain information for program development purposes. After several group meetings they decided that the first step would be to involve other community members in focus group discussions about the issues and then about appropriate next steps. The community members relied entirely on the university researcher to prepare the focus group discussion guide, with the understanding that she would pilot-test it with members of Hispanos Unidos to assess relevance and salience of the issues. After this pilot test the focus group guide was shortened, and a total of six focus group discussions were held with representative community members in their homes to generate information for the mapping activity.

Information from these focus groups was used to design the structure and content of the mapping activity. Members of Hispanos Unidos were interested in knowing where certain behaviors take place and in understanding how youths and their parents see their respective environments (for example, do youths perceive fast-food restaurants as bad or good, and how does this compare with how their parents see them). Mapping was identified as a method for determining where people go in their normal everyday lives so that a program can be designed to fit their current activity patterns. In addition the group discussed and agreed upon integrating the mapping activity with in-depth parent and child interviews, to provide a context for the questions asked during the mapping activity. (See Chapters Four and Twelve for examinations of the use of in-depth interviews.) Members of Hispanos Unidos noted that the mapping activity would be interactive and engaging, yet they also felt that without some context for the questions being asked in the mapping activity (for example, where do people do their shopping?) the data collection process would be awkward. As noted previously, members of Hispanos Unidos relied on the university researcher to determine the best approach for gathering this information, expressing less interest in the process of data collection and more interest in obtaining the information through whatever means possible. Hispanos Unidos members also expressed an interest in serving as participants in this next stage so their maps and voices (via in-depth interviews) could be included in the results.

Selection and Recruitment of Participants. Members of Hispanos Unidos wanted to experience all aspects of this project, both as organizers and as participants. Therefore recruitment of families for the in-depth interviews and mapping activities began with members of Hispanos Unidos who had children who were between thirteen and eighteen years of age, living at home, and residing in the target community. Additional recruitment efforts consisted of members telling friends and family about the opportunity, and the posting of flyers in Mexican grocery stores (*tiendas*) in the area.

Fourteen families (parent-child dyads) participated in the mapping activities and in-depth interviews. All but two of the dyads consisted of a mother and child; two involved the mother, father, and child. The mean age of parent participants was 40 years (SD = 4.05). This sample was similar to the larger Latino population in terms of socioeconomic status and country of origin (75 percent with less than a high school education; 77 percent Mexican). Most of the youths were female (86 percent), with a mean age of 13.3 years (SD = 1.7).

Data Collection. The mapping activity and in-depth interviews with these four-teen families occurred during an evening home visit with each family and were conducted by the PI and one bilingual graduate student research assistant. The parent and the youth were invited to participate in the mapping activity, followed by separate parent and child interviews (in English or Spanish, as appropriate) that assessed activity patterns during the past three days, asked for a twenty-four-hour dietary recall, and sought information about patterns of eating and exercise in the home and at work or school and suggestions for program development. Using a two-page map copied from a city street guide, the youth and the parent were asked to identify the following locations and the modes of transportation used to get to each location:

- Family residence
- Youth's school
- Parent's workplace
- Primary grocery store
- Other locations frequented on a daily or weekly basis

This latter category generally included such places as secondary grocery stores, churches, relatives and friends' homes, parks, and community centers. The youth was asked to place a sticker next to each location found on the map and to use a marker to indicate the route that his or her family takes to get to this location. The research assistant made a note on the map about the type of transportation used to get to each location. During this activity, the youth and the parent were asked to identify locations that may influence their eating and exercise behaviors (for example, a neighborhood park) as well as factors in their lived environments that influence these behaviors (for example, a fast-food restaurant near the parent's workplace or youth's school). The entire data collection protocol lasted approximately two hours, with the PI and research assistant often asked to stay afterward for dinner or *chocolate con pan dulce* (hot chocolate and sweet bread). Families received $35 for participating in the mapping activity and in-depth interviews.

Activities in Progress: Data Analysis, Interpretation, and Application of Results. The original plan was for the university researcher to create a preliminary report on the findings to present in a community forum. However, several members of Hispanos Unidos asked that some of these activities occur in their group meetings. For example, they expressed an interest in creating a large community map depicting common places where youths and adults access food and engage in exercise. This decision may reflect a greater comfort with the research process or greater interest in seeing how mapping and interview data get synthesized, or both. After two meetings during which members talked about how many families were interviewed and reviewed information collected, the next stage was placed on hold because several key members of Hispanos Unidos returned to their country of origin. The Hispanos Unidos group planned to reconvene when these individuals returned to the United States. At that time the group will plan a community forum to review the data and begin synthesis. The expectation is that a preliminary report will be created, and then all families who participated in the mapping activity can be invited to see the results and plan action steps. Before ceasing the data analysis meeting, one Hispanos Unidos member thoughtfully noted that she felt the information would be useful because *"me enseño donde podemos implementar el programa y donde [nuestros hijos] necesitan ayuda"* ("it showed me where we might want to implement the program and where kids need the most help").

CHALLENGES AND LIMITATIONS

Some individuals may not be accustomed to drawing maps or using two-dimensional maps to characterize their environment (Steegmann & Hewner, 2000). The use of maps may not be consistent with cultural norms or practices (Siar, 2003). In the Hispanos Unidos en la Prevención de Obesidad project, participating families often requested several explanations of the mapping activity. This may reflect lack of exposure to using maps or possibly an ineffective protocol for describing the purpose and methods of mapping their activities. Our experiences suggest that more work is needed to improve the use of mapping techniques with community members who have had less access to higher education and who may not be socially or culturally oriented to using maps to describe and depict their experiences in their lived environment.

Mapping social and environmental influences requires a commitment of time and resources to this activity. In the Your Crib study, youths were asked to spend three days logging their activities. Colored pencils, copies of city maps, and large drawing paper were needed to create the synthesized map. In the Hispanos Unidos en la Prevención de Obesidad project, copies of colored street maps, stickers, and colored pens were needed to complete the mapping activity. In addition the mapping activity added approximately thirty minutes to the home visit. Our review of the literature suggests that other resources may be needed, such as mapping software to synthesize information. Researchers and community partners alike should identify the added value of incorporating a mapping activity, considering the expenses associated with preparing maps.

Similarly, mapping techniques do not typically occur in isolation from other data collection methods. This also has implications for the resources needed. Our decision to use focus groups and in-depth interviews was driven by the community members involved and the way the mapping activity was implemented.

A process of focus group interviews followed by a three-day activity record and then mapping was deemed most appropriate for youths in the Your Crib project because it provided an opportunity to discuss barriers to and facilitators of healthy eating and exercise before beginning the mapping exercise. In the Hispanos Unidos en la Prevención de Obesidad project, the mapping activity occurred immediately before the in-depth interview, to provide a context for the subsequent discussion about environmental influences on eating and exercise behaviors. From a research perspective, it provided an opportunity to determine what type of information was best garnered from the mapping activity as compared to the in-depth interviews.

Our immediate process evaluation of the mapping activities indicated that participants in both projects enjoyed the mapping activity, in particular the interactive aspect of finding the location of their activities on a map. This allowed them to develop awareness of the patterns in their daily activities, the distance they covered during a typical day and a typical week, and the physical boundaries of their activities. The visual display of information was easy and exciting for the participants to understand. However, in the Your Crib project, the youths did not enjoy keeping a written log of their daily activities and suggested other media (such as, videotape recording) as an alternate way to capture similar information. As outlined in various chapters in this book, well-established methods exist for informing program development in partnership with community members. The use of mapping techniques, though less well-informed, appears to be an effective method for individuals to better understand environmental influences on health.

LESSONS LEARNED AND IMPLICATIONS FOR PRACTICE

Our review of the published literature and implementation of mapping techniques with two communities led us to consider why and when to use mapping techniques in a community-based participatory research project. Because mapping requires additional resources and effort, knowing why and when to map social and environmental influences are two important considerations for future research endeavors.

The single most important question members of a partnership should ask is, Why use mapping techniques? Researchers are often driven to use multiple methods for exploratory purposes without considering the impact that mapping social and environmental influences may have on community members. Poverty, limited access to educational and employment opportunities, and other social, cultural, and political factors constrain many communities from achieving real structural change. Highlighting factors external to, and often out of the control of the individual, family, or community, may increase this sense of helplessness. It is our recommendation that mapping these influences for problem definition and intervention development purposes should be used so that partnership members can consider the implementation of intervention strategies that target change at the environmental level and that are not limited to increasing community members' awareness of real disparities as a motivator for change or simply improving community members' ability to navigate these unhealthy environments.

Research conducted to date has used mapping techniques to better understand social and environmental influences in order to better define the problem and inform program development. In the two projects discussed in this chapter, this view guided our use of mapping techniques. However, researchers and community partners should also consider using mapping as a form of process evaluation following an intervention. For example, participants involved in an intervention could map changes in children's access to soft drinks and candy in their local and extended community environments. This type of process evaluation would highlight the most effective strategies for successful change in a given context and would inform the allocation of resources and policies.

CONCLUSION

Designing interventions to prevent disease, improve health, or increase access to health care requires an understanding of social and environmental influences. Although several formative research techniques can be used to inform intervention development (Ayala & Elder, 2001), mapping these influences provides unique information and creates an opportunity for members of a partnership to better understand contextual factors in their lived environments. Using mapping techniques to define the problem may be our best approach for engaging community members in understanding the person-environment fit.

References

Atlas.ti, Version 4.2. (2000). Berlin: Scientific Software Development.

Ayala, G. X., & Elder, J. P. (2001). Verbal methods in perceived efficacy work. In S. Sussman (Ed.), *Handbook of program development for health behavior research and practice.* Thousand Oaks, CA: Sage.

Babbie, E. R. (1979). *The practice of social research* (2nd ed.). Belmont, CA: Wadsworth.

Bandura, A. (1986). *Social foundations of thought and action. A social cognitive theory.* Upper Saddle River, NJ: Prentice Hall.

Barry, K., & Britt, D. W. (2002). Outreach: Targeting high-risk women through community partnerships. *Women's Health Issues, 12*(2), 66–78.

Bickes, J. T. (2000). Community health assessment using computerized geographic mapping. *Nurse Educator, 25*(4), 172–173.

Breslow, L. (1996). Social ecological strategies for promoting healthy lifestyles. *American Journal of Health Promotion, 10,* 253–257.

Bronfenbrenner, U. (1979). *The ecology of human development.* Cambridge, MA: Harvard University Press.

Cohen, D., Scribner, R., & Farley, T. (2000). A structural model of health behavior: A pragmatic approach to explain and influence health behaviors at the population level. *Preventive Medicine, 30,* 164–154.

Coulton, C. J., Korbin, J., Chan, T., & Su, M. (2001). Mapping residents' perceptions of neighborhood boundaries: A methodological note. *American Journal of Community Psychology, 29*(2), 371–383.

Cowell, J. M., & Cowell, M. E. (1999). Immunization rates: A community assessment approach for diagnosis. *Journal of School Nursing, 15*(5), 40–43.

Cravey, A. J., Arcury, T. A., & Quandt, S. A. (2000). Mapping as a means of farm-worker education and empowerment. *Journal of Geography, 99*(6), 229–237.

Cravey, A. J., Washburn, S. A., Gesler, W. M., Arcury, T. A., & Skelly, A. H. (2001). Developing socio-spatial knowledge networks: A qualitative methodology for chronic disease prevention. *Social Science & Medicine, 52*(12), 1763–1775.

Dowda, M., Ainsworth, B. E., Addy, C. L., Saunders, R., & Riner, W. (2001). Environmental influences, physical activity, and weight status in 8- to 16-year olds. *Archives of Pediatrics & Adolescent Medicine, 155,* 711–717.

Emmel, N. D., & O'Keefe, P. (1996). Participatory analysis for redefining health delivery in a Bombay slum. *Journal of Public Health Medicine, 18*(3), 301–307.

Emmons, K. M. (2000). *Health behaviors in social context.* In L. F. Berkman & I. Kawachi (Eds.), *Social epidemiology* (pp. 242–266). New York: Oxford Press.

French, S. A., Story, M., & Jeffrey, R. W. (2001). Environmental influences on eating and physical activity. *Annual Review of Public Health, 22,* 309–335.

Ghys, P. D., Jenkins, C., & Pisani, E. (2001). HIV surveillance among female sex workers. *AIDS, 15*(Suppl. 3), S33–S40.

Gordon, A., & Womersley, J. (1997). The use of mapping in public health and planning health services. *Journal of Public Health Medicine, 19*(2), 139–147.

Johnson, H. B., Ved, R., Lyall, N., & Agarwal, K. (2003). Where do rural women obtain postabortion care? The case of Uttar Pradesh, India. *International Family Planning Perspectives, 29*(4), 182–187.

Marín, G., & Marín, B. V. (1991). *Research with Hispanic populations.* Thousand Oaks, CA: Sage.

Miles, M. B., & Huberman, A. M. (1994). *Qualitative data analysis.* Thousand Oaks, CA: Sage.

Moos, R. H. (1987). Person-environment congruence in work, school, and health care settings. *Journal of Vocational Behavior, 31*(3), 231–247.

Morland, K., Wing, S., Roux, A. D., & Poole, C. (2002). Neighborhood characteristics associated with the location of food stores and food service places. *American Journal of Preventive Medicine, 22*(1), 23–29.

Morrow, B. H. (1999). Identifying and mapping community vulnerability. *Disasters, 23*(1), 1–18.

Nemoto, T., Operario, D., Takenaka, M., Iwamoto, M., & Le, M. N. (2003). HIV risk among Asian women working at massage parlors in San Francisco. *AIDS Education and Prevention, 15*(3), 245–256.

Phillips, R. L., Kinman, E. L., Schnitzer, P. G., Lindbloom, E. J., & Ewigman, B. (2000). Using geographic information systems to understand health care access. *Archives of Family Medicine, 9*, 971–978.

Romero, A., Robinson, T. N., Kraemer, H. C., Erickson, S. J., Haydel, F., Mendoza, F., et al. (2001). Are perceived neighborhood hazards a barrier to physical activity in children? *Archives of Pediatrics & Adolescent Medicine, 155*, 1143–1148.

Siar, S. V. (2003). Knowledge, gender, and resources in small-scale fishing: The case of Honda Bay, Palawan, Philippines. *Environmental Management, 31*(5), 569–580.

Steegmann, A. T., & Hewner, S. J. (2000). Mapping toxin exposure risk due to children's play: A case study. *Environmental Research, 84*(3), 265–274.

Sterk, C. E. (2002). The Health Intervention Project: HIV risk reduction among African-American drug users. *Public Health Reports, 117*, S88–S95.

Stokols, D. (1996). Translating social ecological theory into guidelines for community health promotion. *American Journal of Health Promotion, 10*(4), 282–298.

Taylor, D., & Chavez, G. (2002). Small area analysis on a large scale: The California experience in mapping teenage birth "hot spots" for resource allocation. *Journal of Public Health Management and Practice, 8*(2), 33–45.

U.S. Census Bureau. (2000). *Summary of social, economic, and housing characteristics.* Washington, DC: U.S. Government Printing Office.

Veale, A., & Dona, G. (2003). Street children and political violence: A socio-demographic analysis of street children in Rwanda. *Child Abuse and Neglect, 27*, 253–269.

Walters, J. S. (1997). *Exploring local knowledge in tropical coastal ecology: Participatory resource assessment in a Philippine fishing community.* PhD dissertation, University of Hawaii.

Wang, C. C. (1999). Photovoice: A participatory action research strategy applied to women's health. *Journal of Women's Health, 8*(2), 185–192.

CHAPTER TEN

Community-Based Participatory Research and Ethnography

The Perfect Union

Chris McQuiston, Emilio A. Parrado, Julio César Olmos-Muñiz,
and Alejandro M. Bustillo Martinez

Racial and ethnic disparities in health are well documented (Flaskerud & Kim, 1999), yet they are not explained merely by lack of health insurance or income (Weinick, Zuvekas, & Cohen, 2000). Research that explores the multiple and complex issues related to culture, ethnicity, and health disparities is urgently needed (Flaskerud & Winslow, 1998; Weinick et al., 2000). As U.S. demographics change, learning about ethnic and cultural variations among subgroups is increasingly important. Researchers are challenged to move beyond "matching" their methodology to their research question and to practice matching their methods to the cultural group under study as well (McQuiston, Larson, Parrado, & Flaskerud, 2002).

Research strategies and partnerships can address cultural and ethnic variations in health and illness as well as the needs of recent immigrants. The challenge of matching methods to cultural groups includes developing strategies to increase community participation in the research process (Flaskerud & Nyamathi, 2000; McQuiston, Choi-Hevel, & Clawson, 2001).

Acknowledgments: This research was funded by the National Institute of Nursing Research, grants NR08052-03 and NR08052-02S2. The authors would like to thank Amanda Phillips Martínez and Leonardo Uribe for all their help in the community and with translation and transcription. We would also like to thank El Centro Hispano, Horizonte Latino, the Latino community in Durham, North Carolina, and the Center for Innovation in Health Disparities Research at UNC–Chapel Hill School of Nursing.

In this chapter we demonstrate our conception of how to conduct ethnography as community-based participatory research (CBPR). The resulting combination, community-based ethnographic participatory research (CBEPR), explicitly blends community with ethnography, focuses on culture and cultural interpretation, and uses a CBPR process. We begin with an introduction to ethnography and a look at ethnography and CBPR combined, followed by an example of a study that used an ethnographic survey, participant observation, and analysis and interpretation of data to examine gender, migration, and HIV risks among Mexican migrants living in Durham, North Carolina. We conclude with lessons learned and implications for CBEPR.

A GENERAL DESCRIPTION OF ETHNOGRAPHY

There are numerous definitions of ethnography, and ethnography may be conducted in various forms, for example, semistructured or unstructured interviews, surveys, or other elicitation techniques (Tedlock, 2000). A consistent theme, however, is that ethnography is "always informed by culture" (Boyle, 1994, p. 160) and involves rigorous observation and communication in the "field" to ensure accuracy of data (LeCompte & Schensul, 1999b; Vidich & Lyman, 1994). *Culture* refers to commonalities among groups or patterned life ways (Reynolds & Leininger, 1995). Ethnographers attempt to describe these commonalities (culture) systematically, identifying shared systems of meaning. According to Geertz (1983), "the interpretive study of culture represents an attempt to come to terms with the diversity of the ways human beings construct their lives in the act of leading them" (p. 16). Interpreting culture is facilitated by participant observation in the field (where people live, work, attend events, and so forth). Participant observation may vary in terms of how much the ethnographer actually participates (for example, the ethnographer may just be present at a health fair or may help to organize it). However, regardless of the approach to participant observation, the record of the event, referred to as *field notes,* is a contextualized and systematic description (LeCompte & Schensul, 1999a). For the purpose of the study described here, we define *ethnography* as research with an immigrant population based on participant observation of life in a natural setting utilizing the researcher as a major instrument of the research (LeCompte & Schensul, 1999a).

Traditional ethnography focuses on obtaining knowledge, often resulting in a publication developed solely by the ethnographer (Chambers, 2000). Many ethnographers are now choosing to embrace a more collaborative model, one that lends itself to participatory research. Terms describing this type of ethnography include *collaborative, community-based, narrative, reciprocal,* and *dialogic* (Austin, 2003; Lassiter, 2000; Mannheim & Tedlock, 1995; Stringer et al., 1997).

These labels represent a more egalitarian approach to research, with the participants providing ongoing dialogue about the emerging ethnographic text. The approaches to accomplish this goal may differ and some may be more collaborative than others, but there is a common theme among collaborative models of ethnography that represents a shift in thinking away from a hierarchical approach in which the researcher as a participant observer authors alone an account (an ethnography) of the "other" (Schensul, Weeks, & Singer, 1999).

Studies that combine ethnography and CBPR may be carried out, for example, by partnerships established as community-university-agency partnerships (Austin, 2003) or as university-Native American partnerships (tribal relationships) (Chrisman, Strickland, Powell, Squeochs, & Yallup, 1999). University faculty may also be joined by graduate students in such studies (Stringer et al., 1997). A common thread is the desire to fully include nonacademics in multiple levels of the ethnographic study and to work collectively on real-life problems.

METHODS WITHIN METHODS

From an ethnographic perspective, community-based participatory research offers an approach to conducting culturally competent research that aims for a cultural interpretation of research findings and that uses community members as researchers (Meleis, 1996; Sawyer et al., 1995). CBPR includes community members as researchers in all aspects of the research process, including the development of research concepts, the conduct of the research, and the interpretation of the findings (Israel et al., 2003). Community-based ethnographic participatory research closes the gap between ethnography and community. With this method community members are trained as ethnographers. Therefore they are not just helping with interpretation as would be the case with collaborative ethnography but they are also collaboratively determining how and what data will be collected, collecting the data, and collectively interpreting the data. In this case, cultural interpretation gives meaning to the ways in which Latino experiences and perceptions are shaped by the cultural background and structural position of Latino immigrants in U.S. society. Because the ethnographer is interested in the cultural interpretation (Schwandt, 1994) of the data, working with community members as research colleagues allows collective debate about data and what these data mean within the context of the culture of the group participating in the study.

In the following section we describe an ethnographic approach to CBPR undertaken to provide information for the development of culture-specific interventions and to produce data for model and theory development. (See Chapters Four and Five for further discussion of community-based participatory approaches to the development of conceptual models and community assessments.) Using a CBPR approach, we triangulate multiple methods, including an *ethnosexual survey,* participant observation, fieldwork, and qualitative data from participatory group meetings.

COMMUNITY ETHNOGRAPHERS

The purpose of this discussion is to demonstrate the use of CBEPR methods by describing the three separate stages of Gender, Migration and HIV Risks Among Mexicans, a study funded by the National Institute of Nursing Research (NINR). Each stage used different methods to implement a CBEPR approach. In the first stage community and academic participants developed the conceptual basis for a grant proposal. Preliminary ethnographic data were gathered and used to write the background and significance sections and part of the preliminary studies section of the grant proposal. In stage two, community and academic researchers, or more specifically, ethnographers, developed and refined an ethnosexual survey to be used in the study, and community participants were trained in ethnographic methods and conducted the surveys. In stage three, community participants engaged in interpretation of the research findings.

Study Background

Latino community members and academics worked collaboratively on all components of the Gender, Migration, and HIV Risks Among Mexicans study that aims to compare prevalent sexual behaviors among Mexican men and women in Durham, North Carolina, and four sending communities in Mexico, and to identify and describe the impact of migration on the gender structures of labor, power (imbalances within relationships), and gender-specific norms among the Mexican population. The specific objectives of the community group have been to increase capacity on the individual, group, organizational, and community levels as partners collectively develop an understanding of community needs and strengths related to gender, migration, and HIV risk. These objectives mirror the mission statement of El Centro Hispano (ECH), the Latino advocacy agency that is a key partner in this CBEPR effort.

Study Setting

Durham County, North Carolina, is an urban area with a strong economy and numerous construction, hotel, restaurant, and landscaping jobs. These jobs often require few or no English skills and draw Latinos to the area. The Latino immigrant population in Durham grew exponentially from 2,054 in 1990 to 17,039 (8 percent of the total population) in 2000 (Schmidley, 2001). In addition, in 2000, Durham had the most unbalanced sex ratio among immigrant Latinos aged twenty to twenty-nine of any metropolitan area in the country

(Suro & Singer, 2002), with approximately 2.5 men for every woman. New arrivals to the area typically have few resources and work low-entry jobs without health insurance, and many live in crowded, substandard housing. The combination of migratory stress, limited resources, and predominately male migration puts these immigrants at increased risk for HIV/AIDS (McQuiston & Uribe, 2001; Hondagneu-Sotelo, 2003).

Study Participants

Eight community members, from Mexico and Honduras, and two staff members at ECH were involved in the first stage of the project, along with four academic members of the team. Two of the academic team members were from the United States, one from Colombia, and one from Argentina. This group met bimonthly for three months to conceptually develop the proposal. Initially, El Centro Hispano's role was to participate in the conceptual development of the grant proposal and discuss its members' collective experience in the community. Working in this partnership required ECH to make a space for a project that was not directly tied to an intervention. At this point ECH had some difficulty visualizing how the research could lead to interventions. As the project progressed, ECH viewed it as a valuable resource and requested data from the project to inform ECH's grant proposal writing for subsequent projects.

It was helpful that the community participants knew the academic researchers from collaborating on a previous HIV prevention project. Four of the community participants had been trained as lay health advisers (LHAs) for the project Protegiendo Nuestra Comunidad (Protecting Our Community) and the other four had attended additional community training for HIV prevention facilitated by trained LHAs and academics (McQuiston et al., 2001; McQuiston & Uribe, 2001). They viewed research examining HIV/AIDS in the context of migration, and gender as a priority. Their awareness and their experiences with the academic team members over a five-year period greatly facilitated the CBEPR process in the project.

The second and third stages of this project occurred after funding for the study was obtained. During the first stage, the working group was intentionally small, but then participants wanted to hear more diverse views to make sure the project team was on the right track. Four additional women and two men recommended by ECH and the existing community members were invited to participate, with the final community group totaling fourteen community members. The community participants in stages two and three were from Mexico (ten), Honduras (one), Peru (two), and Colombia (one). This group named itself Horizonte Latino (Latinos Moving Forward). The relationship of Horizonte Latino with ECH was fluid, with shared membership of academics on ECH committees, and ECH staff and board members as participants in Horizonte Latino.

Study Meetings

All the collaborative meetings were conducted in Spanish at ECH. Team members agreed on the best time to meet and reviewed what the group process would be. The roles and responsibilities, philosophy, purpose, and process of collaboration, which were agreed on and used with the initial group, were reviewed when new people were asked to join. The context of the team's empowerment philosophy and methodology (looking, critically reflecting, and acting), based on the concepts of Paulo Freire (1970, 1973), was discussed.

This philosophy assumes that community participants have an understanding of behavior within the context of their culture and that they bring insights to the research that their academic partners may not have (McQuiston et al., 2001). Community participants live in the neighborhoods in which the research takes place, and in the case of Horizonte Latino members, have experienced migration and the numerous challenges it holds, including the interface of their own culture with that of the dominant U.S. culture. They observe and experience the influence of the dominant culture on their own values, beliefs, behaviors, and relationships and observe the effects of "settling in" to the United States on community members around them. As researchers and ethnographers, they learn to tease out the cultural meaning of what they have learned as participant observers and the learnings from study findings, and they analyze what these data mean to them as well as the implications of these data for the Latino community.

THE CBEPR PROCESS EXEMPLIFIED

There were three stages in this CBEPR process: developing the proposal, moving from concept to process, and analyzing the findings.

Developing the Proposal

The conceptual development of the grant proposal was accomplished through collaborative meetings in which academic facilitators asked community participants to identify root causes of HIV/AIDS in their community (Hope & Timmel, 1995). The project team divided into two (or sometimes three) small groups. These groups were divided by gender for discussions of sensitive topics. Each small group identified a community member facilitator who kept the group on task. The facilitator was given a task (by the academic facilitator): for example, to ask the group to define HIV in the Latino community or to describe what contributes to the problem and what results from the problem. A scribe was asked to write the group's "findings" on a flip chart, and a presenter was asked to present the group's results to the entire group (Arnold, Burke, James, Martin, & Thomas, 1995). After the small groups had finished their discussions, the presenters posted their findings and summarized the discussions. Many of the concerns the groups shared were related to the process of migration, and participants frequently grounded these discussions in both time and place. For example, when discussing values and beliefs—specifically, issues of gender roles for men and women—the participants would frequently talk about "here" (the United States) and "there" (Mexico). Roles "here" and roles "there" signaled changes in gender roles as part of the migration experience.

Following these discussions the entire group looked at the flip charts for the common themes across the small groups. Typically, there was much agreement, and the participants readily discussed areas of consensus. When themes arose that were not common across groups, participants discussed them and made a decision about what to keep and what to leave out. At times the academic facilitator would help to summarize what the entire group had agreed on or disagreed on up to that point. Decisions were made through group discussion and consensus. After final agreement was achieved, the concepts were included in the grant proposal. Thus the concepts for the study came from the community members. Putting all these concepts together for a fundable study was an academic task, which was presented conceptually to the larger group for approval.

Over the course of six two-hour meetings, the major causes of HIV identified by the group included sexual behavior (the use and availability of commercial sex workers), alcohol or other drug use, lack of education or information about HIV and resources, migration (including limited opportunities available to migrants owing to their concentration in low-wage, poorly paid work), gender roles, and cultural beliefs and values. The group had identified both structural and cultural causes of HIV risk and the interface between the two. For example, they suggested that the uneven sex ratio (more male than female immigrants) and the availability of commercial sex workers (CSWs) and a culture that does not always condemn marital infidelity among men could increase HIV risk in their community.

Moving from Concept to Process

In this stage the project team prepared a survey, trained participants to conduct survey interviews, and administered the survey.

Ethnosexual Survey Development and Participant Training. After the community participants identified the main dimensions affecting HIV risks among Latinos, the academic team members developed a draft of a culture-specific ethnosexual survey for collective discussion. The data collected from the collaborative work of the community members in stage one of this project allowed the survey to be ethnographically informed (Schensul et al., 1999). For example, use of CSWs was a concern within the context of alcohol use and *tiempo libre* (free time where you have nothing to do and can get into trouble). The participants also thought that the men studied were vulnerable to use of CSWs owing to depression resulting from migration and social isolation. Therefore all these concepts were addressed in the ethnosexual survey, using both closed and open-ended questions. (See Chapters Five and Twelve for discussions of the development and implementation of closed-ended survey questionnaires in the context of CBPR projects.) Questions were anchored in time and place by asking questions in the context of Mexico and then asking the same questions again in the context of the United States, to address the "here" and "there" questions raised in stage one. At this point project team members met weekly in small groups to read chunks of the survey out loud, and discuss, reflect, and evaluate this material for cultural and linguistic fit. Comments were then presented to the entire group, with further discussion and decisions regarding which questions to include in the survey.

The team expressed concern about the wording of several items and was especially sensitive to the variety of ways respondents from different countries or places of origin (for example, rural or urban) might interpret certain questions or phrases. In several cases the wording was changed. In other cases alternative words for the same concept were included so that when the team's community participants functioned as ethnographers they would have multiple alternative words readily available as they conducted the interviews. Additionally, the community ethnographers were concerned about the sensitive nature of some of the questions, which they felt needed to be introduced in a general manner. Questions about particularly sensitive issues, such as homosexuality and drug use, were deemed too "alarming" to ask directly and were introduced as hypothetical scenarios. The group's numerous suggestions and insights guided revision of the ethnosexual survey.

After the revisions, academic participants trained the community participants in interview techniques, including participant observation and recording field notes for each interview. The academics modeled how to ask questions and follow story lines, how to observe the environment and note the context of the interview, and discussed what to record in the field notes. (See Appendix F for a copy of the field notes guide.) The community participants used role playing to practice interviewing and discussed potential problems related to both asking questions and documenting responses (the interviews were not taped).

They learned that in the field they would follow the respondent's story line, using a conversational narrative approach typical to ethnography and moving back and forth in the guide as the story evolved (Parrado, McQuiston, & Flippen, unpublished manuscript). For example, a respondent might tell an ethnographer that she initially followed her boyfriend to Texas and that she lived and worked there cleaning houses. Later she might say she moved to Durham with her husband. Following the conversational approach, the ethnographer would need to remember the boyfriend in Texas and say something like, "Is the husband you came to Durham with the same as the boyfriend you went to be with in Texas?" The ethnographer would then follow the story line that resulted from the respondent's answer to this question. In this process, several more moves and another boyfriend might be "discovered." All this would take place in a normal conversational manner.

Administering the Survey. Through collaborative discussions and fieldwork around the city of Durham the project team identified thirteen apartment complexes that housed predominantly Latinos. The team then constructed a census of all housing units in these complexes to serve as a sampling frame. From this list of over 2,000 apartments, the team drew independent random samples of men and women to be visited by the male and female interviewers, respectively. Interviewers were given a list of the dwellings selected for the survey and instructed to conduct the survey with the person that answered the door if he or she was Latino, between the ages of eighteen and forty-five, and the same sex as the interviewer. In cases where the person that answered the door did not correspond to the target population, the interviewer asked if someone with such characteristics lived in the apartment and interviewed the first person suggested by the individual answering the door. Dwellings with no residents who met the study criteria were excluded.

Checking In with the Ethnographers. Two academic project members went to ECH once a week to meet with the community ethnographers and review each completed ethnosexual survey with the person who had done the interviewing. In this way an academic ethnographer and a community ethnographer checked each survey for consistency and accuracy of information. The community ethnographer would often point out areas of the survey where the respondent had contradicted himself or herself, struggled with questions, or provided a particularly detailed response.

Once the academic team member and the community ethnographer finished reviewing the survey for consistency and accuracy, they reviewed the field observation form. Community ethnographers took different approaches to the field observations. Some were particularly detailed in their observations of the physical conditions of the apartment and the complex, providing detailed notes of the parking lots and trash, noting whether there were areas for recreation and what the informant's apartment looked like on the inside. Others focused more on the life story and experience. Any verbal observations made by a community ethnographer that were not included in the field notes were jotted down by the academic researcher on the survey at the time of the meeting.

These meetings were important because errors could be caught almost immediately and corrected before the next interview, and the academic team member could provide the community ethnographers with additional training if it was needed. It was also a good opportunity for these researchers to reflect on their experience with particular informants while each interview was still fresh in their minds. In addition to these one-on-one meetings, the project team met as a group monthly to discuss insights and problems and to begin an initial analysis of what it was seeing and experiencing. At this point in the process, information was going back and forth between ECH and Horizonte Latino, and the tension experienced during the initial meetings concerning the relevance of the research to ECH was replaced with a sense that Horizonte Latino had become institutionalized at ECH.

Analyzing the Findings

Ongoing iterative presentation and discussion of the findings allowed the team to assess the study results, reconsider preliminary expectations, provide a cultural understanding of specific findings, and identify new lines of research and intervention. Central to CBEPR is the critical reflection on cultural values of the group members. Viewing findings within the context of culture as well as social structures allowed Horizonte Latino to build a collective ethnographic account of the community that is not just the sum of personal experiences but the product of community ethnographers looking into themselves and discussing their own experiences and ideas in relation to those of the community respondents.

One example of this process was an exploration of the data pertaining to the relationship between migration and women's power. The prevailing image of gender roles in Mexico is that of submissive women and chauvinistic, *machista* men. Prior to data collection and group discussion, both the community and academic ethnographers alike believed that migrant women are, to some extent, liberated once they come to the United States, as the ethos of egalitarianism (real or imagined) prevalent in the United States comes into conflict with the more traditional, patriarchal gender ideologies brought from communities of origin. Current academic literature recognizes the complexity and limits of gender change resulting from immigration but tends to frame it in positive terms akin to liberation (Hondagneu-Sotelo, 2003).

Through a process of critical reflection, the group reexamined the root causes of gender role change with migration within the context of the survey data and personal and collective experiences. As a result of this reflection, both community and academic ethnographers began to take a more varied view, recognizing both positive and negative aspects of the greater freedom offered by life in the United States.

The second author of this chapter conducted a preliminary analysis of the quantitative findings related to gender roles and migration: comparing labor force participation, the division of household responsibilities (housework and family finances), relationship control, and gender attitudes among married Mexican women in Durham, North Carolina, and in Mexico. Prior to presenting the findings to the group, the academic ethnographers explained the statistics needed to understand the data and then presented research questions and a table with empty cells corresponding to numbers and percentages of survey responses to specific questions. Each community ethnographer gave his or her *guess estimate* of the results of each research question and an explanation of that estimate. There was often group discussion about the community ethnographers' varying perspectives on the community. The women shared their experiences interviewing women in the community, and the men shared their experiences interviewing male informants. Therefore their perspectives and data collection experiences varied and were debated. After the group guesses were recorded on a flip chart, academic facilitators presented and explained the survey results. Group discussion followed about the differences between the community ethnographers' perceptions of the community as informed by their experiences with data collection and the data presented. The academic ethnographers used three questions to guide the group discussion of survey results: What is happening here? Why is it happening? and, What program does the community need to address this issue? These questions are based on Freire's problem-posing approach to critical reflection (Hope & Timmel, 1984).

For example, the academic team members asked the group to guess the percentages of married women working and the percentages of husbands sharing household work in the United States and in Mexico. To illustrate how these guesses relate to findings, Table 10.1 presents selected guess estimates and the corresponding observed data from the ethnosexual survey for the household division of labor. What is striking about the information in Table 10.1 is that, in many cases, community ethnographers overestimated the traditional orientation of Mexican women in Mexico and underestimated traditional gender orientations in Durham. Specifically, they tended to think a greater percentage of the women worked in the United States than was actually the case, and they tended to grossly underestimate the percentages of men who assist with housework in both Mexico and Durham.

In elaborating on the lack of correspondence between expectations and estimates, team members provided an ethnographic account of the processes at play. This grounded the immigrant experience within the structural context of the Durham immigrant community. Even though employment opportunities are more plentiful in the United States than in Mexico, they suggested that the constraints imposed by family life might be stronger as the kin-provided child care common in Mexico is not available. Some women in the group also suggested that the poor quality of the jobs available to immigrant women in the United States restricts their employment. The majority of jobs open to these women, who generally lack legal authorization to work and have limited English

Table 10.1. Community Ethnographers' Predictions and Results from the Ethnosexual Survey for Household Division of Labor in Mexico and the United States

	CBPR Predictions				Observed Through
	1 Ethnographer Guessed	2 Ethnographers Guessed	3 Ethnographers Guessed	4 Ethnographers Guessed	Ethnosexual Survey
Married women working					
Mexico	30%	20%	10%	5%	25%
U.S.	60	70	90	80	51
Husbands sharing household work					
Mexico[a]	1	0	5	—	36
U.S.	10–20	15	10	0	37

[a]The numbers of guesses do not add up to ten for this item because not all group members offered a guess.

language ability, are in domestic and other low-skilled service occupations that pay very poorly.

Similar considerations applied to the interpretation of the estimates for the proportion of men assisting with household work. Although most members of the group held a view of Mexican men as being *machista* and very unlikely to assist with household chores, they believed men were considerably more likely to do so in the United States than in Mexico. The ethnosexual survey results showed very little differences across contexts, however, with close to 37 percent of husbands assisting with household work in both Mexico and the United States (Parrado, Flippen, & McQuiston, 2004).

The group suggested that differences in men's work environments in Mexico and the United States might explain why men do not become more involved in Durham, especially because many more women work in Durham than do in Mexico. Women in the United States sometimes feel that it is unreasonable to ask their husbands to do work around the house after working long hours and frequently in manual occupations such as construction.

This example illustrates the importance of the reflective component of CBEPR, including the centrality of group discussions and collective understanding in interpreting the findings. Once presented with survey findings, community ethnographers were confronted with unexpected patterns that led them to examine their own preconceptions and draw from their participant observations in the community to help explain them. This process not only gave depth and context to the quantitative analysis but also broadened the whole group's understanding of the community. The end result of the reciprocal questioning of findings, assumptions, and experiences provided a collective ethnographic account of the findings as well as the group's critical reflections.

REFLECTIONS ON CAPACITY BUILDING

The specific objectives of this community-based participatory research group were to increase capacity on multiple levels as group members collectively developed an understanding of community needs and strengths related to gender, migration, and HIV risk. Ultimately, the participants want to gain additional resources to develop the type of interventions they envision based on what they have learned by working on this project. The academic partners, ECH, and Horizonte Latino have agreed to respond to a program announcement for community-partnered interventions (National Institute of Nursing Research Program Announcement-02-134). Since its inception, Horizonte Latino has included an action phase aimed at identifying the types of interventions the community needs and the ways in which these interventions should be delivered. Thus far

Horizonte Latino has identified an initial list of grant proposal ideas, including the following:

- Programs targeting men at the work site
- A men's group at ECH
- Multiple LHA groups to target large Latino apartment complexes
- Activities for Latinos to do in their free time

The project group will still target HIV/AIDS, but in a very broad context that also considers migration, gender, social isolation, alcohol use, and perhaps domestic violence. ECH will assist the academic team members in grant writing and resources will be shared across institutions. Horizonte Latino will continue its critical role of informing grant development through shared learning.

In addition to the broader picture, Horizonte Latino members have learned multiple research skills such as

- Human subjects training
- Research 101, including random sampling techniques
- Structured and semistructured interviewing skills
- Participant observation and recording field notes
- Group facilitation and organizational skills
- Group process and critical reflection
- Cultural analysis and interpretation

One community participant described the value of the experience as follows:

The story of the group is like a long journey . . . we began brainstorming, then planned the ethnosexual survey. We designed the survey ourselves, discussed each question including which words to use and which words not to use. We decided which questions were good and which were not. Then we went back and checked the survey again, added a few new questions and discarded others. Finally, we went to the apartments to find people, to observe how they live, what the apartments and the surroundings looked like. We learned so many things by going to the apartments. Then we came back to the group meetings and discussed our experiences, what it was like to do the surveys. Many of us were surprised by what we were finding because we witnessed so many things while doing the surveys. We liked this fieldwork and think it was a great idea that the same people who developed the questions for the survey would then reach out and visit the apartments and do the surveys and then come back and discuss our experiences. We could see how the questions we helped to design worked in real life.

ECH staff who are also members of Horizonte Latino have commented on how their dual roles are basically cross-fertilizing and how skills learned in each role are used in both ECH and Horizonte Latino. Academics have had similar experiences as they function on multiple ECH committees and as Horizonte members. The authors believe that initially existing community resources contributed to the success of the project and that now the success of the project has contributed to community resources.

CHALLENGES AND LIMITATIONS

Combining ethnography and CBPR added a level to an already complex and time-consuming process. However, much of what the community ethnographers learned they learned from each other in collaborative meetings. Therefore, what might be viewed as a time-consuming challenge produced the shared learnings that allowed for collective insight and problem solving. However, there are always additional challenges. Differences in educational levels and style meant that some of the ethnographers wrote little and told the stories they gathered to the academic team weekly (the stories were then recorded as field notes by the academics). These differences in approach mean that the project has a wealth of data, but there are some inconsistencies in the type of data recorded for each interview. The academic team members also had to learn and recognize the strengths of the ethnographers to support them.

The collective meetings to discuss data and work on analysis and cultural and structural interpretation were sometimes a challenge because the ethnographers had such compelling stories to tell about their field experiences. The group had to balance staying on task to answer research questions and allowing members to share their stories. Community facilitators became skillful at keeping the group on task while respecting the members' needs to tell stories.

LESSONS LEARNED AND IMPLICATIONS FOR PRACTICE

This section is divided into how group members learned and what they learned. Sometimes a statement from a group member is supplied to give the reader a better understanding of the lessons presented. Many statements represent co-learning and are a melding of insights from both the academic and the community ethnographers.

How Group Members Learned

Group structure. The academics learned that splitting the large group by gender when dealing with culturally sensitive topics facilitated discussions. The community ethnographers said that they felt comfortable in their small groups even though sensitive topics would be shared with the large group.

Ownership. Participating in the research process from its inception was very important to community ethnographers who participated in all aspects of the research and felt ownership of the process. They particularly valued designing the ethnosexual survey. For example, Consuelo said, "I have learned so many lessons . . . the main one is having had the possibility to participate from the beginning, starting from the design of the survey."

What Group Members Learned

Building an understanding of ethnographic methods. The academic members learned that the community ethnographers understood difficult concepts if they were presented in a context relevant to the group's life experiences. Community ethnographers learned that sharing some of their own stories helped survey respondents feel more at ease when discussing sensitive topics such as migration.

Immigrants interviewing immigrants. The ethnographers learned that sharing their own stories of migration helped them build a relationship with the respondents and encouraged openness. As Adriana said, "You need to build a relationship first, a conversation, a shared feeling that we are both going through the same experiences, that we are both immigrants."

Building on capacity at the individual and organizational levels. Inviting LHAs trained in our earlier programs to participate allowed the group to build on existing capacity. This saved the academic members' time and energy and increased the project's likelihood of being successful. Including ECH staff in the group facilitated the flow of information between the ECH and Horizonte Latino and allowed for direct application of skills to ECH. Blanca reported that "I like the way the group is organized because I can use it as a model for my work at El Centro Hispano."

Carrying out CBEPR with a marginalized group. The academic participants felt that the group could not have successfully conducted its research with recently arrived and often fearful immigrants nor could it have fully understood the meaning of much of the data without the community participants. The ethnographic approach the academics took with their community colleagues enriched the experience and facilitated an in-depth cultural and structural interpretation of data.

Taking action. There were many spin-offs from this research, things that were never planned or even thought about. Motivation for action has come through this work. For example, Julio told the group:

> One of the most rewarding experiences for me was my presentation at the [March 2003] CBPR conference [in Chapel Hill] [see McQuiston, Uribe,

Olmos-Muñiz, & Parrado, 2003]. This was the first time that I ever gave a presentation and I did it in English. I did not feel very comfortable, but I took it as a challenge. I felt very good that the audience had a lot of questions and comments for me. This experience helped me to realize what I had learned; it was like suddenly realizing, "here I am" . . . to collect all the ideas that I ever had as I realized that people in the audience had an interest in listening to them. It was like "Open your eyes," and, "Oh! This is what I have to do." From the day after the conference I felt motivated to reach out and talk to men in the community. We founded a group so men would have something to do with their free time. One of the participants from the community had experience in a soccer league so we decided to create one in Durham. Our initial group of eight has grown [to] twenty-seven soccer teams. This is something that makes me feel good, because I always thought that we needed alternatives for the use of free time among Latinos, but it was only . . . after I gave that presentation that I took action.

Collectively writing this chapter. Collectively writing this chapter was a challenge. Both of the community participants who are chapter coauthors work several jobs and have little time. In addition, neither was accustomed to an academic writing style. After we met and discussed the purpose of the chapter and reviewed the guidelines, we decided that the community participants would contribute what they wanted to write within the context of the guidelines and that the first author would be responsible for incorporating their contributions into the chapter. We also used phone calls and e-mails to facilitate our writing. One community participant typed his contribution and the other taped his ideas. The community participants worked in Spanish, and the academics worked in English.

CONCLUSION

Cross-cultural research in an area of health disparities is a challenge for everyone. Adapting community-based participatory research so that a CBPR project can take an ethnographic approach allows a cultural context that considers values, beliefs, and behaviors. This approach is particularly important for studies of immigrants and facilitates a view of both the positive and negative effects of migration. In this case, participant observation and the conversational approach to the ethnosexual survey allowed the project team to learn about the respondents' stories and to see how they live in the community. Participant observation was critical to providing a context for analysis of the data as well as for grant proposal writing efforts. The CBEPR approach reinforced the authors' belief that any culturally competent program or research project with immigrants must be informed by the immigration experience and the cultural values that are in flux as a result of that experience.

In this study, time spent in the community allowed community ethnographers to see firsthand the crowded and sometimes dangerous conditions of the apartment complexes. It also allowed them to see that for some the challenges of migration brought great creativity and the capability to think beyond boundaries and to face adversity with ingenuity. The stories heard reflected courage and strength as Latinos learned to value their homeland, to gain a wider perspective on world issues, and to develop skills to adapt to adversity and challenges. Eventually, these skills will result in less vulnerability and more self-confidence. CBEPR provides a method for deep understanding and identification of the needs and capacity of the community and can lead to action to address the issues identified.

References

Arnold, R., Burke, B., James, C., Martin, D., & Thomas, B. (1995). *Educating for change* (4th ed.). Toronto: Between the Lines.

Austin, D. (2003). Community-based collaborative team ethnography: A community-university-agency partnership. *Human Organization, 62*(2), 143–151.

Boyle, J. S. (1994). Styles of ethnography. In J. M. Morse (Ed.), *Critical issues in qualitative research methods* (pp. 159–185). Thousand Oaks, CA: Sage.

Chambers, E. (2000). Applied ethnography. In N. K. Denzin & Y. S. Lincoln (Eds.), *Handbook of qualitative research* (2nd ed., pp. 851–869). Thousand Oaks, CA: Sage.

Chrisman, N. J., Strickland, C. J., Powell, K., Squeochs, M. D., & Yallup, M. (1999). Community partnership research with the Yakama Indian Nation. *Human Organization, 58*(2), 134–141.

Flaskerud, J., & Kim, S. (1999). Health problems of Asian and Latino immigrants. *Nursing Clinics of North America, 32*(2), 359–380.

Flaskerud, J., & Nyamathi, A. (2000). Collaborative inquiry with low income Latina women. *Journal of Health Care for the Poor and Underserved, 11*(3), 326–342.

Flaskerud, J., & Winslow, B. (1998). Conceptualizing vulnerable populations: Health-related research. *Nursing Research, 47,* 69–78.

Freire, P. (1970). *Pedagogy of the oppressed.* New York: Seabury Press.

Freire, P. (1973). *Education for critical consciousness.* New York: Seabury Press.

Geertz, C. (1983). *Local knowledge: Further essays in interpretive anthropology.* New York: Basic Books.

Hondagneu-Sotelo, P. (2003). Gender and immigration: A retrospective and introduction. In P. Hondagneu-Sotelo (Ed.), *Gender and U.S. immigration: Contemporary trends* (pp. 3–19). Berkley: University of California Press.

Hope, A., & Timmel, S. (1984). *Training for transformation: A handbook for community workers.* Gweru, Zimbabwe: Mambo Press.

Hope, A., & Timmel, S. (1995). *Training for transformation: A handbook for community workers* (rev. ed.). Gweru, Zimbabwe: Mambo Press.

Israel, B., Schulz, A., Parker, E., Becker, A., Allen, A., III,, & Guzman, R. (2003). Critical issues in developing and following community-based participatory research principles. In M. Minkler & N. Wallerstein (Eds.), *Community-based participatory research for health* (pp. 53–76). San Francisco: Jossey-Bass.

Lassiter, L. (2000). Commentary. *American Indian Quarterly, 24*(4), 601–615.

LeCompte, M. D., & Schensul, J. J. (1999a). Analyzing and interpreting ethnographic data. In J. J. Schensul & M. D. LeCompte (Eds.), *Ethnographer's toolkit* (Vol. 5). Walnut Creek, CA: AltaMira Press.

LeCompte, M. D., & Schensul, J. J. (1999b). Designing and conducting ethnographic research. In M. D. LeCompte & J. J. Schensul (Eds.), *Ethnographer's toolkit* (Vol. 1). Walnut Creek, CA: AltaMira Press.

Mannheim, B., & Tedlock, D. (1995). Introduction. In D. Tedlock & B. Mannheim (Eds.), *The dialogic emergence of culture* (pp. 1–32). Urbana: University of Illinois Press.

McQuiston, C., Choi-Hevel, S., & Clawson, M. (2001). Protegiendo Nuestra Comunidad: Empower participatory education for HIV prevention. *Journal of Transcultural Nursing, 12*, 275–283.

McQuiston, C., Larson, K., Parrado, E., & Flaskerud, J. (2002). AIDS knowledge and measurement considerations with unacculturated Latinos. *Western Journal of Nursing Research, 24*(4), 354–372.

McQuiston, C., & Uribe, L. (2001). Latino recruitment and retention strategies: Community-based HIV prevention. *Journal of Immigrant Health, 3*(2), 1–9.

McQuiston, C., Uribe, L., Olmos-Muñiz, J., & Parrado, E. (2003, March). *Horizonte Latino: Participatory action research with Latino community members.* Paper presented at Building Connections for Community Health: Best Practices for Promoting Health Through Participatory Methods in the Workplace and Community, a conference sponsored by the CDC, Chapel Hill, NC.

Meleis, A. (1996). Culturally competent scholarship: Substance and rigor. *Annals of Advanced Nursing Science, 19*(2), 1–16.

Parrado, E., Flippen, C., & McQuiston, C. (2004). Use of commercial sex workers among Hispanic migrants to the Southeastern United States: Implications for the diffusion of HIV. *Perspectives on Sexual and Reproductive Health, 36*(4), 325–347.

Reynolds, C. L., & Leininger, M. M. (1995). Madeline M. Leininger: Cultural Care Diversity and Universality Theory. In C. M. McQuiston & A. A. Webb (Eds.), *Foundations of nursing theory: Contributions of 12 key theorists* (pp. 371–414). Thousand Oaks, CA: Sage.

Sawyer, L., Regev, H., Proctor, S., Nelson, M., Messias, D., Barnes, D., et al. (1995). Matching versus cultural competence in research: Methodological considerations. *Research in Nursing and Health, 18*, 557–567.

Schensul, J. J., LeCompte, M. D., Hess, G. A., Nastasi, B. K., Berg, M. J., Williamson, L., et al. (1999). Using ethnographic data: Interventions, public programming and public policy. In J. J. Schensul & M. D. LeCompte (Eds.), *Ethnographer's toolkit* (Vol. 7). Walnut Creek, CA: AltaMira Press.

Schensul, J. J., Weeks, M., & Singer, M. (1999). Building research partnerships. In M. D. LeCompte, M. Weeks, & M. Singer (Eds.), *Researcher roles and research partnerships* (pp. 85–164). Walnut Creek, CA: AltaMira Press.

Schmidley, A. D. (2001). Profile of the foreign-born population in the U.S.: 2000 (Current Population Reports, Series P23-206). Washington, DC: U.S. Census Bureau.

Schwandt, T. A. (1994). Constructivist, interpretivist approaches to human inquiry. In N. K. Denzin & Y. S. Lincoln (Eds.), *Handbook of qualitative research* (pp. 118–137). Thousand Oaks, CA: Sage.

Stringer, E., Agnello, M. F., Baldwin, S. C., Christensen, L. M., Henry, D. P., Henry, K., et al. (1997). *Community-based ethnography: Breaking traditional boundaries of research, teaching and learning.* Mahwah, NJ: Erlbaum.

Suro, R., & Singer, A. (2002). *Latino growth in metropolitan American: Changing patterns and new locations.* Washington, DC: Center on Urban and Metropolitan Policy and the Pew Hispanic Center.

Tedlock, B. (2000). Ethnography and ethnographic representation. In N. K. Denzin & Y. S. Lincoln (Eds.), *Handbook of qualitative methods* (2nd ed., pp. 455–486). Thousand Oaks, CA: Sage.

Vidich, A. J., & Lyman, S. M. (1994). Qualitative methods: Their history in sociology and anthropology. In N. K. Denzin & Y. S. Lincoln (Eds.), *Handbook of qualitative research* (pp. 23–59). Thousand Oaks, CA: Sage.

Weinick, R., Zuvekas, S., & Cohen, J. (2000). Racial and ethnic differences in access to and use of health care services, 1977 to 1996. *Medical Care Research Review, 57*(Suppl. 1), 36–54.

CHAPTER ELEVEN

What's with the Wheezing?

Methods Used by the Seattle–King County Healthy Homes Project to Assess Exposure to Indoor Asthma Triggers

James Krieger, Carol A. Allen, John W. Roberts,
Lisa Carol Ross, and Tim K. Takaro

Exposure to harmful substances in the environment is associated with many adverse health effects. Allergens and irritating chemicals can worsen asthma (Institute of Medicine, 2000). Lead can decrease IQ and cause elevated blood pressure (Needleman & Gatsonis, 1990). Air pollution can induce respiratory problems and worsen heart disease (Holgate, Samet, Koren, & Maynard, 1999). Pesticides are often neurotoxic, can disrupt hormonal functions, and can cause cancer (Rom, 1998).

Assessment of harmful environmental exposures is crucial to understanding and preventing environmentally linked disease. Numerous exposure assessment methods are applicable to community-based participatory research (CBPR). They have arisen primarily from techniques developed by industrial hygienists to assess hazards in the workplace. The requirements of sampling design, sample collection, laboratory detection and quantification methods, and time-space

Acknowledgments: Primary funding for the project discussed in this chapter was provided by National Institute of Environmental Health Sciences (NIEHS) grants 5 R21 ES09095 and 1 R01 ES11378. Additional support was provided by Seattle Partners for Healthy Communities (a Centers for Disease Control and Prevention–funded Urban Research Center) grant U48/CCU009654-07, the Nesholm Foundation, and the Seattle Foundation. The project community health workers—Carol Allen, Zhoni Gilbert, Jean Jackson, Cindy Mai, Margarita Mendoza, Nilsa Nicholson, Matthew Nguyen, and LaTanya Wilson—worked devotedly with their clients. Carol Allen, Georgiana Arnold, Kristine Edwards, and Lisa Ross coordinated field and research operations.

analysis require the integration of multiple disciplines, including toxicology, physical science, chemistry, engineering, biostatistics, and medicine.

The techniques developed for measuring specific workplace health hazards have been applied in the community setting to some of the same toxicants, although adapted for assessing lower levels of exposure. For example, the outdoor area monitors used by the U.S. Environmental Protection Agency (EPA) to identify pollution airsheds had their origins in the workplace as particulate monitors. Methods of measuring exposures include air, dust, water, and soil sampling and biomarker measurements. Air samplers allow quantification of levels of ozone, sulfur dioxide, nitric oxides, particulates, volatile organic compounds, biohazards (for example fungi, allergens), and other pollutants. Dust samples collected from inside the home are used to determine levels of allergens, lead, pesticides, and other persistent organic compounds, endotoxins, and fungi. Water and soil samples are assessed for heavy metals such as lead or arsenic, persistent organic compounds, and carcinogens. Biomarkers measure levels in bodily fluids of toxic substances such as heavy metals, organic compounds, and antibodies to allergens; they can also assess markers of the body's own inflammatory response to toxicants (American Conference of Governmental Industrial Hygienists, 2004).

Sampling techniques for measuring exposures to toxicants and irritants may be burdensome and require a high degree of study participant cooperation. Therefore a community-based participatory research (CBPR) approach may be especially useful in fostering collaboration between outside researchers and community members to design sampling methods that are acceptable to participants. In this chapter, we describe the application of CBPR to collecting information on exposure to indoor environmental asthma triggers.

ENVIRONMENTAL EXPOSURE ASSESSMENT METHODS AND ASTHMA

Asthma is a common environmental disease triggered by airborne allergens and respiratory irritants. Asthma affects 15 million Americans (7 percent of the population) (Mannino et al., 2002). Prevalence and morbidity among children in the United States have increased dramatically in the past two decades and remain high (Mannino et al., 2002). The causes of increased asthma prevalence are not well understood (Crater & Platts-Mills, 1998). However, a large body of evidence suggests that exposure and sensitization to allergens and irritants found in the indoor environment are major factors in the development and exacerbation of asthma; these allergens and irritants include dust mite allergens, pet danders, tobacco smoke, dampness and molds, cockroach antigens, rodent urine, endotoxins, and viruses (Andriessen, Brunekreef, & Roemer, 1998;

Custovic & Woodcock, 2001; Institute of Medicine, 2000; Phipatanakul, Eggleston, Wright, & Wood, 2000; Zureik et al., 2002).

Given the widespread prevalence of indoor asthma triggers (Arbes et al., 2004), decreasing exposure to them is an important strategy for reducing asthma morbidity. Reduction of exposure to specific triggers in the home, such as dust mite antigen or tobacco smoke, can reduce asthma morbidity (Platts-Mills, Vaughan, Carter, & Woodfolk, 2000; Shapiro et al., 1999; Wilson et al., 2001). In recent years the Healthy Homes model has emerged as a promising approach for reducing exposure to multiple asthma triggers and improving indoor environmental quality (Alliance for Healthy Homes, 2004; Healthy House, 2004; Jacobs, Friedman, Ashley, & McNairy, 1999; Krieger, Song, Takaro, & Weaver, 2005; Morgan et al., 2004). The model includes auditing the home environment, addressing multiple exposures, motivating participants to take low-cost actions, offering advice and tools to reduce exposures, and providing advocacy. We—the Seattle–King County Healthy Homes Project—along with others, have developed and tested the effectiveness of the Healthy Homes model for reducing asthma morbidity among socially marginalized populations, who often live in substandard housing and experience high levels of asthma morbidity and exposure to asthma triggers (Aligne, Auinger, Byrd, & Weitzman, 2000; Krieger, Takaro, et al., 2002; Litonjua, Carey, Weiss, & Gold, 1999; Mannino et al., 2002).

Reduction of exposure to indoor asthma triggers is a major intermediate outcome that can be used for assessing the impact of home interventions on asthma. The most common approach for assessing exposure to allergens (usually dust mite, cat, dog, roach, and rodent) is measuring allergen concentrations in house dust. Investigators collect surface dust from floors and bedding with a vacuum and then employ immunological methods to determine the concentration of allergens (Chapman, Aalberse, Brown, & Platts-Mills, 1988; Luczynska et al., 1989). Specialized vacuums can collect dust quantitatively from measured surface areas, allowing the determination of surface dust loading. *Loading* is a measure of the amount of allergen per unit of area, which may be a more accurate measure of exposure than simply reporting the concentration of allergen in dust (Braun-Fuhrlander et al., 2002; Takaro, Krieger, Song, & Beaudet, 2004).

Measurement of surface dust, however, may convey only a partial picture of exposure to toxicants contained in dust. Roberts and colleagues suggest that dust deeply embedded in carpet serves as a reservoir for surface dust, continually recharging the surface component (Roberts, Clifford, Glass, & Hummer, 1999). The three-spot test can provide a quantitative measure of deep dust (Roberts, Glass, & Mickelson, 2004). Using a vacuum cleaner with a dirt detector light that changes from red to green when nearly all the dust in the carpet is removed, one measures the time in seconds required to obtain green lights on three spots in the carpet three feet apart.

Methods to assess exposure to tobacco smoke include self-reported smoking behavior, observation of evidence of smoking in the home, air sampling for nicotine, and measurement of nicotine metabolites in urine or saliva. Recent evidence suggests that self-reported tobacco use correlates well with ambient nicotine levels as a measure of environmental tobacco smoke (Hovell, Zakarian, Wahlgren, Matt, & Emmons, 2000).

Measurement of indoor mold levels presents special challenges. There is no agreed-upon standard method. Visible mold is assessed by observing the density and area of mold-covered surfaces in the home, using a standardized rating system (Miller, Haisley, & Reinhardt, 2000). Mold in settled dust can be measured with assays that determine fungal biomass (for example ergosterol or other fungal chemical constituents) (Bush & Portnoy, 2001).

The presence of pests such as rodents and roaches is assessed by observational methods as well as measurement of allergen in dust. Investigators set roach traps to count the number of active roaches. They also observe for evidence of roach or rodent presence in the home (for example, eggs, feces, surface staining) and ask study participants if they have seen any of these pests.

SEATTLE–KING COUNTY HEALTHY HOMES PROJECT

The Seattle–King County Healthy Homes Project (HH) employs community health workers in efforts to reduce asthma morbidity among children with asthma living in ethnically diverse, low-income communities. Community health workers (CHWs) are well suited to implementing the HH approach among these households (Butz et al., 1994; Love, Gardner, & Legion, 1997; Swider, 2002). They are members of the community who promote health through education, social support, and advocacy. They have been increasingly involved in environmental exposure reduction projects in marginalized communities in the past decade.

The HH project is being carried out in two phases. In Healthy Homes-I, which concluded in 2001, community health workers made home visits to help participants reduce exposure to indoor environmental asthma triggers. Healthy Homes-II has built on what was learned in the first phase. Community health workers assist participants in reducing exposure to asthma triggers and in improving their skills in managing the medical aspects of asthma control. This chapter will focus on the exposure assessment activities in both phases of Healthy Homes.

The Healthy Homes Project staff recruited children with symptoms of asthma and their families for the HH project from community and public health clinics, local hospitals, and emergency departments and also through referrals from community residents and agencies. A CHW made an initial home visit to each participant, in which the CHW and the home resident conducted a structured home environmental assessment. Each finding from the assessment was used to generate specific actions for the resident and the CHW. The CHW and the resident then prioritized the actions to prepare an action plan. The CHW made four additional visits over a year to provide education and social support, encouragement of participant actions, resources to reduce exposures (allergy control pillow and mattress encasements, low-emission vacuums with dirt finders, commercial-quality door mats, cleaning kits, referrals to smoking cessation counseling, roach bait, rodent traps), assistance with roach and rodent eradication, and advocacy for improved housing conditions. (For more details about the program, see Krieger, Takaro, et al., 2002; Krieger, Song, Takaro, & Weaver, 2005; Public Health—Seattle & King Country, 2004.)

The Healthy Homes Project evaluated HH with a randomized, controlled trial (RCT) (Meinert, 1986). The RCT, widely used in clinical research, is well suited for measuring the health effects of a carefully defined, individual-level intervention. It permits direct assessment of the intervention effect while minimizing threats to internal validity (such as confounding and bias in measurement of outcomes) and removes the effects of external temporal trends. RCTs rarely incorporate a CBPR approach. The Healthy Homes Project found the application of a CBPR approach to be quite helpful, if not essential, in conducting an RCT of the HH intervention.

We designed the organizational structure of the HH project to formalize participation by involved agencies, parents, staff, and researchers and to promote implementation of the CBPR principles developed by Seattle Partners for Healthy Communities (Koné et al., 2000; Krieger, Takaro, et al., 2002; Sullivan et al., 2001). Seattle Partners (a CDC-funded Urban Research Center that comprises community agencies, community activists, public health professionals, academics, and health providers) provided high-level project oversight and guidance for the first phase of the HH project (Krieger, Allen, et al., 2002). The King County Asthma Forum (the local asthma coalition, with community participation from people with asthma, their families, and twenty-one agencies) played a similar role for the second phase. These partnerships approved any major deviations from protocols and budget.

The HH project developed a project steering committee consisting of CHWs, community partners (for example, community health providers, community-based organizations), and researchers. Some committee participants were also members of Seattle Partners or the King County Asthma Forum, whereas others were associated only with the HH project. The committee met monthly during the start-up phase, semiannually during implementation, and every two months during the data analysis process. The committee participated in the development and approval of project protocols and evaluation methods, approved key project staff hires, monitored project progress, suggested questions for analysis, and reviewed and interpreted evaluation results. Committee members made decisions by consensus, and the principal investigator facilitated committee meetings. An operations team from Public Health—Seattle & King County, the fiscal agent, had responsibility for day-to-day operations.

We also formed the HH Parent Advisory Group, consisting of parent representatives of project enrollees. This group reviewed participant recruitment strategies, evaluation tools, intervention protocols, project implementation, and evaluation findings. The steering committee and operations team valued the advice they received from the advisory group and in nearly every case, adopted it. A CHW coordinated the group and represented it on the steering committee. The steering committee experimented with having two parents as committee members but found this was not particularly effective in gaining participant input. Parents were more vocal when they had a separate forum.

The HH intervention significantly reduced asthma-related symptoms and urgent health services utilization and improved caregiver quality of life (Krieger et al., 2005). We observed an increase in participant actions to reduce exposures, and decreases in floor dust loading, excessive moisture, roach activity, and a composite measure of exposure to asthma triggers (Krieger et al., 2005; Takaro et al., 2004).

HOME ENVIRONMENTAL ASSESSMENT IN THE HEALTHY HOMES PROJECT

The home environmental assessment component of Healthy Homes had two goals. The first was to identify exposures in the home in order to develop a home action plan. The second was to collect research data to describe the effect of the intervention on exposures. As described in the following sections, the partners involved in the HH project engaged in a number of activities related to this environmental assessment (for example, deciding what to measure and determining measurement protocols).

Deciding What to Measure

The researchers brought scientific knowledge of indoor asthma triggers and the underlying housing conditions that increase trigger levels. They also offered knowledge of methods of assessing exposure to triggers.

Community members (CHWs, partner agency representatives, and parents of children with asthma) knew which exposures were common in their communities. This information emerged during discussions in the steering committee and parent advisory group and from the experience of the CHWs working with many households. Their insights were useful in prioritizing the exposures to measure. For example, although the researchers initially believed that roaches were not common in the Seattle climate zone, community members knew otherwise and encouraged more extensive roach exposure assessment. The subsequently collected exposure data substantiated the community members' knowledge: 18 percent of the homes had roaches. In addition, the scientific literature emphasized the role pet allergens play in asthma exacerbations, but community members pointed out that most low-income families could not afford to keep pets. Therefore we chose to collect less extensive data on pet exposure.

Local experts in exposure assessment also helped identify measures of exposure. The Washington chapter of the American Lung Association had developed the Home Environmental Assessment List (HEAL) for use by community volunteers in assessing indoor environmental quality (Dickey, 1998). Working with community environmental activists (John Roberts and Phillip Dickey), the Lung Association, and community residents through in-person meetings and e-mail communications, researchers modified the HEAL so that it included more information about asthma triggers and was more culturally appropriate for the HH participants (Krieger, Takaro, et al., 2002).

Exposure Measures

The researchers synthesized these inputs and proposed a set of exposure measures. The project steering committee reviewed the proposal and agreed on the measures listed in Table 11.1: for example, floor surface dust loading, dust mite allergen level, visible mold, and surface moisture. The researchers developed technical protocols to collect data for these measures.

In addition to assessing the exposures themselves, HH assessed the underlying conditions that affect exposure levels, including dust-control behaviors (controlling track-in, vacuuming and cleaning, using allergen-control bedding covers), mold and moisture problems and contributing "structural" factors (condensation, water infiltration and damage, leaks), ventilation (windows, fans, appliances, weatherization, heating, insulation, vapor barriers), structural conditions (carpeting, building age, condition of paint, structural deficits, recent remodeling), food debris and storage, trash, clutter, heating system filters and ducts, heating and cooking sources, location of garage, use and storage of hazardous and toxic products, and tap and washing machine water temperature. These measures were identified through a participatory process similar to that already described for selecting exposure measures.

Data Collection Methods

The project collected exposure data by completing a home environmental audit, collecting dust samples, and measuring deep carpet dust with the three-spot test.

Table 11.1. Exposure Assessment Measures

Exposure	Measure	Reference
Floor surface dust loading	μg of fine dust per m^2	Roberts, Clifford, Glass, & Hummer, 1999
Carpet deep dust loading	Three-spot dirt sensor test (seconds)	Roberts, Glass, & Mickelson, 2004
Dust mites	ELISA (μg of allergen per g dust, μg per m^2)	Luczynska et al., 1989
Fungi in settled dust	Ergosterol (μg per g dust, μg per m^2)	Miller & Young, 1997; Axelsson, Saraf, & Larsson, 1995; Saraf, Larsson, Burge, & Milton, 1997
Visual mold	Cm^2 covered; mold intensity scale	Miller, Haisley, & Reinhardt, 2000
Surface moisture	Surface moisture probe (percentage)	
Home dampness	Presence of visible mold, water damage, or condensation	Dales, 1991; Dales, Burnett, & Zwanenburg, 1991; Pasanen et al., 2000; Strachan, 1988
Global moisture score	Observer-rated moisture using 1–10 Likert scale	
Roaches	MaxForce traps (number of roaches trapped); participant and community health worker observation; ELISA (μg of allergen per g dust, μg per m^2)	Mollet et al., 1997; Pollart et al., 1991
Pets	Self-report and observation: pets in home, access to child's bedroom; ELISA (μg of cat and dog allergen per g dust, μg per m^2)	Chapman, Aalberse, Brown, & Platts-Mills, 1988; de Groot, Goei, van Swieten, & Aalberse, 1991
Tobacco use: caregiver	Self-report of use: frequency/ quantity; site(s) of smoking; use of smoking jacket	Glasgow et al., 1998; Coghlin, Hammond, & Gann, 1989
Tobacco use: others in household	Self-report of use: frequency/ quantity; site(s) of smoking; use of smoking jacket	
Viral respiratory infections	Symptoms by self-report	
Toxic products in home/ brought home from work	Inventory by interview and observation; work history	U.S. Department of Health and Human Services, 1995
Global indoor environment appearance	Observer rating using 1–10 Likert scale	

Home Environmental Checklist. The CHWs used the Home Environmental Checklist (HEC) to obtain data for many of these measures. The HEC was a structured audit of the indoor environment. Involving CHWs and participants in development of the HEC was important for ensuring its feasibility. Drawing from the Home Environmental Assessment List mentioned previously, researchers developed an initial draft of the HEC and revised it based on comments made during meetings with CHWs and steering committee members. For example, a community partner pointed out that renters might lack the knowledge to answer some questions about their homes (for example, whether vapor barriers were present in crawl spaces) and suggested that it would be better to rely on data collectors' observations for these variables. The CHWs then pilot-tested the draft HEC in each other's homes and reported their suggestions to the researchers, who made further modifications. Then the CHWs tested the next draft in the homes of five parent advisory group members and gave further feedback to the researchers. For example, some parents found the wording of the question, "Have you had roaches in your home?" offensive and were more comfortable when the question was reworded as, "Have you had any problems with roaches in your home?" a small change, but one the parents felt placed less blame on the participant. Parents also suggested prefacing collection of data on pet exposure with the statement that any information about pets in the home would be kept confidential, because the parents knew that many pets were in violation of the terms of a rental agreement. In addition, the CHWs suggested changing the format and item order of the HEC to coordinate the flow of data collection with the sequence of inspection during the home visit (for example, assessing outdoor features before indoor features). CHW input was collected during regular staff meetings held every two weeks attended by CHWs, researchers, and project managers, and during special meetings to review drafts. Asking CHWs to provide written feedback was less effective for obtaining useful input.

Once the English version was finalized, the researchers contracted for translation of the HEC into Spanish and Vietnamese, followed by back translation and then a review by a local native speaker of the translated HEC to ensure accuracy and cultural equivalence of the document. CHWs then pilot-tested the translated versions, and researchers made additional refinements based on the pilot test results.

The HEC was completed jointly by the participant and the CHW as they walked through the home at the first visit. Discussions at staff and parent advisory group meetings revealed several benefits of including the participants in the data collection process: participants were able to observe and learn about adverse exposures, the awkwardness of having an "inspector" walk around the home unattended was avoided, and CHWs and participants agreed about the presence of exposures. (The HEC is available at www.metrokc.gov/health/asthma/healthyhomes.)

Dust Sampling. Community data collectors learned how to collect dust samples. The researchers simplified standard dust collection methods as a result of pilot testing prior to project initiation. Further modifications were made in response to comments from the data collectors as they gained experience in the field (for example, it was decided to discontinue the use of metric numbers in the data collection and to create presized sampling templates to replace measuring and taping of the sampling area). The data collectors also provided feedback to project engineers on how the dust-sampling vacuum could be improved. The engineers used this information when they redesigned the vacuum to improve ease of use.

Three-Spot Dust Test. We used the three-spot test, described previously, as a quantitative yet participatory method for participants to assess the amount of dust in their carpets. Each participant received a vacuum cleaner with dirt-finder. At each visit, the CHW conducted the test and offered feedback to the participant. Participants also conducted the test on their own. CHWs observed that the positive feedback from the green light appeared to motivate more effective vacuuming.

Data Collectors

Project partners had lively discussions about who could best collect data. Advantages that may accrue when professional, experienced research staff collect data include fewer missing data, less bias and more neutrality in posing questions, less need for training and monitoring, and greater adherence to collection protocols. However, community members who collect data may obtain more accurate and honest responses and greater engagement by respondents. Community data collectors may be particularly successful in collecting data in marginalized communities because they share community, culture, and life experiences with the participants and are readily welcomed into the home (Love et al., 1997; Swider, 2002). Ultimately, HH used community members (both CHWs and others) to collect exposure data. (See Chapter Six for a discussion of the development of an interviewer training manual for community members.)

IMPROVING EXPOSURE ASSESSMENT WITH A CBPR APPROACH

Using a CBPR approach improved exposure assessment in a number of arenas: cross-cultural issues, quantity and complexity of data, and data collection.

Cross-Cultural Issues

HH participants were members of diverse cultural groups. When collecting data, the CHWs found that different groups had different boundaries of privacy that affected what they were comfortable discussing or showing about their homes. It was best to ask directly about certain stigmatizing exposures (for example, roaches or tobacco use) with some groups and best to rely more on observation with other groups. Members of some groups were more likely to "clean house" before the exposure assessment visit, which could affect the assessment. The CHWs learned how to explain the importance of not engaging in more intensive cleaning, because of its impact on the assessment.

To address these differences, the CHWs needed to perform their work with cultural competence (Kleinman, Eisenberg, & Good, 1978; Manson, 1988), and the researchers needed to accept some flexibility in implementing data collection protocols. When possible, the project matched the ethnicities of CHWs (African American, Latina, and Vietnamese) and participants (54 percent of the participants shared ethnicity with their CHWs). In addition, all the CHWs lived in the targeted geographical area. CHWs communicated in the primary language of nearly all participants and used interpreters for the few who needed this service. When educational materials were not available in the participant's language, the CHWs participated in developing "homegrown" resources.

The ability of the CHWs to connect with participants through shared culture and ethnicity facilitated development of trust, which in turn made participants more willing to engage in data collection. When a CHW worked with a participant whose culture differed from hers, it was especially valuable to talk person-to-person about neutral subjects (for example kids, food, weather) before moving into collecting data. The added communication helped build trust and cooperation.

Quantity and Complexity of Data

The project experienced tension between the researchers' desire for more data and more complex data collection methods and the participants' and CHWs' desires for a simpler approach. The researchers' interest in collecting comprehensive data covering multiple domains led to long versions of the HEC. The CHWs and participants pointed out that if the HEC were too long, participants would grow weary and not respond reliably to questions. The data collectors were uncomfortable in asking too much of the participants. Eventually, compromises on both sides resulted in a shorter HEC that still satisfied researcher needs for collecting the most important data. The final product reconciled multiple perspectives on questionnaire length and content, which increased the acceptability and feasibility of data collection.

The participatory approach led the project to use exposure measurement methods that relied on simple types of observation and data collection in addition to the more traditional, complex quantitative sampling methods used by many research studies. We wanted methods that could be used by CHWs and participants for developing action plans in the home. The researchers felt comfortable with this approach because evidence suggests that interviews and visual inspection can provide valid measures of home environmental conditions when compared with quantitative assessments (Dharmage et al., 1999).

Data Collection

The project staff found that frequent review and reinforcement of protocols and field observation were valuable for ensuring the quality of the data collected by community staff. For example, researchers assumed that community staff would adhere to dust collection protocols, but did not adequately consider the impact of the staff's lack of prior experience on doing so. Initially, researchers found dust samples on shelves or among project paperwork, which potentially affected the accuracy of the samples. Regular training and field observations helped address this issue. The principal investigator met regularly with the CHWs to review cases and protocols. The research coordinator performed quarterly quality-control field visits to observe dust collection, give feedback, and answer questions.

In the early stages of this work, Public Health-Seattle & King County (the project's administrative and fiscal sponsor) had contracted out the data collection and CHW components of HH to a community-based organization. However, difficulties arose with coordination of field and research activities and with the quality of data collection. A concerted effort to resolve these issues did not succeed, and the steering committee decided to transfer these activities to the public health department in order to meet project goals.

LESSONS LEARNED AND IMPLICATIONS FOR PRACTICE

The application of a CBPR approach in the context of a randomized, controlled trial resulted in a project that was well adapted to community values and realities. The perspectives of the community partners, staff, and participants led to data collection methods that were practical and culturally appropriate. The benefits in terms of logistics and participant satisfaction were evident. Field staff reported that after data collection protocols were modified based on their suggestions, data collection took less time and participants were pleased with a shorter visit. Whether there were additional benefits in the form of improved data quality was difficult to ascertain, although this appears to be the case. For example, we observed that after dust collection protocols were modified based on field staff suggestions, adherence to the protocols increased. After revising the HEC to incorporate parent and staff feedback, data completeness increased.

Each community-based participatory research project comes with its unique set of challenges and rewards (Krieger, Collier, Song, & Martin, 1999; Krieger et al., 2000; Krieger, Allen, et al., 2002). Much depends on the styles and attitudes of partners, how relationships develop, available time and resources, and the degree of congruence in vision and goals. There is always a need for mutual learning and accommodation. (See Chapter Three for a discussion of group processes appropriate for fostering partnership maintenance.) Yet what we experienced in the HH project has been similar to what we have encountered across all our projects. The following paragraphs summarize these lessons learned and their implications for practice.

Striking a balance between scientific rigor and practicality is healthy. Researchers need to contain their zeal for collecting detailed data across every conceivable domain. In most cases excessive data do not contribute to the final analyses, burden respondents unnecessarily, and waste staff time. Measures that require overly complex data collection methods can result in poor quality data.

Community members provide a valuable perspective on what data are feasible and useful to collect. The community staff pointed out that baseline data collection was taking over two hours and that both staff and participants were becoming fatigued. The researchers initially resisted shortening data collection protocols and instruments. They believed that with training and experience, the staff would become more proficient or that more skilled staff would have to be found. However, with time the researchers saw that it was the complexity of the data collection process that was the cause of the fatigue. The researchers simplified procedures and gained more respect for the skills of the staff.

However, community members do not always know what is needed to establish the scientific validity of an evaluation. They may not be aware of the information that potential funders value as evidence of effectiveness.

It is common practice in exposure assessment research to adhere to the initially established data collection protocols throughout the study. This maximizes the consistency of data collected over time. However, most traditional exposure assessment research takes place in predictable, controlled environments. The community context is much more heterogeneous and fluid. As a result, researchers must be flexible. Protocols, and even data collection instruments, may need to be modified before the data collection is completed to reflect new knowledge acquired during study implementation. For example, the CHWs observed that participants were guessing, not paying close attention, or answering inconsistently when responding to questions requiring recall over a defined time period. Researchers added prompts and began using visual cues (for example, calendars with pictures of seasons) to assist participants in answering. In addition, the questions initially used to assess exposure to environmental tobacco smoke did not appear to be determining exposure accurately, despite prior pilot testing. The CHWs observed that the questions were not sufficiently sensitive to pick up smoking by others in the household. Following this observation, the questions were revised. Any loss in the ability to make "pure" baseline and exit comparisons may be outweighed by the higher quality of the exit data.

An inclusive, participatory process has value but is time consuming. The participatory process is iterative, requires much communication and negotiation among partners, and is affected by personalities and relationships. For example, the CHWs and researchers negotiated many of the details of the way the CHWs would collect kitchen dust samples. Initially, the researchers wanted to collect dust from multiple locations, including behind the refrigerator. The CHWs found this too difficult, so this location was dropped, and dust was sampled from other locations in the kitchen. As data collection proceeded, the researchers noticed that the amount of dust collected from the kitchen was too small for analysis. The CHWs suggested additional sites that were relatively easy to access (such as under the sink and near trash receptacles), and the researchers agreed to include them.

Another instance of negotiation involved redesign of the specialized vacuum cleaners used to collect dust samples. In the Healthy Homes-I Project, the vacuum was awkward to carry, complicated to clean, and broke easily. The researchers' insistence on using it nearly led to a revolt among staff; due to the vacuum, they identified dust collection as the least desirable part of their job. Working with feedback from the CHWs, one of the authors (Roberts) developed a new version of the vacuum that was easier to use.

A participatory process facilitates recruitment. Exposure assessment is often burdensome and invasive for study participants, making it challenging to recruit them. We would not have been able to identify the 800 households eligible for participation in the HH project without community collaborators. Community organizations will refer potential participants to research projects they believe have value. Potential participants are more likely to enroll when they learn of the research project from a trusted source. The ability of a CBPR approach to facilitate recruitment may enhance participation in other exposure assessment research projects.

Mutual accountability is necessary. Researchers and community partners must agree on standards for productivity and quality in data collection and do their best to meet them. This can be tricky, especially when partners have not worked together before and discover their expectations are not the same. The project ran into difficulties collecting dust samples early in its life when the research coordinator noticed that the sampling vacuum was not being adequately cleaned between samples (allowing cross-contamination) and that samples were not being properly labeled and stored. Researchers had not adequately explained the importance of these steps in dust collection, and the community partner organization responsible for collecting samples did not maintain adequate quality assurance mechanisms. The steering committee learned that it was simpler and more reliable to have samples collected by community staff under the direct supervision of researchers than to have the supervision come from a community partner organization with limited experience in environmental sampling.

Environmental exposure assessment methods can be burdensome and invasive and have the potential to cause labeling and embarrassment. Some community partners raised concerns that potential participants would decline participation or spread the word that HH was a project to avoid if data collection were too burdensome, embarrassing, or disrespectful of privacy. Given that collecting data involved going into the home and seeing how much dust was on the floors, looking into cabinets for roaches, and asking if people exposed a child with asthma to secondhand smoke, potential participants might have refused to permit environmental sampling or might have cleaned up their home prior to an assessment visit to avoid embarrassment.

The CBPR approach made exposure assessment more acceptable. The ability of community staff to establish rapport with participants and engage in nonjudgmental relationships helped to overcome these concerns. For example, the CHWs learned that "having tea" with Vietnamese participants prior to collecting data facilitated the data collection process. In addition, including community members in the design of environmental sampling methods made these methods more likely to meet community standards of acceptability.

Extensive quality control and frequent reinforcement of protocols is required when using community members as data collectors. Collecting exposure assessment data in a standard, rigorous manner is a learned skill, especially when it involves technical skills and requires precision. The HH staff became increasingly proficient in collecting data. However, their lack of prior experience required research staff to provide more initial and ongoing training than might have been the case had professionals been employed. Likewise, researchers had to invest more time in reviewing the quality of data as it was collected and provide more intensive feedback to staff. At times the data collectors were frustrated with the researchers' insistence on adherence to protocols and consistent documentation. Explaining the rationale behind the protocols to the collectors on several occasions helped convince them that standardization and consistency were important.

When researchers shared data from Healthy Homes-I with community staff, these staff members saw the impact of missing data on the analysis. Some staff obtained more complete data in Healthy Homes-II, an example of a benefit arising from applying the CBPR principle of sharing data and analysis with community members. Mutual benefits also accrued, as the data collectors developed a new set of marketable skills and the researchers obtained better data.

Training community members leads to long-term jobs and opportunities. Staff hired from the community gained living-wage jobs with benefits along with specialized skills and knowledge. They have been able to transition to new projects as funding for earlier ones ended. Researchers have benefited by having a skilled and motivated group of staff with whom to work.

Hiring community members as project staff strengthens community participation in research. A theme running across many of these lessons is the valuable role played by community staff (data collectors and CHWs) in representing community perspectives on exposure assessment. Community staff, like other community partners, were knowledgeable about their communities. Yet they also had firsthand experience in conducting assessment activities, allowing them to provide insights about exposure assessment not available from other partners. They could also participate in project decision making more regularly because they had daily contact with research staff.

Incentives are important to successful recruitment. Both monetary and resource incentives proved highly useful for encouraging enrollment in HH and participation in the time-intensive data collection process. Participants received $25 gift cards for groceries upon completion of data collection and kept the vacuums and other resources mentioned earlier. HH is known as the "asthma vacuum project" among community members. Another incentive reported by parent advisory group members was the satisfaction they felt in seeing their actions benefit their children and in knowing that other families would benefit from the research. Providing benefits to the participants and communities involved is another principle of CBPR.

Community participation helps in the application of generalized scientific knowledge to the needs of a specific community. Knowledge derived from scientific literature and nationally developed guidelines might not apply in a local context. Some scientific knowledge is generalizable and some is not. The knowledge of community members is critical when deciding how to apply and adapt this general information to the local community.

CONCLUSION

In conclusion, an approach to exposure assessment developed through a participatory process involving community members, local experts, and researchers led to exposure data that were collected in a culturally competent manner and were of increasing quality over time. These data provide support for the Healthy Homes approach (Krieger et al., 2005; Takaro et al., 2004) and are proving useful in advocating for more widespread recognition of the important role community health workers can play in interventions to reduce indoor triggers for asthma. Although conducting an exposure assessment using a CBPR approach was challenging at times, we believe that the use of a CBPR approach improved the overall research design as well as the accuracy of the data and findings.

References

Alliance for Healthy Homes. Home Page. Retrieved July 26, 2004, from http://www.aeclp.org

Aligne, C. A., Auinger, P., Byrd, R. S., & Weitzman, M. (2000). Risk factors for pediatric asthma: Contributions of poverty, race, and urban residence. *American Journal of Respiratory and Critical Care Medicine, 162,* 873–877.

American Conference of Governmental Industrial Hygienists. (2004). *Documentation of the TLVs® and BEIs® with Other worldwide occupational exposure values* [CD-ROM]. Cincinnati: Author.

Andriessen, J. W., Brunekreef, B., & Roemer, W. (1998). Home dampness and respiratory health status in European children. *Clinical & Experimental Allergy, 28,* 1191–1200.

Arbes, S. J., Jr., Cohn, R. D., Yin, M., Muilenberg, M. L., Friedman, W., & Zeldin, D. C. (2004). Dog allergen (Can f 1) and cat allergen (Fel d 1) in US homes: Results from the National Survey of Lead and Allergens in Housing. *Journal of Allergy and Clinical Immunology, 114,* 111–117.

Axelsson, B. O., Saraf, A., Larsson, L. (1995). Determination of ergosterol in organic dust by gas chromatography-mass spectrometry. *Journal of Chromatography B Biomed Appl., 7*(666), 77–84.

Braun-Fuhrlander, C., Riedler, J., Herz, U., Eder, W., Waser, M., Grize, L., et al. (2002). Environmental exposure to endotoxin and its relation to asthma in school-age children. *New England Journal of Medicine, 347,* 869–877.

Bush, R. K., & Portnoy, J. M. (2001). The role and abatement of fungal allergens in allergic disease. *Journal of Allergy and Clinical Immunology, 107*(Suppl.), 430–440.

Butz, A. M., Malveaux, F. J., Eggleston, P., Thompson, L., Schneider, S., Weeks, K., et al. (1994). Use of community health workers with inner-city children who have asthma. *Clinical Pediatrics, 33,* 135–141.

Chapman, M. D., Aalberse, R. C., Brown, M. J., & Platts-Mills, T. A. (1988). Monoclonal antibodies to the major feline allergen Fel d I. II: Single step affinity purification of Fel d I, N-terminal sequence analysis, and development of a sensitive two-site immunoassay to assess Fel d I exposure. *Journal of Immunology, 140,* 812–818.

Coghlin, J., Hammond, S. K., & Gann, P. H. (1989). Development of epidemiologic tools for measuring environmental tobacco smoke exposure. *American Journal of Epidemiology, 130,* 696–704.

Crater, S. E., & Platts-Mills, T. A. (1998). Searching for the cause of the increase in asthma. *Current Opinion in Pediatrics, 10,* 594–599.

Custovic, A., & Woodcock, A. (2001). On allergens and asthma (again): Does exposure to allergens in homes exacerbate asthma? *Clinical & Experimental Allergy, 31,* 670–673.

Dales, R. E. (1991). Respiratory health effects of home dampness and molds among Canadian children. *American Journal of Epidemiology, 134,* 196–203.

Dales, R. E., Burnett, R., & Zwanenburg, H. (1991). Adverse health effects among adults exposed to home dampness and molds. *American Review of Respiratory Disease, 143,* 505–509.

de Groot, H., Goei, K. G., van Swieten, P., & Aalberse, R. C. (1991). Affinity purification of a major and a minor allergen from dog extract: Serologic activity of affinity-purified Can f I and of Can f I-depleted extract. *Journal of Allergy and Clinical Immunology, 87,* 1056–1065.

Dharmage, S., Bailey, M., Raven, J., Cheng, A., Thien, F., Rolland, J., et al. (1999). A reliable and valid home visit report for studies of asthma in young adults. *Indoor Air, 9,* 188–192.

Dickey, P. (Ed.). (1998). *Master Home Environmentalist training manual.* Seattle, WA: American Lung Association of Washington.

Glasgow, R. E., Foster, L. S., Lee, M. E., Hammond, S. K., Lichtenstein, E., & Andrews, J. A. (1998). Developing a brief measure of smoking in the home: Description and preliminary evaluation. *Addictive Behaviors, 23,* 567–571.

Healthy House. Healthy House Links. [Environmental Health Watch Web site]. Retrieved July 26, 2004, from http://www.ehw.org/Links/LINK_Healthy_House.htm

Holgate, S. T., Samet, J. M., Koren, H. S., & Maynard, R. L. (Eds.). (1999). *Air pollution and health.* San Diego, CA: Academic Press.

Hovell, M. F., Zakarian, J. M., Wahlgren, D. R., Matt, G. E., & Emmons, K. M. (2000). Reported measures of environmental tobacco smoke exposure: Trials and tribulations. *Tobacco Control, 9*(Suppl. 3), III 22–28.

Institute of Medicine. (2000). *Clearing the air: Asthma and indoor air exposures.* Washington, DC: National Academies Press.

Jacobs, D. E., Friedman, W., Ashley, P., & McNairy, M. (1999). *The Healthy Homes Initiative: A preliminary plan.* Washington, DC: U.S. Department of Housing and Urban Development, Office of Lead Hazard Control.

Kleinman, A., Eisenberg, L., & Good, B. (1978). Culture, illness, and care: Clinical lessons from anthropologic and cross-cultural research. *Annals of Internal Medicine, 88,* 251–258.

Koné, A., Sullivan, M., Senturia, K., Chrisman, N., Ciske, S., & Krieger, J. (2000). Improving collaboration between researchers and communities. *Public Health Reports, 115,* 243–248.

Krieger, J. W., Allen, C., Cheadle, A., Higgins, D., Schier, J., Senturia, K., et al. (2002). Using community-based participatory research to address social determinants of health: Lessons learned from Seattle Partners for Healthy Communities. *Health Education & Behavior, 29,* 361–381.

Krieger, J. W., Castorina, J., Walls, M., Weaver, M., & Ciske, S. (2000). Increasing influenza and pneumococcal immunization rates: A randomized controlled study of a senior center–based intervention. *American Journal of Preventive Medicine, 18,* 123–131.

Krieger, J. W., Collier, C., Song, L., & Martin, D. (1999). Linking community-based blood pressure measurement to clinical care: A randomized controlled trial of outreach and tracking by community health workers. *American Journal of Public Health, 89,* 856–861.

Krieger, J. W., Song, L., Takaro, T., & Weaver, M. (2005). The Seattle–King County Healthy Homes Project: A randomized, controlled trial of a community health worker intervention to decrease exposure to indoor asthma triggers among low-income children. *American Journal of Public Health, 95,* 652–659.

Krieger, J. W., Takaro, T. K., Allen, C., Song, L., Weaver, M., Chai, S., et al. (2002). The Seattle–King County Healthy Homes Project: Implementation of a comprehensive approach to improving indoor environmental quality for low-income children with asthma. *Environmental Health Perspectives, 110*(Suppl. 2), 311–322.

Litonjua, A. A., Carey, V. J., Weiss, S. T., & Gold, D. R. (1999). Race, socioeconomic factors, and area of residence are associated with asthma prevalence. *Pediatric Pulmonology, 28,* 394–401.

Love, M. B., Gardner, K., & Legion, V. (1997). Community health workers: Who they are and what they do. *Health Education & Behavior, 24,* 510–522.

Luczynska, C. M., Arruda, L. K., Platts-Mills, T. A., Miller, J. D., Lopez, M., & Chapman, M. D. (1989). A two-site monoclonal antibody ELISA for the quantification of the major Dermatophagoides spp. allergens, Der p I and Der f I. *Journal of Immunological Methods, 118,* 227–235.

Mannino, D. M., Homa, D. M., Akinbami, L. J., Moorman, J. E., Gwynn, C., & Redd, S. C. (2002). Surveillance for asthma—United States, 1980–1999. *MMWR Surveillance Summaries, 51,* 1–13.

Manson, A. (1988). Language concordance as a determinant of patient compliance and emergency room use in patients with asthma. *Medical Care, 26,* 1119–1128.

Meinert, C. (1986). *Clinical trials.* New York: Oxford University Press.

Miller, J. D., Haisley, P. D., & Reinhardt, J. H. (2000). Air sampling results in relation to extent of fungal colonization of building materials in some water-damaged buildings. *Indoor Air, 10*(3), 146–151.

Miller, J. D., & Young, J. C. (1997). The use of ergoterol to measure exposure to fungal propagules in indoor air. *American Industrial Hygiene Association Journal, 58*(1), 39–43.

Mollet, J. A., Vailes, L. D., Avner, D. B., Perzanowski, M. S., Arruda, L. K., Chapman, M. D., et al. (1997). Evaluation of German cockroach (Orthoptera: Blattellidae) allergen and seasonal variation in low-income housing. *Journal of Medical Entomology, 34*(3), 307–311.

Morgan, W. J., Crain, E. F., Gruchalla, R. S., O'Connor, G. T., Kattan, M., Evans, R., III, et al. (2004). Results of a home-based environmental intervention among urban children with asthma. *New England Journal of Medicine, 351,* 1068–1080.

Needleman, H. L., & Gatsonis, C. A. (1990). Low-level lead exposure and the IQ of children: A meta-analysis of modern studies. *Journal of the American Medical Association, 263,* 673–678.

Pasanen, A. L., Rautiala, S., Kasanen, J. P., Raunio, P., Rantamäki, J., & Kalliokoski, P. (2000). The relationship between measured moisture conditions and fungal concentrations in water-damaged building materials. *Indoor Air, 11,* 111–120.

Phipatanakul, W., Eggleston, P. A., Wright, E. C., & Wood, R. A. (2000, December). National Cooperative Inner-City Asthma Study: Mouse allergen: II. The relationship of mouse allergen exposure to mouse sensitization and asthma morbidity in inner-city children with asthma. *Journal of Allergy and Clinical Immunology, 106,* 1075–1080.

Platts-Mills, T. A., Vaughan, J. W., Carter, M. C., & Woodfolk, J. A. (2000). The role of intervention in established allergy: Avoidance of indoor allergens in the treatment of chronic allergic disease. *Journal of Allergy and Clinical Immunology, 106,* 787–804.

Pollart, S. M., Smith, T. F., Morris, E. C., Gelber, L. E., Platts-Mills, T. A., & Chapman, M. D. (1991). Environmental exposure to cockroach allergens: Analysis with monoclonal antibody-based enzyme immunoassays. *Journal of Allergy and Clinical Immunology, 87*(2), 505–510.

Public Health—Seattle & King Country (2004). Asthma resources: Healthy Homes I Asthma Project. Retrieved January 2004, from http://www.metrokc.gov/health/asthma/healthyhomes

Roberts, J. W., Clifford, W. S., Glass, G., & Hummer, P. G. (1999). Reducing dust, lead, dust mites, bacteria, and fungi in carpets by vacuuming. *Archives of Environmental Contamination and Toxicology, 36*(4), 477–484.

Roberts, J. W., Glass, G., & Mickelson, L. (2004). A pilot study of the measurement and control of deep dust, surface dust, and lead in ten old carpets using the 3-spot test while vacuuming. *Archives of Environmental Contamination and Toxicology, 48*(1), 16–23.

Rom, W. N. (Ed.). (1998). *Environmental and occupational medicine* (3rd ed.). Philadelphia: Lippincott-Raven.

Saraf, A., Larsson, L., Burge, H., & Milton, D. (1997). Quantification of ergosterol and 3-hydroxy fatty acids in settled house dust by gas chromatography-mass spectrometry: Comparison with fungal culture and determination of endotoxin by a limulus amebocyte lysate assay. *Applied and Environmental Microbiology, 63*(7), 2554–2559.

Shapiro, G. G., Wighton, T. G., Chinn, T., Zuckrman, J., Eliassen, A. H., Picciano, J. F., et al. (1999). House dust mite avoidance for children with asthma in homes of low-income families. *Journal of Allergy and Clinical Immunology, 103,* 1069–1074.

Strachan, D. P. (1988). Damp housing and childhood asthma: Validation of reporting of symptoms. *British Medical Journal, 297,* 1223–1226.

Sullivan, M., Koné, A., Senturia, K. D., Chrisman, N. J., Ciske, S. J., & Krieger, J. W. (2001). Researcher and researched-community perspectives: Toward bridging the gap. *Health Education & Behavior, 28*(2), 130–149.

Swider, S. M. (2002). Outcome effectiveness of community health workers: An integrative literature review. *Public Health Nursing, 19,* 11–20.

Takaro, T., Krieger, J. W., Song, L., & Beaudet, N. (2004). Effect of environmental interventions to reduce asthma triggers in homes of low-income children in Seattle. *Journal of Exposure Analysis and Environmental Epidemiology, 14*(Suppl. 1), S133–S143.

U.S. Department of Health and Human Services. (1995). *Report to Congress on Workers' Home Contamination Study, conducted under the Workers' Family Protection Act (29 U.S.C. 671a)*. Retrieved March 2005, from http://www.cdc.gov/niosh/contamin.html

Wilson, S. R., Yamada, E. G., Sudhakar, R., Roberto, L., Mannino, D., Mejia, C., et al. (2001). A controlled trial of an environmental tobacco smoke reduction intervention in low-income children with asthma. *Chest, 120*, 1709–1722.

Zureik, M., Neukirch, C., Leynaert, B., Liard, R., Bousquet, J., & Neukirch F. (2002). Sensitisation to airborne moulds and severity of asthma: Cross sectional study from European Community respiratory health survey. *British Medical Journal, 325*, 411–414.

PART FIVE

DOCUMENTATION AND EVALUATION OF PARTNERSHIPS

In Part Five (Chapter Twelve), we focus on the CBPR phase of documenting and evaluating, on an ongoing basis, the progress of the partnership toward achieving a collaborative process. Given the fundamental importance of partnership formation and maintenance to CBPR, as illustrated by the chapters in Part Two of this book, it is essential to document and evaluate the effectiveness of the process methods used by a partnership (Israel et al., 2003; Lasker, Weiss, & Miller, 2001; Schulz, Israel, & Lantz, 2003; Sofaer, 2000; Wallerstein, Polacsek, & Maltrud, 2002; Weiss, Anderson, & Lasker, 2002).

Using a partnership's CBPR principles as a guide, an evaluation can determine the intermediate outcomes that the partnership can attend to in order to refine and improve its progress toward an effective collaborative process and, ultimately, the accomplishment of long-term outcomes (Lantz, Viruell-Fuentes, Israel, Softley, & Guzman, 2001; Rossi, Freeman, & Lipsey, 1999; Schulz et al., 2003; Weiss et al., 2002). Examples of intermediate partnership outcomes include fosters co-learning and capacity building, involves equitable participation and sharing of influence and power among all partners, and achieves balance between knowledge generation and action. Although the emphasis in Part Five is on assessing a partnership's attainment of intermediate outcomes, it is important to recognize that evaluating the long-term outcomes of a CBPR partnership, such as achieving intervention objectives, is another critical aspect of the evaluation phase. Numerous methods (for example, surveys or focus group interviews) are appropriate for documenting progress toward attainment of both intermediate and long-term outcomes.

In Chapter Twelve, Israel, Lantz, McGranaghan, Kerr, and Guzman present a conceptual framework for evaluating the process and impact of CBPR partnerships and discuss the application of this framework by the Detroit Community-Academic Urban Research Center. This conceptual framework identifies the role of several dimensions that affect the extent to which a partnership achieves its ultimate outcomes. Particular emphasis is placed on assessing "structural characteristics," "group dynamics characteristics," and "intermediate measures of partnership effectiveness." To document and monitor change in these dimensions, the chapter authors used two data collection methods: in-depth, semistructured interviews and closed-ended survey questionnaires. They provide insightful details on the structures and procedures used to engage academic and community partners in evaluating the process and impact of their CBPR partnership. They give particular attention to the participatory process of designing and conducting the evaluation, feeding back and interpreting findings, and applying the results to refine and improve the partnership's adherence to CBPR principles. The authors also examine the challenges and limitations, the lessons learned, and the implications for the use of these methods, all of which are applicable to documenting and evaluating both partnership formation and maintenance and the longer-term outcomes of a CBPR effort.

References

Israel, B. A., Schulz, A. J., Parker, E. A., Becker, A. B., Allen, A., & Guzman, J. R. (2003). Critical issues in developing and following community-based participatory research principles. In M. Minkler & N. Wallerstein (Eds.), *Community-based participatory research for health* (pp. 56–73). San Francisco: Jossey-Bass.

Lantz, P., Viruell-Fuentes, E., Israel, B. A., Softley, D., & Guzman, J. R. (2001). Can communities and academia work together on public health research? Evaluation results from a community-based participatory research partnership in Detroit. *Journal of Urban Health, 78*(3), 495–507.

Lasker, R. D., Weiss, E. S., & Miller, R. (2001). Partnership synergy: A practical framework for studying and strengthening the collaborative advantage. *Milbank Quarterly, 79*(2), 179–205.

Rossi, P. H., Freeman, H. E., & Lipsey, M. W. (1999). *Evaluation: A systematic approach* (6th ed.). Thousand Oaks, CA: Sage.

Schulz, A. J., Israel, B. A., & Lantz, P. (2003). Instrument for evaluating dimensions of group dynamics within community-based participatory research partnerships. *Evaluation and Program Planning, 26*, 249–262.

Sofaer, S. (2000). *Working together, moving ahead: A manual to support effective community health coalitions.* New York: Baruch College School of Public Affairs.

Wallerstein, N., Polacsek, M., & Maltrud, K. (2002). Participatory evaluation model for coalitions: The development of systems indicators. *Health Promotion Practice, 3*(3), 361–373.

Weiss, E. S., Anderson, R. M., & Lasker, R. D. (2002). Making the most of collaboration: Exploring the relationship between partnership synergy and partnership functioning. *Health Education & Behavior, 29*(6), 683–698.

CHAPTER TWELVE

Documentation and Evaluation of CBPR Partnerships

In-Depth Interviews and Closed-Ended Questionnaires

Barbara A. Israel, Paula M. Lantz, Robert J. McGranaghan,
Diana L. Kerr, and J. Ricardo Guzman

As the number of research and intervention partnerships has increased to address the complex set of determinants associated with public health problems, particularly health disparities, numerous challenges, as well as benefits, of a collaborative approach have been identified (Butterfoss, Goodman, & Wandersman, 1993; Green, Daniel, & Novick, 2001; Israel, Schulz, Parker, & Becker, 1998; Minkler & Wallerstein, 2003; Roussos & Fawcett, 2000). Specifically, researchers have gained an enhanced understanding of the time needed to develop and maintain such partnerships and to show an impact on health outcomes (Israel et al., 1998; Roussos & Fawcett, 2000; Weiss, Anderson, & Lasker, 2002). Therefore it is particularly important that partnerships document and evaluate early on the

Acknowledgments: The authors appreciate the involvement of all of the partners involved in the Detroit Community-Academic Urban Research Center, who have contributed greatly to the success of the partnership described in this chapter and to enhancing the authors' understanding of CBPR and research methods for evaluating CBPR (Butzel Family Center, Community Health and Social Services Center, Community In Schools, Detroit Department of Health and Wellness Promotion, Detroit Hispanic Development Corporation, Detroiters Working for Environmental Justice, Friends of Parkside, Henry Ford Health System, Kettering/Butzel Health Initiative, Latino Family Services, Neighborhood Service Organization, Southwest Counseling and Development Services, University of Michigan Schools of Public Health, Nursing and Social Work, and Warren/Conner Development Coalition). Support for the work described here was provided in part by the Centers for Disease Control and Prevention's Urban Health Centers Initiative (Grant U48/CCU515775). (See www.sph.umich.edu/urc for more details.) The authors also thank Sue Andersen for her assistance in preparing the manuscript.

extent to which and the ways in which their partnership process is effective—in adhering to key principles of collaboration for example (Israel et al., 2003; Lasker, Weiss, & Miller, 2001; Schulz, Israel, & Lantz, 2003; Sofaer, 2000; Wallerstein, Polacsek, & Maltrud, 2002; Weiss et al., 2002). A determination of whether and how effectively a partnership is collaborative and participatory (for example, in its project implementation process), and whether and how effectively it achieves its intermediate or impact objectives (for example, those considered essential to attaining ultimate health outcomes), can occur long before it is possible to assess the partnership's impact on health (Rossi, Freeman, & Lipsey, 1999; Schulz et al., 2003). Such information can be used by the partnership to improve its actions and in turn the achievement of its ultimate goals (Lantz, Viruell-Fuentes, Israel, Softley, & Guzman, 2001; Schulz et al., 2003; Weiss et al., 2002).

There are many different types of evaluation—such as process, impact, outcome, participatory, formative, and summative (Israel et al., 1995; Patton 2002; Springett 2003)—and multiple data collection methods—quantitative and qualitative—that can be used for evaluating partnerships (Patton, 2002; Reichardt & Cook, 1979; Schulz et al., 2003; Weiss et al., 2002). The purpose of this chapter is to examine the use of two data collection methods, in-depth, semistructured interviews and closed-ended survey questionnaires, for assessing the process and impact of the collaborative dimensions of community-based participatory research (CBPR) partnerships. We will present a conceptual framework for assessing CBPR partnerships, followed by a brief description of each of these two data collection methods. The application of these methods by the Detroit Community-Academic Urban Research Center will be presented as a case example. Emphasis will be placed throughout on the participatory process used in designing and conducting these methods and in feeding back and interpreting data collected from these two methods for an evaluation of a CBPR partnership. We will examine the challenges and limitations, lessons learned, and implications for the use of these methods.

CONCEPTUAL FRAMEWORK FOR ASSESSING CBPR PARTNERSHIPS

There are a number of theoretical and conceptual models that provide useful frameworks for understanding and assessing how partnerships operate (for example, Butterfoss & Kegler, 2002; Lasker & Weiss, 2003; Schulz et al., 2003; Sofaer, 2000). In our own work we have placed particular emphasis on the importance of a given partnership's adhering to the principles of CBPR—for example, displaying a collaborative, equitable partnership in all phases of the process (see Chapter One in this volume and Israel et al., 1998, 2003)—and the recognition that success in following these principles and achieving long-term outcomes is dependent on the effectiveness of the group in using its resources and satisfying the needs of group members (Schulz et al., 2003). Therefore the development of the evaluation instruments to be discussed here was based upon an extensive review of the group process literature (Johnson & Johnson, 1982; Shaw, 1981) at the time in which the initial tools were developed in 1985 as part of another participatory action research project (Israel, Schurman, & House, 1989). We selected the priority aspects of groups to assess (such as shared leadership; open, two-way communication; and high levels of trust) based on the characteristics of effective groups delineated by Johnson and Johnson (1982). (See Chapter Three for a discussion of group facilitation strategies that can be used to foster the achievement of these characteristics.)

As shown in Figure 12.1, these characteristics of effective groups have been placed in the context of a conceptual framework for understanding and assessing partnerships (adapted from Sofaer, 2000; Schulz et al., 2003; with additional points from Lasker & Weiss, 2003). (Portions of the description of the model were adapted from Schulz et al., 2003.) Briefly, the extent to which a partnership achieves its ultimate outcomes or outputs (for example, collaborative problem solving or improved community health) is influenced by intermediate measures or characteristics of partnership effectiveness (for example, extent of member involvement and empowerment) that are determined by the partnership's programs and interventions. In turn, these are shaped by the group dynamics of the partnership (for example, communication, conflict resolution, and shared goals), which are also influenced by structural characteristics of the partnership (for example, membership and formalization). All these factors in the framework are shaped by environmental characteristics (for example, geographical and cultural diversity and socioeconomic determinants of health). The items included in the closed-ended survey questionnaire and the in-depth interview protocol that we used were informed by this framework, with particular emphasis on assessing the dimensions of "structural characteristics," "group dynamics characteristics," and "intermediate measures."

GENERAL DESCRIPTION OF DATA COLLECTION METHODS

A number of qualitative and quantitative data collection methods can be used to gather information to evaluate the CBPR partnership process (Denzin & Lincoln, 2000; Nardi, 2002; Patton, 2002). It is our premise that the evaluation questions and priorities (identified through a participatory process) are what should determine the type of evaluation being conducted and the data collection methods being employed. Given the conceptual framework described earlier and the evaluation objectives that have emerged in our work, we have relied

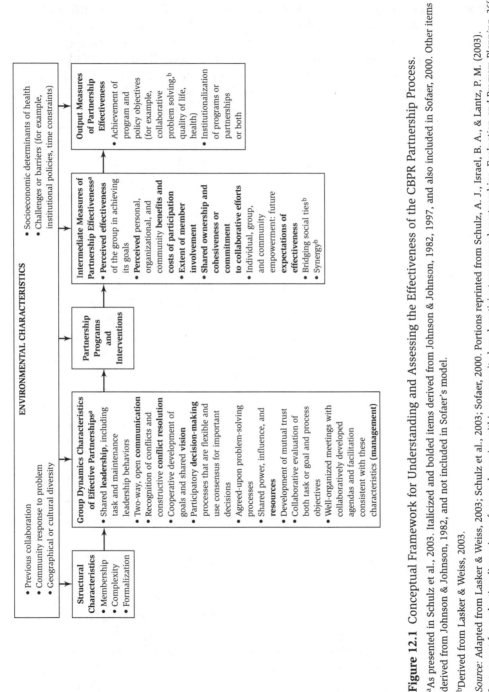

Figure 12.1 Conceptual Framework for Understanding and Assessing the Effectiveness of the CBPR Partnership Process.

[a]As presented in Schulz et al., 2003. Italicized and bolded items derived from Johnson & Johnson, 1982, 1997, and also included in Sofaer, 2000. Other items derived from Johnson & Johnson, 1982, and not included in Sofaer's model.

[b]Derived from Lasker & Weiss, 2003.

Source: Adapted from Lasker & Weiss, 2003; Schulz et al., 2003; Sofaer, 2000. Portions reprinted from Schulz, A. J., Israel, B. A., & Lantz, P. M. (2003). Instrument for evaluating dimensions of group dynamics within community-based participatory research partnerships. *Evaluation and Program Planning, 26*(3), 249–262. Copyright (2003), with permission from Elsevier.

primarily on two types of data collection methods: *in-depth, semistructured interviews* and *closed-ended survey questionnaires.*

In-Depth, Semistructured Interviews

There are a number of approaches to the design of one-on-one, qualitative interviews, and different authors use different terms and definitions in describing them, such as *informal conversational interview* and *standardized open-ended interview* (Patton, 2002). Among the areas in which key distinctions occur across these approaches are the comparative degree of formality or informality, the decision to use fully specified questions or to use topic guidelines, and the degree of flexibility in phrasing questions (asking all respondents the same questions or employing some variation). One of the strengths of all these approaches is the emphasis on asking open-ended questions, with follow-up probes as necessary, that allow the respondent to provide an in-depth explanation of the issues being addressed (Patton, 2002). In addition to the way the questions are asked, such aspects as whom to interview, where to conduct the interview, note taking, tape recording, informed consent and confidentiality, cross-cultural dimensions, and data analysis approaches (Patton, 2002) have to be considered in conducting qualitative interviews.

The focus of this chapter is on the use of the in-depth, semistructured interview, which is aimed at gaining an in-depth understanding of a given phenomenon without imposing any categorization of responses that might limit the inquiry (Fontana & Frey, 2000). (See Chapter Four for a discussion of the use of in-depth key informant interviews.) In-depth, semistructured interviews use a standard set of prespecified, open-ended questions, with follow-up probes to obtain the desired depth of understanding, and allow questions to be asked somewhat differently, if necessary. The advantages of this approach are that all participants are asked similar questions, hence increasing comparability and completeness of responses; there is a degree of flexibility in adapting the questions to particular individuals and contexts; interviewer effects are reduced (when more than one interviewer is involved); and evaluation users may review and shape the interview protocol (Patton, 2002). The disadvantages are that the wording of questions might constrain the relevance of the questions and answers and the comparability may be reduced if all questions are not asked in exactly the same way (Patton, 2002).

Closed-Ended Survey Questionnaires

The closed-ended survey questionnaire is one of the most frequently used methods for gathering information in a systematic and quantitative fashion (Fink & Kosecoff, 1998; Fowler, 2001; Nardi, 2002). Although questions may be asked in different ways, with different response categories, the key dimensions are the use of a predetermined set of questions that are asked of all respondents and the provision of a set of specified response categories into which the respondents' answers have to fit (Fink & Kosecoff, 1998; Nardi, 2002). In addition to the questions themselves, a number of other dimensions of survey questionnaires have to be considered: whom to interview and how the individuals are selected, use of face-to-face or self-administered modes, informed consent and confidentiality, language and translations, number of respondents needed for purposes of statistical power, and use of a cross-sectional or longitudinal approach (Fowler, 2001; Nardi, 2002). (See Chapter Five for an examination of a random sample survey conducted using a CBPR approach.)

APPLICATION OF METHODS TO DETROIT COMMUNITY-ACADEMIC URBAN RESEARCH CENTER

In this section we present a case example, involving the Detroit Community-Academic Urban Research Center, of the use of in-depth, semistructured interviews and a closed-ended survey questionnaire for evaluating the partnership. The partnership's background, goals and objectives, design issues, and implementation steps are discussed in the following sections.

Partnership Background

The Detroit Community-Academic Urban Research Center (URC) is a CBPR partnership of community-based organizations, public health and health care institutions, and academia (the note at the beginning of the chapter lists the organizations). The URC partnership began in 1995, with core funding from the Centers for Disease Control and Prevention (CDC), as part of that agency's Urban Research Centers Initiative (Higgins, Maciak, & Metzler, 2001). The URC is governed by a board that meets monthly and is made up of representatives from each of the partner organizations. During the first two years of its existence, the board adopted a set of CBPR principles that guide its work, and it determined the partnership's mission, goals and objectives, its operating norms and values, and the public health priorities it would address (Israel et al., 2001).

At the first meeting of the board, members engaged in a facilitated discussion in which they identified factors that contributed to effective groups they had belonged to, and they discussed and adopted specific factors as the operating norms that they wanted the URC board to follow (Israel et al., 2001). These norms included: mutual respect, everyone participates, shared leadership, conflicts are brought up and discussed, everyone listens, meetings not dominated by a few members, members agree to disagree, and decisions are made by consensus (Israel et al., 2001). These norms are very similar to the characteristics of effective groups identified in the literature (Johnson & Johnson, 1982, 1997; see also Chapter Three in this volume) and depicted in Figure 12.1. These norms were distributed in print at a subsequent board meeting, were periodically reviewed, and were used to guide the development of the items in the closed-ended questionnaire used to evaluate the CBPR partnership process (for example, items on leadership, participation, and decision-making procedures).

The URC operates primarily in selected neighborhoods in east and southwest Detroit in which approximately 125,000 community members reside. The eastside is predominantly African American and the southwest area of the city is where the largest percentage of Latinos reside.

Goals and Objectives of the URC

The overall goal of the URC is to establish and maintain an effective partnership to conduct community-based participatory research. Specific objectives include: to conduct CBPR projects as identified by the partner organizations; to increase knowledge about the principles and conduct of CBPR; and to educate policymakers and funders on the public health policy implications of the knowledge gained through CBPR projects.

The URC has received over $27 million in federal and foundation funding to conduct over sixteen CBPR projects. Each of these URC-affiliated projects has its own steering committee, comprising representatives from some of the same partner organizations as are involved on the URC board as well as organizations of relevance to the particular focus of the project. Project topics have included diabetes management and prevention, environmental factors associated with childhood asthma, access to health care, and social determinants of health.

Evaluation Design and Role of the Evaluation Subcommittee

The overall research design for the URC evaluation is the case study. A case study provides an in-depth analysis of the different aspects of a program and is an appropriate design for assessing an ongoing, complex phenomenon in its real-life context (Yin, 1984). The URC evaluation approach is both participatory and formative (Israel et al., 2001; Lantz et al., 2001), involving program participants and staff in multiple components of the evaluation process (Cousins & Earl, 1992; Springett, 2003). Members of the URC board have played a critical role in the design, implementation, interpretation, and dissemination of the evaluation results. Thus this evaluation approach adheres to the URC's CBPR principles (Israel et al., 2001, 2003). This participatory approach recognizes that the board members' active involvement in the evaluation enhances the relevance and increases the usefulness of the results.

Funding for the URC began in October 1995, and the first meeting of the board was held in December 1995. Board members participated in the selection of the person who was to serve as the evaluator. The person selected, a University of Michigan School of Public Health (SPH) faculty member, started attending board meetings in the middle of the first year. After attending two meetings, she presented to the board some ideas regarding different directions that an evaluation could take and proposed that an evaluation subcommittee be established. The overarching purpose of the subcommittee was to create a mechanism through which some of the board members would participate outside the monthly meetings in the development of an evaluation plan, which would subsequently be recommended to the entire board. The intent was that subcommittee members would meet in person and by conference call in order to discuss potential evaluation questions and strategies, assist the evaluator in crafting an evaluation proposal, review draft documents and data collection instruments, and help lead discussion of proposed evaluation efforts at full board meetings.

While URC board members were committed to evaluation and believed it to be important, given the other demands and constraints on their time, no nonacademic partners volunteered initially to participate on the evaluation subcommittee when the evaluator solicited volunteers at two different board meetings. Subsequently, the evaluator contacted two board members representing community-based organizations and asked them individually if they would be willing to join the subcommittee, and they both agreed. They had prior experience with evaluation research in their organizations and were vocal, active members of the board. Thus, during the URC's first year, the evaluation subcommittee was established, made up of representatives from academia (the evaluator, another SPH faculty member on the URC board, and a graduate student research assistant), one representative from a community-based organization in eastside Detroit, and one from southwest Detroit. After several years, as the board became more established, the subcommittee was less involved as a separate entity, and the evaluator brought evaluation issues to the entire board for discussion and resolution.

In addition to being participatory, the evaluation design is formative, which means that the results of the evaluation have been shared with the board members on an ongoing basis, and the board members have been involved in the interpretation and application of the evaluation findings (Patton, 2002; Rossi et al., 1999). The evaluation approach also applies both process and impact evaluation (Israel et al., 1995; Patton, 2002). A *process evaluation* assesses the extent to which a program has been carried out as planned and with the level of quality intended (Israel et al., 1995). An *impact evaluation* assesses the extent to which a program is effective in achieving changes in targeted mediators (Israel et al., 1995).

As described earlier, two main objectives of the URC board are to increase the knowledge of and use of CBPR and to improve health through the conduct of CBPR projects in eastside and southwest Detroit. Having an effect on and assessing ultimate health outcomes takes considerable resources over a long period. Therefore the evaluation approach used focuses on impact indicators, or *targeted mediators,* that are more readily assessed and provide a logical link or pathway between the intervention (that is, the URC processes and core activities) and the ultimate outcomes. The identification of the explicit targeted mediators and how they are connected is referred to as a *logic model* in evaluation research (CDC, 1999; Yin, 1984). Although the evaluation was not guided by a logic model per se, the in-depth interview guide and survey questionnaire were informed by the conceptual framework presented in Figure 12.1.

As is typical in case studies, multiple methods for data collection (quantitative and qualitative) and multiple sources of information have been used to understand the process by which the URC has developed and worked toward meeting its objectives, to provide feedback on an ongoing basis to board members, and to assess the impact of the URC. The use of multiple methods increases the types of information collected (Patton, 2002; Yin, 1984) and enhances the validity of the conclusions by revealing areas in which there is convergence across data and areas in need of further investigation because findings do not converge (Denzin & Lincoln, 2000; Israel et al., 1995).

As suggested by Yin (1984), three principles of data collection for case studies have been used in evaluating the URC:

1. Use multiple sources of evidence, also referred to as *triangulation*

2. Develop a well-organized database

3. Maintain a chain of evidence that is consistent with the conceptual framework for the partnership (Figure 12.1)

The set of data sources used includes in-depth, semistructured interviews; closed-ended survey questionnaires; field notes of URC board meetings; documents and correspondence generated by the URC; and minutes from board and subcommittee meetings (Lantz et al., 2001).

In-Depth, Semistructured Interviews

Development of Interview Protocol. During the first year of the board's operation (1996), the evaluation subcommittee met two times outside of monthly board meetings to discuss evaluation design issues. The subcommittee decided that it wanted to obtain in-depth information from board members and that individual, face-to-face interviews would be the most effective way to do so. The subcommittee members discussed the advantages and disadvantages of the use of in-depth, semistructured interviews (as outlined in the literature and described earlier) and decided that this was the approach they wanted to use. They decided that a standard set of open-ended questions would be identified, with appropriate follow-up probes, with the understanding that the evaluator would be flexible in the actual asking of the questions, changing wording as appropriate and eliminating questions if necessary.

The evaluator shared with the evaluation subcommittee members a draft of questions based on both their discussions of topics that they wanted to be included and the characteristics of partnerships as outlined in the literature (as depicted in Figure 12.1). These draft questions were discussed and then revised based on the guidance of the subcommittee. For example, subcommittee members wanted a clear distinction between benefits gained by individuals and those gained by organizations when gathering information regarding perceived benefits of participating in the partnership, and questions were added accordingly. The topics that were covered in the interview questions included expectations and hopes for the first year and whether they were met; major accomplishments, barriers, and challenges and recommendations for meeting them; personal knowledge or skills gained; tangible benefits from an organization's affiliation with the URC; and examples of exchanges of information or assistance or support between partner organizations (see Appendix G for the interview protocol).

These in-depth interviews were conducted again with members of the URC board in 1999 and 2002. Many of the same questions were asked, and in 1999, based on discussions with the evaluation subcommittee and the URC board as a whole, questions were added to address several topics of particular interest. The new topics covered factors that facilitated accomplishments, establishment of new relationships among partner organizations, assessment of the role of the Centers for Disease Control and Prevention (CDC), and recommendations to other partnerships on what went well and what to do differently (see Appendix G). Some of these topics were added because the URC was participating with the CDC and two other URC sites in a cross-site evaluation that year (Metzler et al., 2003). In 2002, one of these "new" topics (factors that facilitated accomplishments) was retained in the interview protocol, and several other topics were added, based on discussions with the URC board, that were especially germane to the board at that time. These topics addressed benefits of the URC to the community and ways to improve benefits; costs to or problems for an individual or an organization because of affiliation with the URC, and considerations if funding were to end and options for future funding (see Appendix G).

Data Collection. The first set of interviews was conducted in late 1996 with current board members ($n = 15$), former board members ($n = 3$), and staff ($n = 5$), for a 100 percent response rate (Lantz et al., 2001). The second set was conducted in late 1999 with current board members ($n = 15$) and staff ($n = 3$), for a 100 percent response rate (Lantz et al., 2001). The third set was conducted in 2002 with 16 board members and staff, for an 84 percent response rate.

The interviews were conducted by the evaluator with a graduate student assistant and were documented through verbatim field notes that they each took. The interviews conducted in 2002 were also tape-recorded. The interviews averaged one hour in length and for board members were carried out most frequently in the member's place of work. The interviewees signed a consent form and were guaranteed confidentiality.

Data Analysis. The two sets of written notes taken at each interview were reconciled and then transcribed (Lantz et al., 2001). In 2002, audiotapes were used as a backup to supplement the handwritten notes taken during the interview. Using a qualitative data analysis approach of *open coding* (Strauss and Corbin, 1990), the transcripts were reviewed systematically by the evaluator and her assistant, and categories that captured embedded concepts or meanings were identified from within the interviews as a whole as the data were reviewed (not beforehand) and then compared across the interviews (Patton, 2002). The results of the qualitative data analysis were also stratified by subgroup (university-based and Detroit-based board members) to identify similarities and differences in responses. Due to the small numbers and issues of confidentiality, the results were not further subdivided, for example, by responses from Detroit-based community-based organization partners and from health service provider partners.

Data Feedback, Interpretation, and Discussion. Several months after the completion of the first set of interviews, the evaluator presented the results to the evaluation subcommittee members for their review and comment. Using their input, the evaluator developed a six-page report of evaluation results that she presented to the entire board at one of its monthly meetings. The findings were organized according to the topics covered in the interview protocol, for example, expectations, accomplishments, and challenges and barriers. The results were presented for all of the interviews combined, except where there were meaningful differences in the ways university-based and Detroit-based board members responded. For example, several university respondents reported that their main expectations for the first year of the partnership related to the goals of establishing a common agenda and developing processes and infrastructure for the board. However, only two Detroit partners expressed similar expectations; the majority of community partners stated that their primary expectation was to see new CBPR projects implemented during the first year, particularly in southwest Detroit.

The results of the interviews conducted in 1999 and 2002 were organized by question and presented by the evaluator to the board, using a PowerPoint presentation format. In addition, from her overall analysis of the data the evaluator identified a set of "issues for ongoing discussion" that were highlighted and discussed by the board. For example, an issue addressed in both 1999 and 2002 was the degree to which people believed resources were fairly distributed among organizations participating in the URC. During the data collection process for the evaluation, a number of respondents raised concerns regarding perceived inequities in financial and other benefits of URC participation, with the main concern being that the academic partner seemed to be benefiting disproportionately when compared to the community partners. Information regarding this concern was presented to the board and became a springboard for ongoing discussions and action on a number of related issues (Lantz et al., 2001).

Program Changes Based on In-Depth Interview Results. Although the focus of this chapter is on the data collection methods themselves and their application within the context of CBPR, and not on the results per se, given the important formative evaluation dimension of this approach, an example is provided here of how the results of the in-depth interviews were used to guide changes in the URC. One finding from the first set of interviews was a suggestion by several of the Detroit partners that they would like to see the partnership expand to include a broader range of community partners. When this was reported to the board, it was decided that this issue should be considered in more depth. Over several meetings the board discussed the potential benefits and disadvantages of adding new community partners and reached a consensus that it did not want to do so at that time but that it wanted to revisit the issue a year later. In the subsequent wave of interviews, this topic was again identified, and at that point the board decided it wanted to add new community-based organizations to the partnership.

In addition to bringing about program changes, the interview findings were also used to identify and disseminate lessons learned and recommendations for conducting CBPR. Several articles have been published based on these data (Israel et al., 2001; Lantz et al., 2001; Metzler et al., 2003), and numerous presentations have been made at professional meetings. In addition, technical assistance and invited workshops have been provided that draw on these evaluation results. All the dissemination activities have included community partners and academic partners as coauthors and copresenters. Although the university partners have most often assumed the role of writing the first drafts of publications and presentations, given that they are expected to write and are compensated for writing as part of their jobs, the community partners have played key roles in team discussions deciding on the initial content and in the subsequent reviewing and editing of manuscripts and presentations. (See Chapter Thirteen for a discussion of dissemination issues in a CBPR context.)

Closed-Ended Survey Questionnaire

Development of Survey Questionnaire. At the end of the URC's first year, during the evaluation subcommittee's discussions of the design of the evaluation, subcommittee members decided that in addition to the semistructured, in-depth interviews, they also wanted to use a closed-ended survey questionnaire with the board members. The purpose of the survey was to assess, in a standardized fashion, the partners' impressions about and attitudes toward different aspects of the URC partnership's efforts (Lantz et al., 2001). Drawing on the operating norms generated and adopted by the board from characteristics of effective groups (described earlier), on the literature on partnership effectiveness factors (as discussed and depicted in Figure 12.1), and on the CBPR principles and specific objectives of the URC, and building on a questionnaire initially developed and revised in the context of two other participatory research efforts (Israel et al., 1989; Schulz et al., 2003), the evaluator drafted a questionnaire that was initially reviewed and revised by members of the evaluation subcommittee. (See Appendix H for the survey questionnaire.) The questionnaire uses mostly Likert scale response categories (for example, ranging from "strongly agree" to "strongly disagree") and, in accordance with Figure 12.1, includes items related to

- Structural characteristics, such as meeting organization, facilitation, and staffing

- Group dynamics characteristics, such as leadership and open communication

- Intermediate measures of partnership effectiveness, such as effectiveness in achieving the group's goals, general satisfaction, benefits of participation, and sense of ownership or belonging to the group (Schulz et al., 2003)

The survey questionnaire has been administered at four different times, with each version including all the items on the initial questionnaire. Additional items were included in subsequent years to assess more specifically levels of trust, decision-making procedures, the degree to which CBPR principles are followed, role of the funder, and accomplishments or impact of the group (see Appendix H).

Data Collection. The survey questionnaire was mailed to all board members, along with a postage-paid return envelope, in 1997, 1999, 2001, and 2002, and response rates were 100 percent, 100 percent, 95 percent, and 86 percent, respectively. Across the years the board numbered approximately twenty individuals, representing ten organizations and institutions. The self-administered questionnaire took about fifteen to twenty minutes to complete.

Data Analysis. The analysis of the data from the survey questionnaires was carried out by the evaluator and involved descriptive statistics (that is, frequency distributions and comparison of means). For each of the surveys the data were analyzed for the entire sample and for the two main subgroups: university-based board members and Detroit-based board members. Given that the overall number of board members is so small ($n = 20$), no statistical tests of significance were computed when comparing results across the subgroups. Rather, the results were examined to identify any patterns that were different across the two main partner groups. Similarly, comparisons of the frequency distributions for all respondents for the same questionnaire items were made across the years that the surveys were conducted.

Data Feedback, Interpretation, and Discussion. The results of the analysis of both the initial survey administration and the initial in-depth interviews were included when the evaluator shared the evaluation findings with the evaluation subcommittee and developed the first feedback report (described earlier) and subsequently shared the findings with the board. At this time the frequency distributions for all the questionnaire items were provided to the board, along with a verbal summary of the key findings. In subsequent years, at a regularly scheduled board meeting, the evaluator provided the frequency distributions for all the items and presented PowerPoint slides of key findings across major question categories (for example, perceptions of trust, decision making, general satisfaction, and perceived impact). Major differences that were found over time and between the university partners and the Detroit partners were highlighted. For example, in 1999, 53 percent of the board members agreed with the statement, "I have adequate knowledge of the URC budget, URC resources, and how resources are allocated," and in 2001, 70 percent agreed. In further examination by subgroup in 2001, it was noted that 100 percent of the university respondents agreed, whereas only 43 percent of the Detroit partners agreed. The board engaged in a series of discussions following the presentation of these results. One result of these discussions was the decision to present budget and other financial information to board members on a more regular schedule and in a manner that is transparent and allows time for discussion.

Program Changes Based on Survey Questionnaire Results. A number of program changes have been made over the years based on the results of the closed-ended survey questionnaires (Lantz et al., 2001; Schulz et al., 2003). For example, the survey asked whether (1) "certain individuals' opinions get weighed more than they should" and whether (2) "one person or group dominates at URC board meetings." In 1997 and 1999, the responses of those who agreed or strongly agreed with the first statement were 50 percent and 53 percent, respectively. In 1997 and 1999, the same responses to the second statement came from 28 percent and 42 percent of the group, respectively. There was no clear pattern regarding the person or group thought to dominate, but in discussion of these results at the board meeting, concern was expressed that changes needed to be made and that everyone needed to pay attention to fostering more equitable levels of participation. The facilitator of the board meetings tried consciously to encourage all members to participate actively at these meetings. In 2001 and 2002, the responses to the first statement were considerably lower (18 percent and 13 percent, respectively), as were the responses to the second statement (24 percent and 19 percent, respectively).

In addition to spurring these program changes, the findings have been used to contribute to the literature on CBPR (Israel et al., 2001; Lantz et al., 2001; Schulz et al., 2003) and have been incorporated into presentations at professional meetings and into invited workshops. This use of the data is particularly important given that one of the stated objectives of the URC is to increase and disseminate knowledge about the principles of CBPR and how to conduct such research.

CHALLENGES AND LIMITATIONS

In the course of our evaluation activities, we have identified challenges and limitations in the use of both in-depth interviews and closed-ended questionnaires. Although in-depth interviews provide rich information that can contribute to an enhanced understanding of the phenomenon being investigated, they are extremely labor and time intensive and require considerable skill on the part of the evaluator. The time needed to conduct the analysis is particularly challenging in that it means the results may not be presented until several months after the data have been collected, which can be frustrating for the partners because they are waiting for the results and because changes can occur over that time period that might make the results less relevant.

Two of the difficulties related to the use of closed-ended questionnaires are associated with the method itself. First, the use of closed-ended questions limits both the responses that can be provided and the issues that can be addressed (Schulz et al., 2003). Furthermore, the wording and interpreting of the questions themselves can be problematic. It is likely that not everyone interprets each question or the response categories in the same way. As one community member emphasized at a board meeting, some people are not going to indicate the best or most positive response category for most items simply because they believe "there is always room for improvement. This doesn't mean, however, that we have big problems."

Given the small number of members in most partnerships and the turnover that occurs, several challenges and limitations arise in the data analysis of closed-ended questionnaires. First, only simple descriptive statistics can be used, and it is not possible to apply tests of statistical significance to assess whether there have been any changes over time (Schulz et al., 2003). Second, we chose to assess change in the group as a whole over time by aggregating the results across respondents at two points in time, rather than tracking change in individual respondents over time. Although such an approach is useful for capturing what is occurring within the group over time, if there are any changes it is not possible to determine whether they are due to changes in group membership or events that have happened in the group or events that may have had an impact on some members of the group but not others (Schulz et al., 2003).

A second challenge that relates to partnership size and data analysis applies to the use of interviews as well as questionnaires. It is the inability to analyze the data by many different subgroupings. It is critically important to guarantee confidentiality, and the analysis of data by small subgroups would run the risk of exposing the responses of individual group members (Schulz et al., 2003). Hence, although we were able to analyze the data for two categories, university-based and Detroit-based partners, we were not able to further examine the data by Detroit-based health providers and Detroit-based community-based organizations. There might have been some important differences there that we were not able to identify. Similarly, it would be valuable to analyze the results based on other factors that might contribute to the responses, such as the length of time someone has been a member and his or her level of participation in the group, and this may not be possible with the small numbers involved (Schulz et al., 2003).

A third challenge, and one that also applies to both data collection methods, is the time constraints on the partners involved. Participating in the in-depth interviews in particular, but also completing the closed-ended questionnaire, can place time pressures on the partners' already busy schedules. This can cause additional strain on the evaluator who may have to be persistent with members in order to collect the data, which can in turn create tension in the relationships between the evaluator and the members.

Related to this point is the concern that the role of the evaluation subcommittee, the time spent by the members, and the level of participation of those members were all diminishing over time. Some of this was due to the time constraints on all the members, and the difficulty of attending yet another meeting. Over time, the board as a whole served more in this participatory role, and the evaluator brought questions to the entire board rather than the subcommittee.

Another specific area of concern was the subcommittee's and the board's lack of involvement in the data analysis. In accordance with the URC's principles of CBPR, the board promotes the involvement of all partners "as appropriate in all major phases of the research process" (Israel et al., 2001, p. 19). Although the evaluator certainly considers it "appropriate" for the community partners to be involved in the data analysis, a decision was made not to do so in this instance due to the confidential nature of the responses. Given the small number of respondents for both the closed-ended questionnaire and the in-depth, semistructured interviews, it would not have been possible for community partners to review and analyze the data without identifying who the respondents were, and this would have violated confidentiality. Importantly, as described earlier, the evaluation subcommittee and board members were actively involved in a number of meetings in which the results of the data were fed back and the members engaged in discussions to interpret the findings.

Finally, although these two data collection methods have provided a wealth of information for assessing the URC partnership process, there may be important dimensions that they do not measure. For example, as indicated in Figure 12.1, drawing on the work of Lasker and colleagues (Lasker & Weiss, 2003; Lasker et al., 2001), we consider *synergy,* defined as the actions and products that a partnership can create when its members combine their skills and resources, to be an intermediate measure of partnership effectiveness. However, to date, we have not directly measured this concept with either the interview protocol or the survey questionnaire.

LESSONS LEARNED AND IMPLICATIONS FOR PRACTICE

Given the strengths and limitations of the evaluation approach presented here, we recommend the use of multiple methods (for example, both closed-ended survey questionnaires and in-depth, semistructured interviews) as a way to complement and enhance the knowledge gained from any one method. It is often suggested that these methods can be used sequentially, for example, qualitative interviews may be conducted first and used to inform the development of closed-ended survey questionnaires, or qualitative interviews may be conducted after a survey is administered to assist in explaining the meaning of the quantitative data (Denzin & Lincoln, 2000; Israel et al., 1995). It is also frequently suggested that these methods can be used simultaneously, allowing triangulation with the results of both methods to assess convergence as well as differences in the findings (Denzin & Lincoln, 2000; Israel et al., 1995). With the evaluation of the URC board, the initial interviews and questionnaires were conducted within several months of each other, and the data were analyzed and the results presented at the same time. The two methods were used nearly a year apart in subsequent years. This approach was beneficial in that there was an assessment annually that obtained useful information, using one method or the other, and it was not as demanding on everyone's time as annual in-depth interviews would have been. Furthermore, the closed-ended survey questionnaires provided standardized data, which could be compared over the years, and the in-depth interviews allowed issues that were not covered in the survey questionnaire to be identified and discussed. In addition to these two methods, we also collected and analyzed other data (for example, field notes of meetings) that further enhanced the quality and validity of the findings (Lantz et al., 2001).

As depicted in Figure 12.1, a general set of issues is applicable across partnerships, and these issues can guide the development of interview protocols and survey questionnaires. It is important that a partnership develop its own conceptual framework or logic model, and the specific questions asked need to be tailored to the context and the culture of the partnership. For example, with the URC board, the collectively determined operating norms that grew out of group members' experiences with effective groups suggested many of the questions included in the closed-ended questionnaire. This joint process also served to enhance the partners' buy-in and sense of ownership when it came to the evaluation (Schulz et al., 2003). It is also necessary to recognize that the instruments themselves and the questions asked are part of an iterative process, with revisions and additions made over time as the partnership evolves.

This tailoring of the evaluation to the specific partnership is particularly critical for partnerships that include members from diverse communities and ethnic groups. Given the long-standing inequities that exist and the understandable mistrust of research in communities of color (Israel et al., 1998), an assessment of the partnership process needs to examine, for example, the extent to which community partners are engaged on an equal power basis (Wallerstein, 1999), the reasons and incentives for members to "come around the table," how and why diverse interests work together for common goals, and the challenges and opportunities provided by the partnership for serving different interests in diverse communities.

The use of an evaluation approach that is participatory is particularly important in the context of a CBPR partnership. The active involvement of all partners in the evaluation is consistent with the core principles of CBPR. Every partnership needs to decide how it wants this participatory process to occur. For example, it may be decided that an evaluation subcommittee is needed to work closely with the evaluator or that the entire partnership will serve in that capacity. Furthermore, a partnership may decide that it is interested primarily in influencing and being involved in the data collection, interpretation, and dissemination activities but not in data entry and data analysis per se. What is critical here is that the partnership as a whole makes these decisions, rather than the evaluator or academic partners.

Related to this concern, the formative component of the evaluation, with its emphasis on ongoing feedback and group interpretation of the data, is particularly germane when evaluating a CBPR partnership. This feedback and interpretation, and any subsequent actions based on the results, need to occur in a timely manner. Given the volume of data collected, it is necessary to be selective in presenting and discussing results in meetings with the partnership as a whole. Here again, the evaluator needs to work with a subcommittee or the entire partnership to determine what criteria to use in selecting the findings to present (Schulz et al., 2003). There are several possible ways to determine what results to feed back:

- Identify items or issues in which substantial changes appear to have occurred between years
- Conversely, select items or issues where there has been considerable stability over time
- Choose differences that occur across subgroups, for example, academic and community partners (Schulz et al., 2003)

The evaluation of a CBPR partnership's process and impact needs to begin as soon as possible and continue throughout the duration of the partnership. It is important to recognize that the collection of baseline data, in the traditional sense, is not possible because by the time of the first data collection point, a partnership may well have been working together for a year or more. Therefore it is valuable to begin documenting the efforts of the partnership (for example, through field notes of meetings) as soon as possible. In addition, the first major data collection point (for example, in-depth interviews or a survey question-naire) becomes a key time with which all subsequent data results can be compared. The ongoing collection of data using similar methods then provides beneficial information for assessing the partnership's progress over time. With the URC board, we have now been able to compare the responses to closed-ended questions over four points in time, and it has been quite compelling to see, for example, that whereas 72 percent of the board in 1997 indicated that they agreed or strongly agreed that the board had been effective in achieving its goals, this number increased in 1999 to 95 percent and was 100 percent in both 2001 and 2002. In addition, the first time that the in-depth interviews were conducted, one of the major "challenges" identified was bringing the southwest and eastside communities together for a common purpose. When the interviews were conducted subsequently, one of the major "strengths" identified was that the Latino community (southwest Detroit) and the African American community (eastside Detroit) were working together on common issues for the first time in the history of the city. Thus it is clear that the use of these data collection methods needs to extend beyond capturing only a snapshot at one point in time to capturing multiple points in order to assess the dynamic, evolving partnership process and its impact.

The application of these two data collection methods requires an investment in time and resources on the part of the partnership. Ideally, where external funding is involved, some of the costs can be budgeted for up front. Although this might be seen as taking resources away from other program functions of the partnership, the knowledge gained and changes made can contribute greatly to the effectiveness of the partnership. Here again, this needs to be a topic that is discussed openly by the partners. Furthermore, given that the resources needed often involve the group members' time, the partnership needs to decide the extent to which and the ways in which this time commitment can be managed and members compensated for it.

CONCLUSION

Given the growing emphasis on the use of partnership approaches, particularly CBPR, to address health problems and eliminate health disparities, the evaluation of the partnership process is critical for improving partnership functioning and enhancing the likelihood of partnership success. In this chapter we have examined the use of two methods for these purposes, in-depth interviews and closed-ended survey questionnaires, using the Detroit Community-Academic Urban Research Center as a case example. There are a number of useful resources, measurement instruments, workbooks, and Web-based materials available for partnership evaluation purposes (for example, Fawcett et al., 2000; Francisco, Paine, & Fawcett, 1993; Goodman & Wandersman, 1994; Hardy, Hudson, & Waddinton, 2003; Ontario Healthy Communities Coalition, 1999; Sofaer & Kenney, 1996; Sofaer, 2000; Wallerstein et al., 2002; Weiss et al., 2002). The critical component is that all members of the partnership play a key role in the evaluation process (design, implementation, interpretation, dissemination, and so forth), and that the methods used are developed in accordance with the local context, culture, and goals of the partnership. As more such evaluations are conducted, researchers and communities will gain an increased understanding of the factors that contribute to effective community-based participatory research partnerships, and the strategies for affecting these factors in ways that contribute to improved health and quality of life.

References

Butterfoss, F. D., Goodman, R. M., & Wandersman, A. (1993). Community coalitions for prevention and health promotion. *Health Education Research, 8*(3), 315–330.

Butterfoss, F. D., & Kegler, M. (2002). Toward a comprehensive understanding of community coalitions: Moving practice to theory. In R. J. DiClemente, R. A. Crosby, & M. C. Kegler (Eds.), *Emerging theories in health promotion practice and research: Strategies for improving public health* (pp. 157–193). San Francisco: Jossey-Bass.

Centers for Disease Control and Prevention. (1999). Framework for program evaluation in public health. *MMWR, 48*(RR-11), 1–40.

Cousins, J. B., & Earl, L. M. (1992). The case for participatory evaluation. *Educational Evaluation and Policy Analysis, 14*(4), 397–418.

Denzin, N. K., & Lincoln, Y. S. (Eds.). (2000). *Handbook of qualitative research* (2nd ed.). Thousand Oaks, CA: Sage.

Fawcett, S. B., Francisco, V. T., Schultz, J. A., Berkowitz, B., Wolff, T. J., & Nagy, G. (2000). The Community Tool Box: A Web-based resource for building healthier communities. *Public Health Reports, 115,* 274–278.

Fink, A., & Kosecoff, J. (1998). *How to conduct surveys: A step-by-step guide.* Thousand Oaks, CA: Sage.

Fontana, A., & Frey, J. H. (2000). Interviewing: The art of science. In N. K. Denzin & Y. S. Lincoln (Eds.), *Handbook of qualitative research* (pp. 361–376). Thousand Oaks, CA: Sage.

Fowler, F. J. (2001). *Survey research methods* (3rd ed.). Thousand Oaks, CA: Sage.

Francisco, V. T., Paine, A. L., & Fawcett, S. B. (1993). A methodology for monitoring and evaluating community health coalitions. *Health Education Research, 8*(3), 403–416.

Goodman, R. M., & Wandersman, A. (1994). FORECAST: A formative approach to evaluating community coalitions and community-based initiatives. *Journal of Community Psychology* (CSAP special issue), pp. 6–25.

Green, L. W., Daniel, M., & Novick, L. F. (2001). Partnerships and coalitions for community-based research. *Public Health Reports, 116*(Suppl. 1), 20–31.

Hardy, B., Hudson, B., & Waddington, E. (2003). *Assessing strategic partnership: The partnership assessment tool.* London: Nuffield Institute for Health.

Higgins, D. L., Maciak, B. J., & Metzler, M. (2001). CDC Urban Research Centers: Community-based participatory research to improve the health of urban communities. *Journal of Women's Health and Gender Based Medicine, 10*(1), 9–15.

Israel, B. A., Cummings, K. M., Dignan, M. B., Heaney, C. A., Perales, D. P., Simons-Morton, B. G., et al. (1995). Evaluation of health education programs: Current assessment and future directions. *Health Education Quarterly, 22*(2), 364–389.

Israel, B. A., Lichtenstein, R., Lantz, P. M., McGranaghan, R. J., Allen, A., Guzman, J. R., et al. (2001). The Detroit Community-Academic Urban Research Center: Development, implementation and evaluation. *Journal of Public Health Management and Practice, 7*(5), 1–19.

Israel, B. A., Schulz, A. J., Parker, E. A., & Becker, A. B. (1998). Review of community-based research: Assessing partnership approaches to improve public health. *Annual Review of Public Health, 19,* 173–202.

Israel, B. A., Schulz, A. J., Parker, E. A., Becker, A. B., Allen, A., & Guzman, J. R. (2003). Critical issues in developing and following community-based participatory research principles. In M. Minkler & N. Wallerstein (Eds.), *Community-based participatory research for health* (pp. 56–73). San Francisco: Jossey-Bass.

Israel, B. A., Schurman, S. J., & House, J. S. (1989). Action research on occupational stress: Involving workers as researchers. *International Journal of Health Services, 19*(1), 135–155.

Johnson, D. W., & Johnson, F. P. (1982). *Joining together: Group theory and group skills* (2nd ed.). Upper Saddle River, NJ: Prentice Hall.

Johnson, D. W., & Johnson, F. P. (1997). *Joining together: Group theory and group skills* (6th ed.). Needham Heights, MA: Allyn & Bacon.

Lantz, P. M., Viruell-Fuentes, E., Israel, B. A., Softley, D., & Guzman, J. R. (2001). Can communities and academia work together on public health research? Evaluation results from a community-based participatory research partnership in Detroit. *Journal of Urban Health, 78*(3), 495–507.

Lasker, R. D., & Weiss, E. S. (2003). Broadening participation in community problem solving: A multidisciplinary model to support collaborative practice and research. *Journal of Urban Health, 80*(1), 14–60.

Lasker, R. D., Weiss, E. S., & Miller, R. (2001). Partnership synergy: A practical framework for studying and strengthening the collaborative advantage. *Milbank Quarterly, 79*(2), 179–205.

Metzler, M. M., Higgins, D. L., Beeker, C. G., Freudenberg, N., Lantz, P. M., Senturia, K. D., et al. (2003). Addressing urban health in Detroit, New York, and Seattle through community-based participatory research partnerships. *American Journal of Public Health, 93*(5), 803–811.

Minkler, M., & Wallerstein, N. (Eds.). (2003). *Community-based participatory research for health.* San Francisco: Jossey-Bass.

Nardi, P. M. (2002). *Doing survey research: A guide to quantitative research methods.* Boston: Pearson Allyn & Bacon.

Ontario Healthy Communities Coalition. (1999). *Pathways to a healthy community: An Indicators and Evaluation Tool Kit user guide.* Toronto: Author.

Patton, M. Q. (2002). *Qualitative evaluation and research methods* (3rd ed.). Thousand Oaks, CA: Sage.

Reichardt, C. S., & Cook, T. D. (1979). Beyond qualitative versus quantitative methods. In T. D. Cook & C. S. Reichardt (Eds.), *Qualitative and quantitative methods in evaluation research* (pp. 7–32). Thousand Oaks, CA: Sage.

Rossi, P. H., Freeman, H. E., & Lipsey, M. W. (1999). *Evaluation: A systematic approach* (6th ed.). Thousand Oaks, CA: Sage.

Roussos, S. T., & Fawcett, S. B. (2000). A review of collaborative partnerships as a strategy for improving community health. *Annual Review of Public Health, 21,* 369–402.

Schulz, A. J., Israel, B. A., & Lantz, P. M. (2003). Instrument for evaluating dimensions of group dynamics within community-based participatory research partnerships. *Evaluation and Program Planning, 26*(3), 249–262.

Shaw, M. E. (1981). *Group dynamics: The psychology of small group behavior* (3rd ed.). New York: McGraw-Hill.

Sofaer, S. (2000). *Working together, moving ahead: A manual to support effective community health coalitions.* New York: Baruch College School of Public Affairs.

Sofaer, S., & Kenney, E. (1996). *A survey tool for coalition self assessment.* Washington, DC: Center for Health Outcomes Improvement Research, George Washington University Medical Center.

Springett, J. (2003). Issues in participatory evaluation. In M. Minkler & N. Wallerstein (Eds.), *Community-based participatory research for health* (pp. 263–288). San Francisco: Jossey-Bass.

Strauss, A., & Corbin, J. (1990). *Basics of qualitative research: Grounded theory procedures and techniques.* Thousand Oaks, CA: Sage.

Wallerstein, N. (1999). Power between evaluator and community: Research relationships within New Mexico's healthier communities. *Social Science & Medicine, 49*(1), 39–53.

Wallerstein, N., Polascek, M., & Maltrud, K. (2002). Participatory evaluation model for coalitions: The development of systems indicators. *Health Promotion Practice, 3*(3), 361–373.

Weiss, E. S., Anderson, R. M., & Lasker, R. D. (2002). Making the most of collaboration: Exploring the relationship between partnership synergy and partnership functioning. *Health Education & Behavior, 29*(6), 683–698.

Yin, R. K. (1984). *Case study research: Design and methods.* Thousand Oaks, CA: Sage.

PART SIX

FEEDBACK, INTERPRETATION, DISSEMINATION, AND APPLICATION OF RESULTS

Part Six focuses on four components of the "final" phase of the CBPR process—feedback, interpretation, and dissemination of research findings and the application of findings to guide the development of interventions and policy formation. Feedback and interpretation of findings involve all research partners and participants in reviewing results from data analysis in order to share their reactions and possible corrections as well as their interpretation of what the results may mean in the context of their community. As Stoecker (2003) notes, although it is optimal for data analysis to be done collaboratively by all research partners, at the very least data analysis should be done with strict accountability to the community. Such accountability can be ensured by feeding back results to the community to engage them in reacting to the findings, including correcting findings and offering their interpretation of what these findings mean for their community.

Equally important to the CBPR process is the dissemination of findings to all research partners and communities through multiple venues and in ways that are understandable, respectful, and useful (Israel, Schulz, Parker, & Becker, 1998). Moreover, dissemination of results is an increasing requirement of funding agencies (Green et al., 2003; Ammerman et al., 2003) and an expectation of study participants and their communities (López, Parker, Edgren, & Brakefield-Caldwell, 2005). Nonetheless, broad dissemination activities can be challenging for academic partners, who may have to go beyond their usual bounds of scientific journals and audiences (Chávez, Duran, Baker, Avila, & Wallerstein, 2003; Flaskerud & Anderson, 1999). Dissemination can also be challenging for community members, who may have little time or training, or both, to develop guidelines for, plan, and conduct dissemination activities.

Finally, the translation and application of research findings for intervention development and policy formation is a crucial link to CBPR's commitment to action. As noted by Themba and Minkler (2003), one of the critical differences between CBPR and other research approaches is CBPR's commitment to action and to fostering social changes as an integral part of the research process.

In Part Six, Chapters Thirteen through Seventeen collectively illustrate the four elements of data feedback, interpretation, dissemination, and application of research findings. They show how various data collection methods used within CBPR relate to these four elements. The data collection methods used include group interview and dialogue, photovoice, document review, survey question- naire, focus group interview and secondary data analysis. These chapters also describe process methods that were used to ensure active participation of all partners in the activities of this phase.

In Chapter Thirteen, Parker, Robins, Israel, Brakefield-Caldwell, Edgren, and Wilkins describe the development and application of guidelines for the dis- semination of results from the Community Action Against Asthma project in Detroit, Michigan. The authors offer valuable detail on how and why the part- nership members decided they needed guidelines for dissemination and created a structure to develop both the guidelines and procedures for disseminating results. The guidelines provide a useful template for other partnerships to con- sider and adopt. The authors present concrete examples of procedures and mechanisms to feed back specific components of the research findings to project participants, build in structured time for participants to interpret these findings, and share the results more broadly with community members. The authors also highlight both the successes and challenges of implementing the dissemination guidelines, and the lessons learned throughout the process.

In Chapter Fourteen, Baker and Motton focus on their use of in-depth group interviews in the Planning Grant project and describe the stages involved in col- lecting data and then using these data to develop action within a CBPR effort. They present a case example of the Planning Grant partnership project in rural southeast Missouri, which conducted a series of group interviews with the Bootheel Heart Health Coalitions over an eleven month period. The authors highlight the following steps in conducting in-depth group interviews: the role of community and academic partners in developing the interview guide, par- ticipant recruitment, data collection and analysis, feedback on findings, inter- pretation of findings, and planning action based on the findings. Their description of the processes used to feed the findings back to participants and seek their interpretation is particularly insightful and will be most helpful to other CBPR partnerships. In addition, the authors describe how the partnership applied the findings, as the basis of an action planning process, to prioritize community issues for which to develop and implement change strategies. The authors provide a compelling description of the challenges and lessons learned in undertaking in-depth group interviews in the context of the CBPR Planning Grant project.

In Chapter Fifteen, López, Eng, Robinson, and Wang describe the use of photovoice as the principal data collection method for a CBPR project with African American women breast cancer survivors in rural eastern North Carolina. Photovoice is a participatory method in which community members use cameras to take photos that represent and communicate to others their experiences (Wang & Burris, 1994). The authors present a brief overview of photovoice, including the origins and previous applications of this method. Their case example is the Inspirational Images project, an academic-community partnership formed to enable breast cancer survivors to explore and voice their survivorship concerns so that appropriate interventions could be developed to address them. The authors' description of how they conducted photovoice and disseminated their findings, using a CBPR process, offers unique insights into combining research with empowerment education methods. They provide practical detail on planning and conducting a forum to disseminate photovoice findings to "influential advocates" (such as local policy and decision makers) and engage them in a discussion of initiating the next action steps. Their examination of challenges and lessons learned is also most instructive. For example, their discussion of when and how to invite influential advocates to the forum and considerations of the drawbacks of the option they took will assist other partnerships in addressing this issue.

In Chapter Sixteen, Freudenberg, Rogers, Ritas, and Nerney describe their work in participatory policy research (PPR), which is a CBPR approach to analyzing the impact of policies on public health and applying the findings to catalyze action to change harmful policies. As the case example the authors present the Community Reintegration Network (CRN), which advocates for citywide changes in policies related to community reintegration of individuals returning from a municipal jail system to urban, low-income communities in New York City. The authors provide a thoughtful description of some of the key aspects of PPR, such as its emphasis on involving all stakeholders, especially those traditionally excluded from the policy process; beginning with community perceptions of the problem, and thus framing the policy questions broadly and across various sectors and levels of government; and embracing both analysis and action rather than stopping once analysis is completed. Their detailed description of how the CRN partnership applied the following PPR methods to affect policy is particularly valuable: reviews of relevant professional, mass media, government, and advocacy literatures; interviews with government policymakers, administrators, and advocates; and surveys of various constituencies. The authors conclude with a frank discussion of the limitations and challenges of using PPR, the lessons learned, and the implications for the use of PPR by others.

In Chapter Seventeen, the final chapter, Morello-Frosch, Pastor, Sadd, Porras, and Prichard focus on using the method of secondary data analysis to identify and change policies that adversely affect communities. Their case example is the Southern California Environmental Justice Collaborative, a community-academic partnership that combines (1) research on regional economic development and environmental health, public policy advocacy, and community organizing and (2) research using secondary data sources to document and address Southern California's demographic and geographical distributions of pollution. The authors offer valuable detail on activities to disseminate findings, providing examples of successful efforts to link research with community organizing and advocacy activities to promote policy change. They conclude with insights on the challenges and limitations of using secondary data analysis in a CBPR project and the lessons learned by the collaborative.

References

Ammerman, A., Corbie-Smith, G., St. George, D.M.M., Washington, C., Weathers, B., & Jackson-Christian, B. (2003). Research expectations among African-American church leaders in the PRAISE! project: A randomized trial guided by community-based participatory research. *American Journal of Public Health, 93*(10), 1720–1727.

Chávez, V., Duran, B. M., Baker, Q. E., Avila, M. M., & Wallerstein, N. (2003). The dance of race and privilege in community-based participatory research. In M. Minkler & N. Wallerstein (Eds.), *Community-based participatory research for health* (pp. 81–97). San Francisco: Jossey-Bass.

Flaskerud, J. H., & Anderson, N. (1999). Disseminating the results of participant-focused research. *Journal of Transcultural Nursing, 10*(4), 340–349.

Green, L. W., George, M. A., Daniel, M., Frankish, C. J., Herbert, C. J., Bowie, W. R., et al. (2003). Guidelines for participatory research in health promotion. In M. Minkler & N. Wallerstein (Eds.), *Community-based participatory research for health* (pp. 27–52). San Francisco: Jossey-Bass.

Israel, B. A., Schulz, A. J., Parker, E. A., & Becker, A. B. (1998). Review of community-based research: Assessing partnership approaches to improve public health. *Annual Review of Public Health, 19*, 173–202.

López, E.D.S., Parker, E. A., Edgren, K. K., & Brakefield-Caldwell, W. (2005). Lessons learned while using a CBPR approach to plan and conduct forums to disseminate research findings back to partnering communities: A case study from Community Action Against Asthma, Detroit, Michigan. *Metropolitan Universities Journal, 16*(1).

Stoecker, R. (2003). Are academics irrelevant? Approaches and roles for scholars in community-based participatory research. In M. Minkler & N. Wallerstein (Eds.), *Community-based participatory research for health* (pp. 98–112). San Francisco: Jossey-Bass.

Themba, M. K., and Minkler, M. (2003). Influencing policy through community based participatory research. In M. Minkler & N. Wallerstein (Eds.), *Community-based participatory research for health* (pp. 349–370). San Francisco: Jossey-Bass.

Wang, C., & Burris, M. A. (1994). Empowerment through photo novella: Portraits of participation. *Health Education Quarterly, 21*(2), 171–186.

CHAPTER THIRTEEN

Developing and Implementing Guidelines for Dissemination

The Experience of the Community Action Against Asthma Project

Edith A. Parker, Thomas G. Robins, Barbara A. Israel,
Wilma Brakefield-Caldwell, Katherine K. Edgren, and Donele J. Wilkins

Ensuring that findings are disseminated to the communities studied is an important aspect of all public health research endeavors. This is especially true in community-based participatory research (CBPR), because a fundamental tenet of CBPR is to use the knowledge generated to inform action with the community involved in the research (Green et al., 1995; Israel, Schulz, Parker, & Becker, 1998). For this to happen the research design and methods must include a plan for translating and disseminating findings so that these findings can inform and be incorporated into community efforts for change at the individual, organizational, community, and policy levels (deKoning & Martin,

Acknowledgments: The Michigan Center for the Environment and Children's Health (MCECH) is a community-based participatory research initiative investigating the influence of environmental factors on childhood asthma, and is a project of the Detroit Community-Academic Urban Research Center (www.sph.umich.edu/urc). MCECH involves collaboration among the Detroit Department of Health and Wellness Promotion, the University of Michigan Schools of Public Health and Medicine, the Henry Ford Health System, the Michigan Department of Agriculture Office of Pesticides and Plant Management, and the following community-based organizations: Community Health and Social Services Center, Friends of Parkside, Warren-Conner Development Coalition, Kettering/Butzel Health Initiative, Butzel Family Center, Latino Family Services, United Community Housing Coalition, Detroiters Working for Environmental Justice, and Detroit Hispanic Development Corporation. We thank these partners for their contributions. MCECH is funded by the National Institute of Environmental Health Sciences (grants P01-ES09589, R01 ES10688) and the U.S. Environmental Protection Agency (grant R826710-01).

1996; Farquhar & Wing, 2003; Green et al., 1995; Israel et al., 1998). Despite the potential usefulness of creating a dissemination plan, there are few examples in the literature of how to engage all partners in determining the structure and products of the dissemination process. In this chapter, we discuss the experience of the Community Action Against Asthma project of the Michigan Center for the Environment and Children's Health (MCECH) in involving community and academic partners in establishing and then implementing a process aimed at disseminating findings in a timely and understandable fashion to participants, community members, health practitioners, government officials, academics, and policymakers.

OVERVIEW OF THE MCECH AND COMMUNITY ACTION AGAINST ASTHMA PROJECT

The Michigan Center for the Environment and Children's Health is affiliated with an already existing community-academic partnership, the Detroit Community-Academic Urban Research Center (URC) (see Chapter Twelve for a more detailed description of the URC). The URC had identified childhood illnesses related to the environment as a priority area for research. In 1998, the URC board successfully competed for funding from the Children's Environmental Health Research Initiative, awarded by the National Institute of Environmental Health Sciences (NIEHS) and the U.S. Environmental Protection Agency. This five-year award enabled the Detroit URC to establish MCECH as a coordinating structure for the following three studies of childhood asthma:

1. A laboratory-based, mouse model study to determine if the mechanism of chronic pulmonary inflammation due to children's repeated exposure to allergens is mediated by excessive local production of chemokines (the *chemokines* project)

2. An intervention study to reduce environmental triggers for childhood asthma at the household and neighborhood levels

3. An epidemiological study of the relationship between ambient and indoor air quality exposures (for example, ozone and particulate matter) and children's lung function and other asthma-related health indicators

The epidemiological and intervention studies were conducted with the same participant population and guided by the same steering committee (described later) and therefore were combined into one larger project, named Community Action Against Asthma (CAAA). In year two, realizing that there were insufficient funds to implement the neighborhood component of the CAAA intervention due to an initial cut in the MCECH budget, the CAAA Steering Committee applied for and received an additional grant from NIEHS. This project, which was incorporated into the CAAA activities and was thus administered by the steering committee, focused on neighborhood organizing and policy change aimed at reducing triggers for childhood asthma. Many of the community organizing activities of this project involved disseminating results of CAAA's household intervention and epidemiological studies.

The initial funding period for the three MCECH studies (the mouse model project, the household intervention, and the epidemiological study) ended in October 2004. CAAA's neighborhood- and policy-level intervention study is funded through June 2005 and will enable CAAA to continue its dissemination work.

Because the chemokines project was laboratory based, community members were not as involved in it as they were in the other projects. In addition, the steering committee recognized that the results of the chemokines project would not be as interesting to community members as other project results would because this project was not as immediately relevant to community members' lives as the other studies were. Consequently, although the chemokines project fell under the MCECH dissemination guidelines being discussed here, it did not focus its dissemination activities in the community. Thus this chapter will examine the process and structure for interpreting and disseminating CAAA's household intervention and epidemiological research projects.

CAAA followed the set of CBPR principles originally adopted by the URC to guide the research (Israel et al., 1998). The work of CAAA was guided by a steering committee (SC) that included representatives from community-based organizations, health services institutions, and academia (see the note at the beginning of the chapter for a list of the partner organizations). The CAAA SC met monthly and was actively involved in all major phases of the research and intervention, for example, defining the research questions, designing survey instruments; hiring key staff, and designing research and intervention activities such as educational materials and incentives for participants (Edgren et al., in press; Parker et al., 2003). To ensure that CAAA project results were disseminated according to the CBPR principles, the SC established a dissemination committee to develop guidelines and operating procedures for project dissemination.

CAAA was conducted in eastside and southwest Detroit. Eastside Detroit is predominantly African American (more than 90 percent), and the southwest is the part of the city where the largest percentage of Latinos resides (approximately 40 percent Latino, 50 percent African American, and 10 percent white) (U.S. Census Bureau, 1990). The specific aim of the household intervention project was to reduce residents' exposure to the triggers of childhood asthma. The household component consisted of a minimum of nine visits over a one-year period by a *community environmental specialist* or outreach worker, who provided education and materials needed for reduction of exposure to asthma triggers, and referrals for medical care, tenant issues, and smoking cessation. The neighborhood component, as described previously, was funded after MCECH began under a separate grant mechanism and involves community organizers working with community residents and organizations to reduce neighborhood- and community-level physical and psychosocial stressors associated with childhood asthma. The neighborhood component is still ongoing.

The epidemiological study analyzed the relationship between ambient and indoor air quality and children's asthma-related health status. The study included the collection of data on asthma symptoms, lung function, medication use, and health care utilization, together with exposure measures such as ambient PM 10 and PM 2.5 (particulate matter with aerodynamic diameters of <10 microns and 2.5 microns, respectively) and ozone.

FORMATION AND FUNCTIONS OF THE CAAA DISSEMINATION COMMITTEE

During the first year of the CAAA project, steering committee members identified three issues of dissemination. First, they wanted to ensure that dissemination reached both academic and community audiences and in a timely fashion. Second, the SC wanted to build and guide the capacity of all CAAA partners, including but not limited to the academic partners, to communicate results, through a range of channels, as soon as the results became available. Especially in view of the potentially significant policy ramifications of project results, the SC agreed that project findings presented by different partners in different venues needed to be highly consistent. The SC was concerned that without a standardized summary of the findings, information might be presented differently by various SC partners and these differences might be used to discredit the findings. Finally, the SC wanted to ensure that both academic and community representatives would always copresent at conferences and coauthor publications on CAAA methods and findings.

Hence, in the fall of 1999, the SC decided to form the dissemination committee (DC) to develop guidelines for dissemination activities and oversee decisions around dissemination. The SC asked one of the academic principal investigators to serve as chair of the DC and to work with other academic investigators to write the first draft of a set of dissemination guidelines for review and input by the full SC. This draft outlined the potential role of the dissemination committee (for example, outlining core articles, reviewing and approving requests for use of data and access to data, and determining and prioritizing methods of dissemination of findings), suggested criteria for determining coauthorship on academic manuscripts, and proposed that committee membership be composed of five academic and two community partners (representing the different cores and projects of MCECH).

Upon reviewing this draft the SC's community members noted that community representation on the DC needed to be equal to that of academic representation. Thus representation on the DC was set at six academic partners and six community partners.

Recruiting and Selecting Members

The selection processes for the academic and the community members of the dissemination committee differed slightly. After discussion the academic members of the SC decided to ask the leaders of the various MCECH components to be representatives to the dissemination committee. These leaders included the MCECH principal investigator; the intervention, epidemiological, and chemokines project leaders; and the leaders of MCECH's Biostatistics and Exposure Assessment Facilities Cores. This decision was made because these persons would be knowledgeable about the types of data results that would be generated from their projects and also because of a desire to protect the time of those faculty who were more junior in their careers. For the DC community member positions, volunteers from the SC were solicited, with an emphasis on ensuring that there were an equal number of members from both eastside and southwest organizations. Community members who volunteered became members of the DC. Once membership was decided the committee met monthly from January through June 2000. As will be described later, the activities of the DC were assumed by the SC in July 2000.

The dissemination committee decided to hold its meetings before or after steering committee meetings, to make them more convenient for members since all members of the DC were also members of the SC. Dissemination decisions were made through a consensus process used previously by the URC (Israel et al., 2001). Members were asked if they could agree to a proposed decision by at least 70 percent (as opposed to 100 percent). Using this rule, proposed decisions were discussed and modified, if necessary, until all DC members could support the decision by at least 70 percent. The proposed decisions were then added to the next steering committee meeting agenda for discussion and final approval.

Further Developing Dissemination Guidelines and Related Issues

During DC meetings, members discussed and revised the draft dissemination guidelines and related issues and agreed on recommendations to make to the SC, as discussed later, for decisions about

- Developing a process for selection of SC members to participate in conference and meeting presentations
- Further revising and finalizing the dissemination guidelines
- Establishing ground rules for coauthorship
- Drafting a proposed list of core articles and presentations to be developed from the project

Selecting Partners to Copresent at Conferences. At the first meeting of the DC, members discussed the procedure for selecting CAAA partners to copresent at conferences at length. Committee members recognized the importance of presentations at national and local venues as a vehicle not only for disseminating research results but also for emphasizing the CBPR partnership between MCECH researchers and community members. DC members' discussion of including, whenever possible, a community copresenter with an academic copresenter addressed the following issues and suggestions:

- The CAAA dissemination policy should articulate procedures that would avoid resentment among SC members and staff who might like to copresent but were not chosen to do so.
- The selection criteria for copresenters should include level of participation in the project and attendance at the monthly SC meetings, ability to present a quality and informed presentation, and comfort in presenting in a public venue. The committee acknowledged that not all persons participating in CAAA would have public-speaking skills and experience and therefore the DC discussed the possibility of offering training in public speaking.
- Requests to copresent at a conference should be brought to the steering committee meeting for approval. If this were not possible, owing, for example, to time constraints imposed by due dates for abstracts, the person requesting permission to present at the conference would contact all SC members via phone, e-mail, or fax for approval.
- Because CAAA's academic partners often received information about conferences that the community partners did not receive, they had an extra responsibility to notify community partners in a timely fashion to allow adequate opportunities for the DC to follow dissemination policy.

- Two guiding principles for CAAA's dissemination process have been to ensure that all presentations are made with the knowledge and approval of the SC and that the authority of community partners is equal to that of academic partners in deciding who speaks for the whole group.

To ensure equitable copresentation at conferences, one academic partner suggested the adoption of the Rose Bowl Principle. This refers to the policy followed by the Big Ten athletic conference (which includes the University of Michigan) for determining which team will participate in the Rose Bowl football game when two teams have identical records. The policy states that the team that has participated less recently in the Rose Bowl will be selected. Hence, the SC should select copresenters who either have not presented before or have not presented as recently as other potential presenters.

Further Revising and Finalizing Dissemination Guidelines. The DC took approximately three months to develop and further revise the dissemination guidelines, carrying out such tasks as adding a section on procedures for selecting participants to present at conferences, as just described. An ad hoc committee of the DC was formed for the purpose of further revising the guidelines. Members of this ad hoc committee drafted a statement of rationale and operating philosophy, and after approval by the SC, this statement was merged with the already existing description of dissemination procedures. This final document was adopted by the SC and titled the "Philosophy and Guiding Principles for Dissemination of Findings of the Michigan Center for the Environment and Children's Health (MCECH) including Authorship of Publications and Presentations, Policies and Procedures, Access to Data, and Related Matters" (see Appendix I).

Establishing Ground Rules for Coauthorship. The DC wanted to follow standard guidelines for authorship, such as those of the International Committee of Medical Journal Editors, which states that all authors must have made substantial contributions to each of three activities (in either oral or written form): (1) conception and design, or analysis and interpretation; (2) drafting the article or revising it critically for important intellectual content; and (3) review and approval of the final version to be published (International Committee of Medical Journal Editors, 2004). The DC also wanted to make explicit what was meant by a "substantial contribution" in a way that ensured recognition of community as well as academic partners as authors. The definition agreed to was active participation in the conception and design or analysis and interpretation, measured directly by number of hours of input on collecting, processing, and interpreting data; indirectly by time and energy spent supervising a junior researcher in the acquisition, processing, and interpretation of data; or both. Though not stated in the guidelines (perhaps because it was recognized from the start as an implicit requirement of all dissemination activities), all manuscripts must include both community and academic partners as coauthors. As described later, the DC then developed a process for proposing manuscripts for publication and presentations, determining their priority, and identifying the lead and coauthors for each.

Drafting a Proposed List of Core Publications and Presentations to Be Developed from the Project. The DC asked its academic members to draft a proposed list of core articles for publications and presentations on findings from the CAAA project. Core articles were defined as those central to the main hypotheses described in the initial proposal. The SC agreed that once those core articles were determined by the DC, other members of the broader CAAA team could propose additional topics for publication and presentation. Over the course of four months, the academic members drafted a list that went beyond the initially proposed core articles and included thirty-five possible topics in seven broad areas (such as methodology, exposure assessment, and intervention-related). Later, when the teams began writing, they realized that many of these topics were not sufficient for stand-alone articles and they combined topics into a smaller number of manuscripts.

The DC approved the list and expected that the lead author for articles that were data driven would come from the academic members of the research team, because they would be the best versed in the details of study design and analysis. The DC also suggested adding articles on findings that were not data driven, such as lessons learned about different participant incentive options, noting that the lead author for these articles would come from the community members of the research team. The DC acknowledged that even in the CBPR literature, community partners rarely served as the lead author, perhaps, as noted by a community member of the DC, because community partners tend to be "the doers, not the writers." Hence, CAAA's contribution to furthering the influence of CBPR could be to build the capacity of community partners to take the lead in disseminating findings to an academic audience. A category of articles entitled "other qualitative methodological," with seven possible topics, was added to the list to cover these possible manuscripts. As will be discussed later, to date there have been no articles in which the lead author was a community partner. The DC prioritized the overall list of possible articles and identified seven manuscripts that should be completed first. These manuscripts were mostly descriptive and were chosen because they did not require data results (which were not yet available) and they would describe the various aspects of the project so that future manuscripts would not have to include such details on the project methodology and could instead refer to these earlier articles.

Establishing Procedures for Feedback to the Community

The DC also discussed and established initial procedures for dissemination of information to the community. For example, the DC established a process for handling requests from the media in which any inquiries from the media would be directed to the project manager, who would determine which academic and community members it would be best to involve, depending on their expertise and availability. The DC also decided to have a fact sheet about the project and key findings, which would be updated quarterly, as well as a newsletter to disseminate information and to serve as a retention tool for participants (as described later). Processes for some community-wide dissemination activities (such as community forums and meetings with policymakers) were not specified by the DC but were later handled by the SC and will be described in the next section.

TRANSITION OF DC RESPONSIBILITIES TO THE SC

After six months, questions arose during a dissemination committee meeting about whether there was a continuing need for a separate dissemination committee or whether its ongoing functions should be part of the steering committee's responsibilities. Attendance at DC meetings was becoming a problem; sometimes not enough members were present to establish a quorum. Consequently, DC members decided that after dissemination procedures were in place, they would meet less frequently and much of the DC business would be carried out by fax, e-mail, and mail.

With the SC's adoption of the "Philosophy and Guiding Principles for Dissemination," the DC ceased to meet. Although there was never an explicit discussion and decision about disbanding the DC, the SC began handling dissemination issues at its monthly meetings. This occurred due to a combination of the following factors:

- Dissemination processes and procedures were in place, so the SC had a roadmap to use in making dissemination-related decisions

- All but two members of the steering committee were also members of the dissemination committee, so the DC was well represented on the SC

- The time required placed an excessive burden on community members who served on both the DC and SC

- A leadership transition had occurred when the DC chairperson left for a sabbatical and was replaced by another academic member

IMPLEMENTATION OF THE GUIDELINES: EXAMPLES OF DISSEMINATION DECISIONS AND ACTIVITIES

The dissemination activities of CAAA were varied and included presentations and materials focused on academic audiences, the steering committee itself, the broader community, and the participants in the CAAA research projects. Table 13.1 lists the types of dissemination activities carried out by CAAA during the course of the project. The following section describes how the dissemination and steering committees implemented the guidelines in the various dissemination-related activities.

Selecting Representatives for Conferences and Meetings

For the most part the selection of presenters for conferences and meetings followed criteria and procedures as discussed earlier and outlined in the

Table 13.1. Types and Numbers of CAAA Dissemination Activities over Five Years

Type of Dissemination	Number Completed
National conferences, invited presentations	58
State or local conferences, invited presentations	7
Community forum(s)	3
Academic manuscripts	10
Newspaper, Web-based, magazine, radio, or TV interviews	15
Briefings or presentations for elected officials or government employees	3
Newsletters	12
Fact sheets (findings, project description)	6
Web-site development	1
University classroom presentations	10
Presentations to community groups	
• Schools	20
• Community-based organizations	4
Feedback to project participants	
• Lung function (all participants)	280 participants
• Indoor air sampling results (subsample of participants)	15 participants
• Feedback forums	1 for eastside, 1 for southwest

dissemination guidelines (see Appendix I). The selection of academic representatives was often the most clear-cut process, depending as it did on the nature of the meeting and the subject to be presented (for example, results of the intervention, results of the epidemiological study, air quality monitoring). Whenever possible, academic members of the research team who were more junior in experience were selected, to help them gain further experience and recognition.

The DC had worried about potential disagreements over which community representative would make certain presentations, but this did not occur. For example, during the third meeting of the DC, one of the academic researchers notified the members that a community member was needed to copresent with an academic at a national conference on CBPR, sponsored by the National Institute of Environmental Health Sciences. After discussion of the focus of the conference and the presentation that had been requested, one community partner nominated another community partner to present, based on her involvement and knowledge of CAAA and the relevance of her previous work to the presentation. The rest of the committee supported this nomination and the "nominee" agreed to copresent.

In general, selection of attendees for conferences became a more informal process than originally proposed by the DC. For example, for each conference presentation or meeting invitation, the dissemination guidelines spelled out that the SC would develop a list of the people who were eligible, based on their level of participation, their knowledge and experience, and the SC's desire to ensure that a variety of members were offered this opportunity. In actuality, academic members who were either submitting conference abstracts or had been invited to present, would ask for volunteers or would suggest a person (based on the presentation topic) and request SC approval.

Approving Abstracts and Abstract Authorship for Conference Presentations

The DC also discussed the need for a process for submitting abstracts for SC approval before they were officially submitted for review by conference organizers. Noting that abstracts were sometimes "last-minute" submissions, the DC discussed ways to ensure that the abstracts would be reviewed by the SC without jeopardizing their timely submission. The DC suggested that SC members create a list of the conferences and meetings (and their abstract submission deadlines) that the SC would like partners to attend, so that to the extent possible, last-minute approvals and submissions could be avoided. However, this list was never formally developed.

The DC also adopted and implemented the following procedure for abstract submission. The interested person (if other than the lead researcher) first submitted the abstract to the lead researcher of the project that was the subject of the abstract, for his or her approval. The lead researcher would then send the abstract to the steering committee members. If time permitted, this process happened before an SC meeting so that the abstract could be discussed at the meeting. If this were not possible, SC members were asked to respond by telephone or e-mail to say whether they had any questions or concerns with the abstract and whether or not they approved the abstract. This approval process was one of passive consent, that is, if steering committee members did not respond about the abstract, it was assumed that they approved its content and coauthorship.

Selecting Lead Authors and Coauthors for Manuscripts

As noted earlier, the dissemination committee drafted and prioritized a list of core articles for publications and presentations. The steering committee selected lead authors for core articles, from the principal investigators or coinvestigators of the project. Writing teams were then determined, based on the topic and the involvement of SC members in that particular aspect of the project. Once the SC named a writing team, the lead author brought the writing team together either in person or by telephone conference call, at which time he or she either presented a draft outline for discussion by the group or spent this time working with the group to create an outline. The lead author was responsible for writing the first draft, basing it on this outline and discussion and consulting with the coauthors as needed. This first draft was then shared with the coauthors for their review and feedback, and the lead author made revisions in light of the coauthors' comments, repeating this process until the article was ready to be submitted. The early stages of this process usually involved several meetings of the writing team, with the subsequent review and revisions handled via e-mail and regular mail and telephone conversations.

Handling Requests for Use of Data

The DC also developed a procedure for requesting permission to use data from the CAAA project. As part of this procedure, anyone interested in using the data for a purpose other than writing a core article had to complete the "Request for Use of Community Action Against Asthma Data" form. The form required the applicant to answer the following questions.

1. Are you requesting this data for personal or for organizational use? Please explain.

2. Please describe in detail what data you are requesting from CAAA, both with respect to scope and desired format.

3. Please describe in detail for what purposes you wish to obtain this data and how the data will be used. Include in your description how this use of the data will benefit the Detroit community, as appropriate to the intended purpose, and how this use otherwise will follow community-based participatory research principles [a copy of these principles was attached to the form].

If necessary, the requester was asked to come to a SC meeting to further explain the request and answer questions. In addition, all requesters who were allowed to use data were required to come to an SC meeting to present the findings of any analysis performed with CAAA data. To date, three doctoral degree students and one master's degree student have requested and used CAAA data for their theses.

Discussing a New, Affiliated Project and the Way to Handle Dissemination Requirements

Within six months of the DC's formation, an investigator from another university approached the Community Action Against Asthma Steering Committee about collaborating on an additional exposure assessment project. This new project, which was to take place during one of CAAA's seasonal assessments, would require parking a mobile laboratory (contained in a specially modified tractor-trailer) beside one of the primary schools where CAAA was conducting ongoing air quality monitoring using equipment placed on the school roof. The investigator wished to use CAAA data to augment data collected by the mobile laboratory (which would conduct animal experiments assessing the effects of exposures to concentrated pollutants in the air on the animals' lung function). The DC was concerned about how data from the two projects would be shared and wanted to ensure that all results from this new project would be shared with community members in a way that complied with CAAA's dissemination guidelines. The DC recognized that the investigator of the proposed new project did not use a CBPR approach, but felt that he might be open to learning more about and following the principles of CBPR, especially in this project. After much discussion the DC suggested that CAAA draft a letter of agreement that stipulated the requirements for dissemination, and the SC agreed with this suggestion. The letter of agreement included the following requirements: any manuscripts that originated from this new project must include coauthors from CAAA, the CAAA data manager and biostatistician must be informed of any additional analysis undertaken by others, and CAAA must be kept abreast about the work and progress of this new project (through such means as formal presentations of results to the CAAA steering committee). The CBPR principles and the dissemination policies and procedures were attached to the letter of agreement. The new investigator agreed to the requests in the letter of agreement and subsequently presented project results to the SC on several occasions.

Feeding Back to Participants and the Wider Community

Throughout the project both the dissemination committee and later the steering committee were active in developing and implementing mechanisms for feedback to study participants and the larger community. Methods of feedback included fact sheets about the project and general project findings, individualized feedback sheets for project participants (including, in some cases, individualized meetings to explain the results), and a series of forums for project participants and the broader community.

Fact Sheet Development and Distribution. One of the initial decisions of the DC was to create a *fact sheet* about the project. The DC proposed that the fact sheet be developed in layperson's language, updated quarterly, and distributed within the community. The DC felt these fact sheets could serve as the main source of information for informal presentations by SC members and staff in the Detroit community and could also be distributed directly to interested community members, legislators, and government officials. The intent of the fact sheets was to give an overview of the CAAA intervention and exposure assessment projects, share data findings as they emerged, and also include relevant findings from other research projects on similar topics. The DC and later the SC were instrumental in the development of these fact sheets. They provided input on focus and content and ensured that the sheets were understandable and culturally and linguistically appropriate for the intended audiences. (See Appendix J for an example of a fact sheet on particulate matter.)

Individualized Feedback to Project Participants. As part of the exposure and health effects component of the project, lung function assessments were performed twice daily over two weeks in each season, with a handheld, digitized peak flow device. The two academic physician members of the SC worked closely with SC community partners to develop a clear and useful format for sharing this inherently complex data with project participants. The results were also mailed to all physicians of the participating children if the caregivers had requested CAAA to do so.

Individualized feedback on indoor air quality was also presented to the fifteen families who participated in the intensive air sampling component of the exposure and health effects study. The academic partners involved in this component worked with project staff to develop individualized feedback sheets. These sheets showed the levels of particulate matter (PM) 2.5 and ozone in each individual home compared to the aggregate levels of all fifteen homes and to the overall EPA National Ambient Air Quality Standards for outdoor levels of PM 2.5 and ozone. These sheets were shared with the families during a meeting in which the academic partners gave an overview presentation of what they had found, explained the results, and then were available to meet with the families to answer their questions. (See Appendix K for an example of a feedback sheet on air quality provided to a participant in the intensive air sampling component.)

Community Forums. In the fourth year of the project, as preliminary results became available, the steering committee conducted a series of forums to feed back the results to the broader community and the project participants. A subgroup of the SC, consisting of project field staff, two academic partners, and two community partners, developed a proposed plan for the forum and shared it with the SC for input and modification. Initially, the SC planned to have a single forum for both project participants and other interested community groups, but on further discussion the SC chose to hold separate forums. Some of the academic partners suggested that the results should first be presented to the participating families for their information and reactions before being presented to the wider community. Following this suggestion, the SC decided to have two separate forums for participants (one in eastside and one in southwest Detroit) before staging a community forum for the wider community. The SC also felt that having two separate forums would make it easier for participants from these separate intervention areas to attend a forum. These two forums were held on successive Saturdays and lasted two hours each.

The format of the family forums consisted of a welcome by project staff, presentation of intervention and air quality research results by the academic partners, questions and discussion, and a small-group exercise in which the family participants were asked to respond to a set of questions developed by the planning committee and aimed at increasing understanding of the findings. CAAA served refreshments, distributed door prizes, and provided transportation and child care to ensure that participants could attend. The southwest and eastside family forums were attended by twenty-five adults and nineteen adults, respectively. Forum participants included adult caregivers from CAAA participant families and guests of the immediate families (friends and additional family), numerous children who either went to the child-care room or participated in forum activities, and several CAAA staff, researchers, and steering committee members. The community-wide forum was held a few weeks after these two initial family forums and focused more on the results of the air quality and health effects investigations. This emphasis was proposed by the planning committee and approved by the SC, both of whom felt that community members would be more interested in this aspect of the study than in the results of the intervention. Members of community-based organizations, governmental agencies and officials, families who had participated in the study, and individual community residents who had attended previous CAAA events or had worked for CAAA in data collection activities were invited to attend the community-wide forum. This larger forum was attended by forty-one individuals, including CAAA family participants, staff members of locally elected officials (a state representative and a county commissioner), agency representatives, advocacy workers, and community members. Many of these individuals and groups were identified through an assessment performed by the staff of the community organizing component of CAAA with the active involvement of the SC. (For more information on these forums, see López et al., 2005.)

CHALLENGES

The steering committee experienced a number of challenges in creating and implementing guidelines for disseminating research findings in a community-based participatory fashion. We describe these challenges in this section, and in the next section we present the lessons learned about handling these challenges, as well as the implications of these lessons.

Adhering consistently to the dissemination guidelines. One of the challenges CAAA faced involved situations in which academic members of CAAA were invited to speak about the project at national meetings or conferences. When this occurred, the invited person would let the conference organizers know that due to the participatory process of the CAAA partnership, presentations were normally copresented by an academic and a community partner. Often the organization or conference planner would agree to pay for two persons to copresent, but sometimes the organization did not have enough funds to sponsor more than the academic person originally invited. If project funds were not available to pay for the community partner's expenses, the situation was discussed openly at SC meetings. In general, community partners understood the constraints and the academic partner would present alone.

Another challenge involved meeting deadlines for submitting abstracts and responding to invitations to present at conferences when these occurred in between the monthly meetings of the DC (and subsequently the SC). A combination of e-mail, phone, and fax messages was used to communicate between the abstract submitter or the invitee and the rest of the SC. Though not as ideal as a face-to-face discussion at a SC meeting, this system seemed to work fairly well.

A third challenge in adhering to the dissemination guidelines was that of balancing dissemination activities with other project demands. All research projects, including more traditional projects, face this tension between ongoing project implementation and data collection and dissemination activities. Yet the additional dissemination-related activities needed in a CBPR approach can increase the difficulty of achieving a balance between ongoing implementation and dissemination of findings. During the CAAA project, not all the activities outlined in the dissemination guidelines happened as originally planned. For example, although the original intention of the DC was to have all fact sheets updated quarterly, SC members' and project staff's occupation with project implementation activities left little time for further data analysis or even recognition that updating of the fact sheets had fallen behind schedule. Another example is that feedback to the participants about their lung function results happened much later than was originally intended. Much of this delay was due to the ongoing project implementation duties of the members of the research team. The community partners and field staff were understandably frustrated by the delay in presenting these results to participants, and the academic members were frustrated at the lack of resources to make this happen sooner.

Ensuring up-to-date involvement of community partners in the data analysis process. CAAA also faced challenges related to involving community partners in data analysis and informing them of the data analysis steps. As occurs with most research projects, data preparation and analysis was conducted at the partner university and was ongoing from the second through the sixth year of the project. Community partners involved in writing articles and papers usually viewed the data in table form, after preliminary data analyses had been conducted. Given the large amount of data collected, data cleaning and analysis took what seemed to community partners to be a very long time. Although the academic members of the SC gave semiannual reports about preliminary findings, community members of the SC were rarely kept up to date about the progress of data cleaning and analysis. In addition, it became clear toward the end of the project that community members had not been well informed about the complexity of data cleaning and analysis and the time it typically took. This resulted in frustration about the delay in feeding back results to the community and in completing and submitting manuscripts about project results.

Achieving a balance between dissemination and feedback to community and academic audiences. CAAA also faced the challenge of achieving a balance between the dissemination and feedback to the community through such means as fact sheets and forums and the dissemination to academic audiences through such means as journal articles. Israel and colleagues (1998) have identified the considerable time it takes to develop and maintain relationships and to involve all partners in the research process as a challenge for academics participating in CBPR. Although some aspects of preparing for dissemination of results to community members (for example, data analysis and the preparation of visual displays) can also be useful in manuscript development, the time spent disseminating results to community members can be time that is taken away from writing manuscripts. In the fifth year of this project, concerns related to productivity (defined by the funder as manuscript submission and publication) were discussed. SC members considered ways to ensure that academics had the time needed to produce manuscripts while also ensuring that dissemination to the community continued. They discussed having community members of the SC take the lead on presenting at community venues. This strategy had been discussed by the DC (and was the impetus for the development of the fact sheets), but such presentations did not occur. SC members determined that community members serving on the SC would need to receive training on data interpretation and presentation and would need to have additional resources (such as stipends) because these activities would be over and beyond their everyday duties. CAAA intends to pursue this approach in the future.

Ensuring that dissemination is culturally sensitive and competent. Another challenge faced by CAAA was that of ensuring that dissemination took place in a culturally sensitive and competent manner. Given that CAAA worked with two different geographical communities and with white, African American, and Latino participants, issues of culture were important in designing community feedback activities. All project materials, including fact sheets about project results, were produced in English and Spanish. In addition, at the forum in southwest Detroit (which is the area with the largest percentage of Latinos in Detroit) and at the community-wide forum, a Spanish interpreter was present to provide simultaneous interpretation. CAAA also hired an interpreter for the one deaf project participant. To ensure that project materials were appropriate to the African American and Latino cultures with which CAAA was working, SC members and project staff of these ethnicities reviewed all dissemination materials (including presentations at the forum) and offered suggestions to improve them.

Involving partners with differing experience and expertise. As the dissemination committee had recognized at the beginning of the project, not all partners had the same level of experience and expertise in preparing manuscripts or presenting at conferences. Seeking to ensure that persons with less experience and expertise were not excluded, the committee suggested processes for capacity building (for example, conducting mock presentations before the scheduled meeting so persons would gain experience and feedback). In addition, academic partners realized that being a coauthor might be a new experience for some of the partners and considered multiple ways of obtaining comments and ideas on each article from all partners. For example, some partners preferred to suggest changes and edits through direct conversation rather than in writing.

LESSONS LEARNED AND IMPLICATIONS FOR PRACTICE

The CAAA experience offers a number of lessons and implications for the field.

The value of and need for joint academic-community participation in all dissemination activities. The SC found that involvement of academic and community members in all dissemination activities greatly enhanced the efforts of the CAAA project. As expected, community partners brought expertise on venues for community dissemination as well as advice on "breaking it down," as they referred to the process of helping the academic members deliver research results in language that was understandable to community members. Similarly, academic partners brought their experience in writing presentations and publications for academic audiences. Partners also contributed to each other's traditional area of expertise in dissemination-related activities. For example, community members coauthoring manuscripts and copresenting at conferences raised issues about interpretation of results and offered valuable input on content and writing style, which served to make these presentations and manuscripts much stronger. And as noted before, academic members were the ones to raise concerns about presenting results at a community forum before first presenting the results to project participants.

As described in this chapter, the presence of structures (for example, a steering committee and its subcommittees) and processes (for example, frequent meetings, written dissemination guidelines) that fostered relationship building and trust facilitated the joint participation of academics and community members in dissemination activities. We would suggest that all research partnerships develop initial structures and processes for joint collaborative participation as a first step toward such participation in dissemination of research results. (See Chapters Two and Three in this volume for further discussion of ways to ensure joint collaborative participation.)

The need to recognize that dissemination is time consuming and may not be part of the "job description" of all partners and that projects should address how to compensate partners for their time and contributions and how to acknowledge what they do. Stoecker (2003) notes that in a CBPR project, community members may be asked to "participate in ways they aren't interested in or don't have time for" (p. 102). This may be especially true for some aspects of dissemination, such as involvement in coauthoring manuscripts or copresenting papers at national conferences and meetings, because these tasks are not part of the usual duties of most community partners. For example, as described earlier, despite much discussion and actual identification of potential manuscript topics for community members to take the lead on, to date no community member has served as lead author for a manuscript. Thus resources that would enable community members to involve themselves in this type of dissemination need to be identified and provided.

Stoecker's observation may also apply to academic partners. Traditionally, academics are rewarded for their participation in certain scientific dissemination activities, such as peer-reviewed publications and, to a lesser extent, presentations. Other forms of dissemination, such as community presentations, authoring fact sheets about research findings, and individual presentations to project participants, however, are not recognized and rewarded by most tenure and promotion systems or by funding agencies (such as the National Institutes of Health).

To address these issues, research partnerships need to consider dissemination when they are developing the initial proposal. For example, providing stipends for community members that more accurately reflect their desired involvement in dissemination activities may allow them to participate more intensively. In addition, continued efforts are needed on the national level, first, to educate academic institutions on the importance of dissemination activities in the community as a form of translation of research findings and the importance of recognizing this type of dissemination in the tenure and promotion process and, second, to educate funding agencies about the need to acknowledge these types of dissemination activities in evaluating the "productivity" of CBPR projects.

The need to develop an appropriate mechanism for identifying and deciding on dissemination issues and guidelines. When the SC formed the dissemination committee, it was with the understanding that this committee would continue to function throughout the life of the project. As noted earlier, however, the DC ceased to meet after the guidelines were developed and the steering committee took on the duties of the DC. In retrospect the SC was unrealistic in adding another layer of meetings and responsibilities to the work of SC members.

We recommend a more realistic process that would involve forming a short-term, ad hoc committee to focus on developing dissemination guidelines, with the understanding that once the guidelines were developed the partnership's governing body would implement them. We further suggest the incorporation of a standing "update" agenda item on dissemination for each meeting of the partnership, even if no dissemination-related events have taken place. This would encourage ongoing discussion on the progress made in data analysis and foster more open discussion and the education of all partners about what is involved in the data preparation and analysis process.

The need to budget adequate resources for dissemination activities. As suggested earlier, resources to compensate community partners for their participation in dissemination-related activities need to be included in grant proposals. In addition, funds for dissemination activities (for materials and refreshments for community forums, translation of materials into appropriate languages, and interpretation services for forums and meetings) should be included in project budgets. Finally, resources are needed to cover the staff time required to pursue dissemination-related activities.

CONCLUSION

Dissemination of research findings in ways that are understandable and helpful to community members is a crucial component of community-based participatory research. In this chapter we have shared our experience in establishing a process for dissemination of research results using a CBPR approach. Although we have had successes in our dissemination activities, we also acknowledge the challenges we have faced and the need to continually improve upon our efforts. We have been energized by the positive and enthusiastic reaction to our efforts to share the results of our research with the project participants and community members who have made the project possible and to do so in a way that acknowledges the contributions of both community and academic partnership members. This positive reaction has strengthened our belief in the importance of community-academic participation in the dissemination of research findings to the project participants and community members who will most benefit from knowing and applying these results to foster community change.

References

deKoning, K., & Martin, M. (Eds.). (1996). *Participatory research in health: Issues and experiences.* London: Zed Books.

Edgren, K. K., Parker, E. A., Israel, B. A., Lewis, T. C., Salinas, M., Robins, T. G., et al. (in press). Conducting a health education intervention and an epidemiological research project involving community members and community partner organizations: The Community Action Against Asthma Project. *Health Promotion Practice.*

Farquhar, S., & Wing, S. (2003). Methodological and ethical considerations in community-driven environmental justice research: Two case studies from rural North Carolina. In M. Minkler & N. Wallerstein (Eds.), *Community-based participatory research for health* (pp. 221–241). San Francisco: Jossey-Bass.

Green, L. W., George, M. A., Daniel, M., Frankish, C. J., Herbert, C. J., Bowie, W. R., et al. (1995). *Study of participatory research in health promotion.* Ottawa: Royal Society of Canada.

International Committee of Medical Journal Editors. (2004). *Uniform requirements for manuscripts submitted to biomedical journals.* Retrieved July 7, 2004, from http://www.icmje.org

Israel, B. A., Lichtenstein, R., Lantz, P., McGranaghan, R., Allen, A., Guzman, J. R., et al. (2001). The Detroit Community-Academic Urban Research Center: Development, implementation and evaluation. *Journal of Public Health Management and Practice, 7*(5), 1–19.

Israel, B. A., Schulz, A. J., Parker, E. A., & Becker, A. B. (1998). Review of community-based research: Assessing partnership approaches to improve public health. *Annual Review of Public Health, 19,* 173–202.

López, E.D.S., Parker, E. A., Edgren, K. K., & Brakefield-Caldwell, W. (2005). Lessons learned while using a CBPR approach to plan and conduct forums to disseminate research findings back to partnering communities: A case study from Community Action Against Asthma, Detroit, Michigan. *Metropolitan Universities Journal, 16*(1).

Parker, E. A., Israel, B. A., Brakefield-Caldwell, W., Keeler, G. J., Lewis, T. C., Ramirez, E., et al. (2003). Community Action Against Asthma: Examining the partnership process of a community-based participatory research project. *Journal of General Internal Medicine, 18*(7), 558–567.

Stoecker, R. (2003). Are academics irrelevant? Approaches and roles for scholars in community-based participatory research. In M. Minkler & N. Wallerstein (Eds.), *Community-based participatory research for health* (pp. 98–112). San Francisco: Jossey-Bass.

U.S. Census Bureau. (1990). *Statistical abstract of the United States.* Washington, DC: U.S. Department of Commerce, Economics and Statistics Administration.

CHAPTER FOURTEEN

Creating Understanding and Action Through Group Dialogue

Elizabeth A. Baker and Freda L. Motton

In community-based participatory research (CBPR), data collection is seen as an essential part of and integral to taking action (Israel, Schulz, Parker, & Becker, 1998). Focusing on the method of in-depth group interviews, this chapter will examine the stages involved in collecting data and using these data to develop action in a CBPR project. Attending to these stages will enhance the quality, validity, and relevance of the data, and this in turn will contribute to the appropriateness and effectiveness of actions taken (Greenwood & Levin, 1998; Heron, 1996; Mason, 1996; Mishler, 1986).

In order to illuminate these stages, we first review the literature regarding in-depth group interviews and identify the stages in the process. We then present a case study describing a project's experiences in using in-depth group interviews, with emphasis on data feedback, analysis, interpretation, and action. Finally, we discuss some of the challenges, limitations, and lessons learned in using this data collection method in the context of a CBPR effort.

Acknowledgments: The authors would like to acknowledge the contributions of all members of the Bootheel Heart Health Coalitions and particularly the chairs of these coalitions: Rutha Boyd, Tonya Mitchell, Cynthia Pulley, and Dorothy Walton. In addition, the authors would like to thank Laura Brennan Ramirez, Ellen Barnidge, and Julie Bender for their contributions to the project activities described and the development of this chapter. Lastly, we would like to acknowledge the contributions to our thinking from our collaborators at Tulane University (Robert Goodman, now at the University of Pittsburgh, and Adam Becker), the University of Illinois at Chicago (Michele Kelly), and the University of New Mexico (Nina Wallerstein). This project was funded by the Centers for Disease Control and Prevention Research Center, grant U48/CCU710806.

METHOD OVERVIEW: IN-DEPTH INTERVIEWS

In-depth interviews are often described as following one of three approaches: unstructured conversational interview, interview using a general interview guide, or structured, standardized open-ended interview (see Patton, 2002, for an in-depth discussion). In the unstructured conversational interview there is no predetermined set of questions; instead, the interviewer responds to the conditions at hand and pursues various lines of inquiry accordingly. One particular individual or group may be interviewed on multiple occasions. This method allows the interviewer to respond to the specific context and is most useful when an interviewer will be in the community for an extended period of time. This approach is also helpful in gathering insight into the types of questions or issues to pursue in a second or subsequent interview. However, use of the conversational interview makes it difficult to obtain similar types of information from several different groups or individuals. In contrast, when interviews using a general interview guide are carried out, the interviewer uses a general outline of issues to direct the lines of inquiry to be explored. This approach allows similar issues to be addressed across individuals or groups while maintaining a conversational quality or tone in the interview and allowing unique responses across individuals and groups. Lastly, the standardized open-ended approach employs a carefully worded set of questions, so that each interviewer asks each participant the same questions in exactly the same way, thus providing maximum consistency across interviews. Although these methods are often framed as three different approaches, it is also possible to combine aspects of them: for example, one might use a standardized open-ended approach but maintain the flexibility to ask participants somewhat different questions or to probe for more depth depending on their responses (Patton, 2002).

In-depth interviews may be conducted with individuals or with groups and may occur multiple times with the same or new participants. A project may mix and phase the approaches across time to maximize the types of information gathered (Mason, 1996; Mishler, 1986). The use of group interviews, as discussed here, involving a common core of individuals in an iterative process, may enhance participant cohesion and the likelihood that the group will be able to use the information collected to create interventions (Mason, 1996; Mishler, 1986). For an examination of the use of in-depth interviews with individuals see Chapters Four, Ten, and Twelve.

Projects face several considerations in deciding which of these approaches is most appropriate. For example, the standardized open-ended interview method is useful when there are multiple interviewers; however, it allows the least amount of variability and responsiveness. In addition, this approach is least likely to build rapport among individuals or groups. Alternatively, although the conversational interview approach may be helpful for establishing trust and rapport within a CBPR approach, it is often useful to combine it with a more structured process so that project partners will have appropriate data for defining directions for action.

In a CBPR approach all partners are involved in all stages of the research (Baker & Brownson, 1998; Greenwood & Levin, 1998; Israel et al., 1998, 2003; Minkler & Wallerstein, 2003; Mishler, 1986), including developing the data collection methods, recruiting, collecting data, analyzing data, conducting feedback and member checking, interpreting data, and moving from analysis to action. The partners involved in a CBPR effort for public health will vary according to the project and may include academicians, health department personnel, health care providers, members of community-based organizations, and individuals who identify themselves as members of a community relevant to the project (Baker & Brownson, 1998; Israel et al., 1998). In some instances the project may create new alliances; in other instances the project may draw on existing relationships among individuals, groups, and organizations; and in yet other instances, some of the project partners will have worked together previously and others will not. (See Chapter Two for a discussion of developing and maintaining CBPR partnerships.)

The roles that each partner takes in the various stages of the research may vary considerably. It is therefore important for partners to agree to the operational details of the processes used for a particular project, including what data will be collected and how they will be collected; who will review the data collection guides; who will collect the data; from whom data will be collected; who will take part in data analysis, feedback, and interpretation; and who will take the accumulated information and move it toward action. These roles should be made explicit for each project, regardless of the previous history partners may have from working together.

Developing Interview Guide and Recruitment Strategies

CBPR paradigms for data collection recognize that the questions asked and the way they are asked influence the information gathered and thus the actions taken as a result. It is therefore important that any interview guides or standardized questions make sense to and are useful for all partners (Israel et al., 1998; Mason, 1996; Minkler & Wallerstein, 2003; Mishler, 1986). In addition, within the context of a CBPR project, the development of the interview guide is an iterative process in which partners are involved in deciding not only what questions to ask but also how to administer the agreed-upon interview guide. As a result, the interview guide may be administered as part of a larger community assessment or program development process.

A related issue is deciding from whom data will be collected and how these respondents will be recruited. It is important to decide on an appropriate sampling strategy ahead of time. Patton (2002) describes several sampling strategies, ranging from "snowball" to "maximum variation" to "criterion." The best strategy to use depends on the information the partners agree they want to gather. For example, in snowball sampling, recruitment begins with those who are known to be appropriate given the purpose of the interview. and these initial contacts then recommend others they think would be useful interviewees. In other instances recruitment might involve contacting particular agencies or individuals who hold positions in the community and inviting them to be part of the process. If one is interested in group interviews (the focus of this chapter) that build on, and perhaps help to enhance, existing social networks, one might be best served by involving existing coalitions and community or civic groups. In a CBPR context community partners can provide critical information about the best people and groups to contact. Often it is useful to contact individuals by telephone and follow up with a letter confirming the time and place that the interview will be held. The organization or individual making the contact may influence willingness to participate. It may therefore be helpful to have community partners rather than academic partners make the initial contacts.

Data Collection

A facilitator (or co-facilitator) usually conducts the data collection process, initiating and maintaining discussion throughout the group interview. When using a general interview guide, it is possible to ask broad questions and then probe for more information while allowing the specific ordering of the questions to follow the conversation generated within the group (Patton, 2002). It is essential to document the discussion in a way that allows the content and process to be captured. Documentation may take the form of written field notes, audiotapes, or a photographic record (videotapes or still photographs), or any combination of these. It is also essential to obtain informed consent from participants for how the data will be shared and with whom they will be shared.

Analysis

The analysis of group interview data is a process of describing the data, not interpreting the reason for the data (Patton, 2002). The initial coding of data can happen in many ways. Most frequently, tape-recorded interviews are transcribed, keeping as close as possible to the exact words used during the interview. The transcriptions are then divided into meaningful data segments and placed into categories of common themes, using deductive focused or open coding techniques (Patton, 2002; Strauss, 1987). The data in these categories are then compared, using a process of constant comparison, to ensure that they have similar meanings within categories and different meanings across categories (Strauss, 1987; Strauss & Corbin, 1990). It is often beneficial to train and use multiple individuals, people representing both academic and community partners, to code the data. It is also important to pay attention to issues of interrater reliability: that is, the comparability of coding across data analysts (Patton, 2002). Differences in coding may point to problems in the coding scheme. Alternatively, if both academic and community partners have been involved in the coding, coding differences may highlight their different perceptions. Although identifying differences in academic and community perceptions is beneficial, one of the concerns when community partners code raw data is confidentiality. Even when identifiers are removed, community partners can sometimes tell who is speaking by the context and content of the statement. In such instances it is usually best to have community partners work with the data after they have been summarized and coded.

Feedback and Member Checking

Once data have been collected and analyzed, it is important to ensure that the summary of results is accurate and can be used for action planning (Mason, 1996). This requires collecting feedback and conducting what some have called *member checking,* checking with the individuals who took part in the data collection process to make sure that the results of the data analysis reflect the information they supplied (Heron, 1996; Mason, 1996; Seale, 1999). In the context of CBPR it is also important to provide the broader community, not just the participants in the interview process, with the summary information and to engage community members in the feedback process so that data can lead to appropriate action steps (Heron, 1996; Mason, 1996; Seale, 1999).

The best way of summarizing and sharing the results of in-depth group interviews depends on the type(s) of data collected and the participants involved in the process. Data may be shared verbally, in writing, or through pictures or other formats. Regardless of the method, they need to be shared in a way that allows participants to understand, modify, and suggest alternative summaries. The idea is to develop a process through which participants can determine whether the data accurately represent the viewpoints of those who provided them. Feedback and member checking are intended to allow all partners to move toward increased and sometimes new understandings and to ensure the credibility of findings (Guba & Lincoln, 1989; Heron, 1996; Lincoln & Guba, 1985).

Interpretation

Interpretation is the process of moving from a summary of the data to explanatory thinking in a way that suggests paths for action (Heron, 1996). It is helpful in this process to incorporate methods that point to similarities and differences in the data in ways that enable all partners to move beyond specific examples and toward underlying issues and meanings (Brydon-Miller, 2001). In this stage, as in feedback and member checking, it is also helpful to use multiple methods (verbal, written, artistic and expressive) in order to engage all partners in the process.

Several levels of participation may be used as partners complete these inter-pretive steps (Mishler, 1986; Seale, 1999). Some have argued that all partners need to participate in all aspects of the interpretation if the findings are to inform action (Heron, 1996). This joint interpretation enables all partners to develop a thorough understanding of the nature of the relationships of interest. Compared to action based on varying levels of participation, action based on joint inter-pretations may be easier to carry out, because all partners understand why the particular course of action is appropriate (Mason, 1996; Mies, 1983).

However, in order to jointly interpret data, all partners have to learn the skills necessary to engage in this collective process of assigning meaning to the data. Even when presented with this opportunity, there may be some partners who are less likely to contribute at this stage. Some may feel that their time is better spent in other endeavors. Some may feel that their contributions are not suffi-ciently appreciated. Having one partner analyze the data and present the results to the other partners, the most common CBPR method of interpreting data (Seale, 1999), takes far less time and does not require all partners to develop skills that they may or may not see as beneficial. However, when partners are presented with data placed in a framework or categorized, the assumption is often made that all partners understand the categorization language in the same way that the partner who did the interpretation does (Seale, 1999). This assumption is typically inaccurate. In addition, those partners who have not been involved in the initial processes of data analysis and interpretation may not believe or agree with the information presented and may therefore be hesitant to take action based on the findings.

Regardless of the process used to make sense of the data, it is important to integrate the knowledge and understanding that community members have. This enables the development of *local theory* (Elden & Levin, 1991) and makes it more likely that actions taken based on the data will be appropriate for the community.

Moving from Interpretation to Action

Although interpretation of the results may signal the end of the in-depth inter-view process when using traditional methods, CBPR partners expect knowledge generation to be linked with action (Israel et al., 1998). The research processes and methods described throughout this book are cyclical, beginning with reflec-tion, moving to action, and then shifting back to reflection. This cycle suggests that it is important to act based on what one knows at the time and to recog-nize the importance of learning from that action what needs to be done next (Heron, 1996). Because the process stages are always emerging and because dif-ferent individuals and perhaps even different partners may be involved at different times in any CBPR partnership, the results from in-depth interviews and the actions taken in response to these findings may or may not make sense to the individuals responsible for applying what has been learned. Moreover, the "best" action may be difficult to define because there are likely to be multiple perspectives among partners and even within partner organizations and groups. It is necessary to come to terms with and address these differences in order to move toward action.

IN-DEPTH INTERVIEWS IN THE PLANNING GRANT PROJECT

In order to illustrate how in-depth group interviews can be used in the context of a CBPR project, we will present an overview of the Planning Grant project and then outline how this project carried out each of the stages described above. The Planning Grant was conducted through the Saint Louis University School of Public Health (SLU-SPH) Prevention Research Center and included academic partners from SLU-SPH as well as partners from the Bootheel Heart Health Coalitions. These heart health coalitions are located in four economically depressed African American communities in rural southeast Missouri. The coalitions were formed in 1989, with the mission of reducing morbidity and mortality due to cardiovascular disease. They accomplish this mission by implementing programs to reduce risky health behaviors (Brownson et al., 1996, 1997). The coalitions were initially funded by the Centers for Disease Control and Prevention (CDC) through the Missouri Department of Health and later became functions of the Prevention Research Center (also funded by the CDC) at SLU-SPH. Each coalition is facilitated by a volunteer coalition chair who is a member of the community. Members of the coalition usually select the chair. The chair recruits members, facilitates meetings, and helps plan and implement activities.

The initial activities of the coalitions included efforts to change individual attitudes and behaviors as well as the social norms around cardiovascular disease risk factors (particularly smoking, diet, and physical activity). Their collective efforts have expanded in many ways since the partnership between SLU-SPH and the Bootheel Heart Health Coalitions began. The coalitions have increasingly moved from implementing programs defined by others to providing a menu of options for programs to working together to define their own programs. In addition, they are now placing more emphasis on creating changes in the structures of the physical environment that influence behaviors (for example, building walking trails to encourage exercise).

The current project, the Planning Grant, was added to these efforts in response to the requests of coalition chairs and members to learn more about assessment and planning and to expand the efforts of the coalitions to issues beyond cardiovascular disease risk reduction. This Missouri project was carried out as part of a four-site (Missouri, New Mexico, Louisiana, and Illinois)

CDC-funded project conducted through the Prevention Research Centers (PRCs) (for additional information, see CDC, 2005). The aim of this PRC project was to assess the extent to which locally defined dimensions reflected academically derived dimensions of community capacity and social capital (Goodman et al., 1998; Kreuter, Lezin, & Koplan, 1997; Putnam, 1993, 1995). The Planning Grant project thus had this goal, but it also had the goals of building community capacity for planning and engaging in community change projects (hence the name *Planning Grant*). These goals were added because the coalitions demanded that their collective work include the opportunity to use the learning as a springboard for action planning and intervention implementation. As a result the implementation of the Planning Grant included components that were both similar to and unique from the components of the other three PRC project sites.

Type of Interview

The Planning Grant partners used a combination of interview approaches over the course of several meetings with some common and some unique participants in order to gather information and to build community support for action. As described earlier, given the recognition that context influences the information obtained and the desire to move from data collection to action using a collective, or partnership, approach, the interviews were conducted within the existing coalition groups (Mason, 1996; Mishler, 1986). An iterative, in-depth group interview process was used that enabled the gathering of information to be part of, rather than separate from, project planning and action. In addition, the partners' aim was that the community and coalition members would experience the interview process as a way to build community cohesion, consensus, and understanding. Lastly, it was hoped that this process would engage new community members in the coalitions' action planning process.

Developing the Interview Guide

As part of this overall planning grant process, a structured interview guide was created to gather information about factors that facilitate and hinder community efforts in creating change and in working within and across various sectors (such as schools, businesses, and government) of communities: in other words, it was created to learn about dimensions of community capacity and social capital. A draft interview guide was developed by the local academic partners and reviewed by the local community partners in face-to-face meetings. The guide was then shared through teleconferences and e-mail with staff at the other three sites, who also shared their locally defined guides. Modifications to the locally defined guide were suggested that would allow some cross-site comparisons. These recommended changes were discussed with the chairs of each of the four local coalitions in face-to-face meetings. This process resulted in some revisions and at the same time was responsive to the unique needs of the Missouri coalitions. For example, one of the main concerns of the coalition chairs was that some questions asked respondents to discuss their "community" without first asking them how they defined their community. The guide was therefore changed so that participants were first asked to define their community and then asked to refer to this community for the remainder of the interview. (See Appendix L for a copy of the interview guide.)

In regard to conducting these group interviews, the chairs indicated that the process needed to

1. Be integrated into the coalitions' already established meeting patterns (in terms, for example, of length of meeting time, number of individuals attending, and importance of using coalition activities to build community participation and skills)

2. Provide something back to the community instead of just taking from the community

3. Share information with community members in a way that was understandable and usable

4. Provide a blend of both information gathering and action planning

Therefore the overall interview process was broken down into multiple parts that were administered separately over a period of several meetings across all four of the coalition counties.

Recruitment and Data Collection

Given the goal to build community member involvement in coalition planning and activities, the interview process was conducted separately in each of the four counties, with only community members and coalition members from that particular county attending. In counties where a coalition had regularly scheduled meetings, the group interviews were conducted as part of, and hence at the same time and place as, these regularly scheduled meetings.

As they did for all other coalition activities, the coalition chairs recruited individuals to take part in all of the meetings. They invited members of their community who they thought would be interested in attending the meeting as well as those who might be willing to engage in the later planning and action phases of the project. The result was that approximately half of the participants in the group interviews were "regular" members of the coalition and half were individuals who, although familiar with the coalition, did not regularly attend coalition meetings. In each of the four counties, an average of twenty individuals attended each of the meetings in which the interviews were carried out (with the earlier meetings having more attendees than the later meetings).

Meeting 1. During the first meeting, participants formed small groups and created posters representing health in their communities. The academic partners stimulated the process by asking individuals to "create a poster that visually presents the health of your community. This can include both positive and negative aspects of health in your community . . . and you can define health as broadly as you think is appropriate." Participants were divided into small groups of approximately five individuals and provided with poster board, pipe cleaners, glitter, construction paper, felt markers, glue, and scissors. Once the posters were completed, each small group explained its poster to the larger group. After all the presentations the academic partners summarized the common and unique features of the posters and facilitated a brief discussion to determine if any important ideas were missing. Meeting 1 took approximately one hour, and the proceedings of this meeting were documented with field notes and the posters themselves.

Meeting 2. During the second meeting, statistical information on many of the health issues identified in Meeting 1 was presented by the academic partners and discussed by the group. These data had been collected and summarized by the academic partners from public use data sets available through the Internet. These data included school graduation and dropout rates; unemployment rates; and diabetes, cardiovascular disease, and cancer rates. The information was presented along with information on where community participants could find such information for themselves in the future (for example, URL addresses were provided along with copies of some of the introductory Web site screens to illuminate how to navigate the system). Participants then discussed how the coalitions had addressed or could address these issues. Meeting 2 took approximately one hour and was documented through field notes.

Meeting 3. During the third meeting a video of a community development project was shown and used as a springboard for discussion of the ways the heart health coalitions have addressed issues in their own communities in the past and what they might do in the future. Meeting 3 took approximately one and one-half hours and was documented through field notes.

Meeting 4. At the fourth meeting, following the outline in the interview guide described earlier, participants were, first, asked to reflect on how they define their community. They were then asked to describe the strengths and challenges that they face in conducting change efforts in their respective communities, given how they had conceptualized health in the first meeting and the subsequent discussions. Broad questions were asked initially (for example, "What has helped the coalition to implement activities?"), followed by specific questions on the role of various community sectors, again based on the issues discussed in Meeting 1 and the previously generated guide (for example, "How do the businesses in this community help the coalition to implement activities?"). These meetings were facilitated by the academic partners, with the coalition chairs assisting in facilitation, question clarification, and discussion initiation. This co-facilitation role was particularly important in helping community members to see that issues could be raised that might not be considered appropriate or well received in other settings (such as issues of organizational turf, institutional racism, and conflicts with local governmental agencies). Meeting 4 took approximately one and one-half hours and was tape-recorded and transcribed verbatim, with participant consent.

Data Analysis

The meeting transcripts were reviewed to ensure completeness and then coded by two coders who were part of the academic staff, using focused coding techniques (Strauss, 1987; Strauss & Corbin, 1990). The focused coding technique involved using the interview guide questions to establish categories (for example, business, school, and government facilitators and barriers). All information that did not fit in these categories was placed in an "other" category, and then this "other" category was reviewed and sorted into categories identified from the data themselves. This data analysis was done separately for each county.

Data Feedback and Member Checking

Data feedback and member checking was carried out at a fifth meeting in each county. Meeting 5 began with the academic partners presenting participants with written (bulleted) summaries of the results of the data analysis (feedback) and asking them to discuss the accuracy of these summaries and to make changes as appropriate (member checking). These meetings involved not only community members who had taken part in data collection but also community members who had not been part of the previous discussions. Those who had not participated previously either provided validation of the prior conversation or, in some cases, questioned the accuracy of various comments. In addition, those who had participated in the previous meetings identified areas where the summaries did not reflect the discussion. This process enabled the project partners to identify areas where the summaries were inaccurate. For example, during the interviews the participants had discussed the ways in which local businesses both facilitated and hindered community health and coalition activities, and the participants in one county had stated that local businesses facilitated coalition activities by contributing incentives and prizes. However, during the feedback process, it was pointed out that although this *was* what the participants had said, it was not accurate, as businesses had stopped providing these incentives and prizes many years ago. The participants who had provided this information said that they had done so because they thought the partners "wanted" something positive and this was the only thing that came to mind. This discussion and the next part of meeting 5 (described in the following section) were tape-recorded and transcribed, with participant consent.

Interpretation: Responding to Existing Frameworks and Creating New Ones

The remainder of Meeting 5 involved asking the participants to critically reflect on the extent to which the summaries (with the changes made during the first part of the meeting) fit into existing academic dimensions of community capacity, and to expand on these existing conceptualizations as appropriate. This process entailed providing each participant with a list of the community capacity dimensions found in the literature (such as community participation, leadership, skills, resources, connections, sense of community, community history, community power, and community values) and the academically derived definitions of these dimensions (Goodman et al., 1998). After a review and discussion of these dimensions, the participants were asked to collectively assign the locally generated summaries, or categories, from the group interviews to one or more of these dimensions, or *buckets,* and to identify any new dimensions they thought were not reflected in the literature. Large signs with the names of each dimension (bucket) had been put on the walls of the meeting room, each in a different color (community participation in purple, leadership in orange, and so on). The facilitator then reviewed each summary and asked participants to put it in the appropriate bucket by taping the statement on the wall under the sign of their choice (for example, community participation or leadership). Each of these summary statements could be placed in more than one bucket. The participants were then asked to discuss and critically reflect on the reasons why they had assigned the summary statement to a particular bucket, or dimension, thereby further refining the *local operationalization* of that dimension. These discussions were facilitated by the academic partners, with participants joining in by asking each other to clarify why they thought a statement belonged in a particular bucket and in some instances assisting with putting the summary statements on the wall underneath the appropriate sign. Each of the two Meeting 5 discussions took approximately two hours.

Although it is beyond the scope of this chapter to fully report on the findings (see Baker et al., 2002), a key result was that the participants indicated that they found the academically defined community capacity dimensions useful; however, they did not see them as acting independently to influence change. For example, community history was seen as influencing community participation and interorganizational networks, which in turn influenced community power and resources. They also noted that the dimensions inadequately reflected the importance of physical and environmental structures, and more important, did not address what they saw as two primary deterrents to change—institutional racism and lack of economic development.

Action Planning

The project partners in each county then met (Meeting 6) to determine how to use the lessons learned from these analyses for action planning. In each county this involved reviewing the main issues and challenges faced in the local community, along with the capacities they had also identified. They then prioritized the issues so that each coalition determined one main issue to focus on. The criteria used for prioritizing had been developed by the academic partners and presented to each community for changes and additions. The final criteria stipulated, for example, that the issue had been raised during the in-depth interview process, that a number of people were willing to work on the issue, and that the issue moved the coalition toward a focus on social or community factors rather than individual factors. Each coalition decided on an issue that reflected the interests of the majority of the participants. Once an issue was chosen, each coalition brought partners, often including individuals and organizations who had not taken part in the earlier data collection process, into this action phase of the process. A mini-grant was provided by the Planning Grant effort to fund one project per coalition, and community and academic partners worked together to plan and develop a budget for each of the projects. The planning included jointly defining the goal, the specific objectives that would help the coalition achieve the goal, the specific activities that would be conducted to achieve the objectives, and the evaluation strategies that would document the process and accomplishments. The planning process also paid explicit attention to the ways in which the community capacity dimensions discussed earlier influenced particular activities, so that the activities either attempted to build on community strengths or to work around challenges. We will discuss the interpretation and action planning process in one of the coalition counties, Pemiscot County, as an illustrative example.

Following Meeting 5 in Pemiscot County, the academic staff typed up the heading and the summary statements for each community capacity dimension, or bucket. A subsequent review by the coalition members of the placement of the statements in each bucket showed that many of the issues of concern focused on community participation and resources. For example, one issue identified in Pemiscot County was a lack of social integration and an absence of adult men in community activities. The coalition and academic partners held subsequent meetings to further refine this issue. Participants in these discussions stated that the absence of men could be seen, in part, as a function of inadequate job opportunities. These inadequate job opportunities were thought to have the potential to minimize a man's self-worth and hence his sense of having something to contribute to others. The coalition therefore decided to focus on creating a male mentoring program that would develop and offer a GED program. This program would lead to opportunities for vocational training and subsequently the development of local job opportunities specifically for men. The aim was that the men in these programs would begin to see their own strengths and potential and would also discover ways in which they could use these to achieve their personal goals. This would in turn result in improved self-esteem. In light of their new self-perception, these men would be asked to serve as role models and mentors to younger men.

In developing the program the coalition was able to reflect on and use some additional findings from the previous data collection, feedback, and analysis activities. In particular, it was noted that certain institutions (those already part of existing interorganizational networks, for example) were more likely to work with the local community and that others (those in which institutional racism was evident, for example) were less likely to do so. Moreover, the coalition noted that churches and religious institutions were sources of strength, trust, and power in the community and would thus be excellent places in which to begin a new program.

The coalition therefore worked with a local faith-based, nonprofit organization and brought together multiple partners to jointly plan and implement program activities. The coalition was able to bring GED classes to the community. Transportation was provided, and motivational speakers came to the classes to encourage completion of the GED program as well as movement toward other life achievements. As a result of the relationships established by the GED program, participants in that program have been able to increase their computer and job-readiness skills through additional programs provided by various partners. There are currently two GED program sites in the county, with participation ranging from five to twenty students. The men in the GED courses have also been active in mentoring younger men by participating in a "back to school" rally and encouraging them to stay in school.

The outcomes go beyond these specific program activities. For example, various organizations in the local community, including the local housing authority, local businesses, and an outreach ministry, have now worked together in new ways or in ways that had not been seen for some time. The CBPR process intentionally brought together institutions that were identified as community strengths in ways that have enhanced the GED program as well as other programs in the community.

CHALLENGES AND LIMITATIONS

Many challenges and limitations are encountered when using the type of in-depth group interview process described in this chapter in a CBPR project, including the need to deal with individuals' and organizations' lack of understanding of or time for CBPR, to recruit appropriate participants, to maintain consistent participation, to balance coalition activities, and to allow for changes in direction and finances.

Dealing with lack of understanding of or time for CBPR. Although the stages of reflection, action, and further reflection are critical to community-based participatory research, they are not always easy and smooth to implement nor linear in their process. Ideally, all partners would understand the full process prior to initiation of the CBPR project; however, much of the process is developed jointly as the partnership moves forward and thus cannot be fully defined ahead of time. In part individuals create and learn a process by being engaged in it (Greenwood & Levin, 1998). It is our experience that several iterations of and multiple ways of engaging in the process may be required to understand what is involved. Some have argued that this type of cycling is also important for ensuring validity of the findings (Greenwood & Levin, 1998; Heron, 1996). This reality creates challenges in conducting the in-depth interviews and moving toward action in that many individuals may engage in the first stages and then not be interested in further participation in what may be perceived as a loose, noncontrolled process. Moreover, this particular effort took almost three years from initiation to implementation of action steps. Many individuals from a community may not see the benefit of and may become very frustrated with what could be viewed as a drawn-out process. Alternatively, many academic partners may not have the patience, support, or financial ability to work with communities over such a time period to define strategies in this way.

Recruiting appropriate participants. Another challenge is participant recruitment. In the Planning Grant project the coalition chairs recruited all participants. Although this was advantageous given the chairs' knowledge of the community, this approach has certain limitations. For example, although the academic partners indicated what would be involved and the types of participation that would be most appropriate, at times coalition chairs may have invited the people they were most familiar with rather than those who would be most useful in providing diverse perspectives.

Maintaining consistent participation. Maintaining consistency of participant involvement across different stages of the in-depth group interviewing process is a challenge. There are advantages to having the same individuals involved in all stages: for example, it increases participants' understanding of how the process moved from one stage to the next. However, given the numerous demands on people's time, it may not be possible or realistic to obtain this level of involvement over a multiyear period.

Balancing coalition activities. A related issue was balancing the various coalition activities. The interviews and action planning described in this chapter occurred at the same time that coalition members were engaged in other coalition activities, such as health fairs and senior programs. Given that the

communities were small, it was often challenging to ask the people to participate in the processes described here when they were also committed to working on other coalition activities. It was critical to acknowledge these other
activities to ensure that the interviews and action planning did not take away
from other activities and overburden community members.

Allowing for changes in direction and finances. It is important to allow and
plan for the evolution, or unfolding, of this work. For example, over time there
may be a change in the issue on which the partners initially decided to focus.
The initial data and summaries from the in-depth interviews may suggest one
issue that seems appropriate for action, but the analysis, feedback, and interpretation phases of this process may suggest an alternate issue once people have
assessed the barriers or the enthusiasm for addressing the issue. This can lead
to changes in partner interest as well as changes in anticipated budget allocation. This possibility highlights the importance of ensuring that the project
resources are not fully expended at one time and that budget allocations allow
for some unanticipated expenses.

LESSONS LEARNED AND IMPLICATIONS FOR PRACTICE

The partners in the Planning Grant project have learned many lessons by implementing in-depth group interviews and carrying out the subsequent action planning within the context of a community-based participatory research effort.

Trust. First and foremost, as with all CBPR activities, the partners must have
established some element of trust, and all actions must function to build rather
than destroy this trust. Important in this process are partners' familiarity with
each other's environment and language, a willingness to question issues when
they are not clear, and a willingness to clarify issues once they are questioned.
In conducting in-depth interviews, issues of trust influence everything from the
development of the guide to the analysis and interpretation of the data to
the attention paid to the needs of each partner regarding the use of the data (for
example, for publication only or for action).

Co-facilitation. Related to the issue of trust is the important issue of co-
facilitation by academic and community partners during the data collection
and interpretation processes. In the Planning Grant project, the chairs of each
coalition assisted by helping to initiate dialogue during the interview process,
often by raising key issues that community members were not certain could
be raised within the context (for example, racism and a history of neglect
by various local institutions). In addition, the chairs helped to ensure that
the participants understood the intention of the questions by clarifying the
language as needed. The chairs also helped the academic partners understand

the nuances of the participant discussions during data collection and interpretation of the findings.

Language. Another important lesson learned is that even when all partners and community members are speaking the same language, terms used by one party or another are often not understood by everyone. It is therefore important to review the aims and assumptions underlying the in-depth interview guide content with all partners and to ensure that the language used will be understood as intended by participants. In addition, it is important to translate meaning throughout the interactions. During the Planning Grant work, *social capital* and *community capacity* were phrases used by the academic partners to describe various community strengths and how they could be used to create collective action. Even though community members and organizations had a full understanding of the concepts represented by these phrases, they did not use this terminology in their expression of the concepts. Similarly, the community members used *crawdaddying* to describe a form of interpersonal relationship in which one person acts in such a way as to limit another's ability to move forward. Understanding each other's meanings is essential so that all partners can move from data to action with a common understanding.

Adapting to transitions in participation. As noted earlier, there may be frequent transitions in individual involvement and even in partner involvement in each of the stages outlined. It is useful for the partnership to determine methods of orienting people to the project that reflect the need for relationship and trust building. One way to do this is to clarify the language, culture, and processes used in the partnership for each of the new partners or community members as they enter. This is sometimes done informally in the coalition meetings. For example, the chair might comment occasionally on meeting practices, saying, for example, "We usually review our agenda first." At other times this orientation may happen through informal discussions between the chair, other coalition members, and the academic partners and the new members. It is also helpful to regularly and explicitly state how each activity of the coalition fits into the overall process of CBPR.

CONCLUSION

Qualitative in-depth group interviews are a useful method to incorporate into a CBPR endeavor. They can generate knowledge in a way that sets the stage for collaborative learning and action, particularly when collective feedback, member checking, and interpretation are intentionally incorporated into the process. Although the methods described in this chapter provide guidance, it is important to understand that the process is likely to evolve so that it more closely meets the needs of the specific partners. Each partnership is different, and this means that even a defined procedure will be implemented somewhat differently across partnerships. Some groups have a long history of involvement in community change and working in partnerships; other groups may have relied more on outsiders to define programs or may have a history of mistrusting others who enter their communities. All of these prior experiences influence each stage in the conduct of in-depth group interviews. As a result there are no absolutes in determining the right way to engage in each stage, as processes will reflect the context and history of the group. Consequently, when using in-depth group interviews one must become comfortable with some level of uncertainty as the stages unfold. Perhaps the best academic partners can do is to refine the process in ways that acknowledge the context of a given CBPR effort and meet the needs of all partners, while continuing to build individuals' and organizations' capacity to work together to improve individual and community health.

References

Baker, E., & Brownson, C. (1998). Defining characteristics of community-based health promotion programs. *Journal of Public Health Management and Practice, 4*(2), 1–9.

Baker, E., Motton, F., Boyd, R., Mitchell, T., Pulley, B., & Walton, D. (2002). *Using participatory processes to develop measures of social protective factors.* Paper presented at the Conference on Chronic Disease, Prevention and Control, Atlanta, GA.

Brownson, R., Mayer, J., Dusseault, P., Dabney, S., Wright, K., Jackson-Thompson, J., et al. (1997). Developing and evaluating a cardiovascular risk education project. *American Journal of Health Behavior, 21*(5), 333–344.

Brownson, R., Smith, C. Pratt, M., Mack, N., Jackson-Thompson, J., Dean, C., et al. (1996). Preventing cardiovascular disease through community-based risk reduction: The Bootheel Heart Health Project. *American Journal of Public Health, 86*(2), 206–213.

Brydon-Miller, M. (2001). Education, research and action. In D. Tolman & M. Brydon-Miller (Eds.), *From subjects to subjectivities: A handbook of interpretive and participatory methods* (pp. 76–95). New York: New York University Press.

Centers for Disease Control and Prevention, National Center for Chronic Disease Prevention and Health Promotion, Prevention Research Centers. (2005). *Saint Louis University Prevention Research Center.* Retrieved January 2005, from http://www.cdc.gov/prc/centers/stlouis.htm

Elden, M., & Levin, M. (1991). Cogenerative learning: Bringing participation in action research. In W. Whyte (Ed.), *Participatory action research* (pp. 127–143). Thousand Oaks, CA: Sage.

Goodman, R., Speers, M., McLeroy, K., Fawcett, S., Kegler, M., Parker, E., et al. (1998). Identifying and defining the dimensions of community capacity to provide a basis for measurement. *Health Education & Behavior, 25*(3), 258–278.

Greenwood, D., & Levin, M. (1998). *Introduction to action research: Social research for social change.* Thousand Oaks, CA: Sage.

Guba, E., & Lincoln, Y. (1989). *Fourth generation evaluation.* Thousand Oaks, CA: Sage.

Heron, J. (1996). *Co-operative inquiry: Research into the human condition.* Thousand Oaks, CA: Sage.

Israel, B., Schulz, A., Parker, E., & Becker, A. (1998). Review of community-based research: Assessing partnership approaches to improve public health. *Annual Review of Public Health, 19,* 173–202.

Israel, B., Schulz, A., Parker, E., Becker, A., Allen, A., & Guzman, J. (2003). Critical issues in developing and following community-based participatory research principles. In M. Minkler & N. Wallerstein (Eds.), *Community-based participatory research for health* (pp. 53–77). San Francisco: Jossey-Bass.

Kreuter, M., Lezin, N., & Koplan, A. (1997). *National level assessment of community health promotion using indicators of social capital.* Atlanta, GA: Health 2000.

Lincoln, Y., & Guba, E. (1985). *Naturalistic inquiry.* Thousand Oaks, CA: Sage.

Mason, J. (1996). *Qualitative researching.* Thousand Oaks, CA: Sage.

Mies, M. (1983). Toward a methodology for feminist research. In G. Bowles & R. Klein (Eds.), *Theories of women's studies* (pp. 117–139). New York: Routledge.

Minkler, M., & Wallerstein, N. (Eds.). (2003). *Community-based participatory research for health.* San Francisco: Jossey-Bass.

Mishler, E. (1986). *Research interviewing: Context and narrative.* Cambridge, MA: Harvard University Press.

Patton, M. (2002). *Qualitative evaluation and research methods.* Thousand Oaks, CA: Sage.

Putnam, R. (1993). The prosperous community: Social capital and public life. *The American Prospect, 13,* 35–42.

Putnam, R. (1995). Bowling alone: America's declining social capital. *Journal of Democracy, 6*(1), 65–78.

Seale, C. (1999). *The quality of qualitative research.* Thousand Oaks, CA: Sage.

Strauss, A. (1987). *Qualitative analysis for social scientists.* Cambridge, England: Cambridge University Press.

Strauss, A., & Corbin, J. (1990). *Basics of qualitative research: Grounded theory procedures and techniques.* Thousand Oaks, CA: Sage.

CHAPTER FIFTEEN

Photovoice as a Community-Based Participatory Research Method

A Case Study with African American Breast Cancer Survivors in Rural Eastern North Carolina

Ellen D. S. López, Eugenia Eng,
Naomi Robinson, and Caroline C. Wang

Photovoice is a participatory action research method that involves placing cameras in the hands of community people so that they may visually represent and communicate to others their lived experience (Wang & Burris, 1994). One important application of the methodology is to enable participants to use their photographs to elicit emotions, feelings, and insights about topics that may be shrouded in silence. During group discussions participants have the opportunity to comparatively examine their worldviews and the events that have shaped them, and communicate insights about their lives to influential people (Wang, Burris, & Xiang, 1996). The goals of photovoice are to enable people to

1. Record and reflect their personal and community's strengths and concerns through taking photographs

2. Promote critical dialogue and knowledge about important issues through discussion of their photographs

Acknowledgments: We thank all the survivors who took on the responsibility of being coinvestigators during this project. We also extend our gratitude to our colleagues at the North Carolina Breast Cancer Screening Program and the Lineberger Comprehensive Cancer Center who helped forge the way for our work and provided support. This project was supported by the Susan G. Komen Breast Cancer Foundation through a dissertation research award (0100647), and the University of North Carolina at Chapel Hill (UNC-CH) through a University Research Council research grant, a graduate school dissertation fellowship, and a Center for Health Promotion and Disease Prevention traineeship. All project-related research protocol and materials were approved by the UNC-CH School of Public Health Institutional Review Board of Human Subjects.

3. Reach policymakers and decision makers who can influence positive social change through public forums and showings of their photographs (Wang, 1999)

Used in a community-based participatory research (CBPR) approach, photovoice has the potential to enhance the quality and validity of research by drawing on local expertise to generate a new understanding about issues participants deem important. In sharing their knowledge with influential people to whom they might not normally have access, participants may forge relationships through which their insights may come to be used by others to catalyze individual and social change (Israel et al., 1998; Wang & Burris, 1997; Wang, Yuan, & Feng, 1996).

In this chapter we focus on the use of photovoice in the context of a CBPR approach. Following a brief review of the origins, diverse applications, and theoretical underpinnings of photovoice, we present a case example of a CBPR project we conducted using photovoice as the primary method of research. We also share the lessons we learned, and we draw from feedback provided by photovoice participants to describe the implications of the method for CBPR.

THE ORIGIN, USE, AND THEORETICAL UNDERPINNINGS OF PHOTOVOICE

Photovoice was originally codified and applied by Caroline Wang, Mary Ann Burris, and colleagues while they were working in China's Yunnan province with rural village women. Owing to their low social status, these women seldom had access to those who made decisions affecting their lives (Wang & Burris, 1994). Photovoice afforded control to these village women over the ways in which their perspectives and life situations were depicted, discussed, and communicated to others. They reached policymakers and decision makers through public showings and forums during which they presented and interpreted their photographs. The power of their photographs, coupled with text from their critical discussions, helped influence others' decisions to enact beneficial changes, such as the construction of day-care facilities and water tanks in villages and the establishment of educational scholarships for rural girls (Wang & Burris, 1994).

Although it is beyond the scope of this chapter to discuss other photovoice projects comprehensively, the method has been used with diverse populations around the world to achieve participatory goals covering a wide range of issues. Youths, adults, and policymakers in Flint, Michigan, have used photovoice to document and discuss their interpretations of community health (Wang, Morrel-Samuels, Hutchinson, Bell, & Pestronk, 2004), and working-class women living in Belfast, Ireland, have applied this method to explore the relationships between the places they live and their everyday lives (McIntyre, 2003). Others who have used photovoice to amplify their voices include men and women living at a homeless shelter in Ann Arbor, Michigan, who documented their everyday health, work, and life conditions to counteract stigmas and stereotypes about homeless people (Wang, Cash, & Powers, 2000), and Latino adolescents in North Carolina, who examined the influence of immigration (Streng et al., 2004). (Descriptions of other projects may be found at www.photovoice.com)

Photovoice takes its theoretical and practical underpinnings from Freire's empowerment education for critical consciousness (Freire, 1970), feminist theory, and participatory documentary photography (Wang & Burris, 1994). Each approach embodies a distinct set of underlying values; each also acknowledges that the absence of research and information regarding underrepresented groups perpetuates powerlessness. Each approach questions the political and power structures that undermine the expertise individuals have about their own lives and situations, strives to shift control over representation and knowledge generation from those in positions of power to those whose perspectives are seldom seen or heard, and seeks to apply knowledge gained from these perspectives to inform and implement social change. All three approaches identify the visual image as a means to achieve this last goal and as one key component through which groups that have been ignored by society can share knowledge and engage in critical discourse about the social and political forces that influence their daily lives (Ewald, 1996; Freire, 1970; Reinharz, 1992; Solomon, 1995; Wallerstein & Bernstein, 1988; Weiler, 1994).

APPLICATION OF PHOTOVOICE IN A CBPR PROGRAM: THE INSPIRATIONAL IMAGES PROJECT

In this section we present the Inspirational Images Project as a case study of a CBPR collaboration that used photovoice as its principal method. This project partnered academic researchers from the University of North Carolina at Chapel Hill (UNC-CH) School of Public Health, facilitators from a local self-help group for African American breast cancer survivors, funders from the Susan G. Komen Breast Cancer Foundation (Komen), and thirteen African American breast cancer survivors from three counties in rural eastern North Carolina. Through this collaboration, these survivors engaged in a photovoice process that entailed the following:

- Attending a training session
- Documenting their experiences as rural African American breast cancer survivors by means of five photo-assignments
- Participating in seven photo-discussion sessions

- Assessing the trustworthiness of findings that emerged during analysis of discussion transcripts

- Planning and hosting a forum to present findings and forge collaborations with influential people identified as advocates for change

Preparing for the Photovoice Project Using a CBPR Process

What follows is a discussion of the purpose of the project, guided both by testimonies from survivors and by a body of survivorship and quality of life literature. We also describe the goals and objectives of the CBPR partnership, the collaboration with two survivors to pilot the feasibility of using photovoice, and the protocol developed to conduct the Inspirational Images Project.

Background and Purpose. For African American women in rural eastern North Carolina, cultural norms and beliefs promote silence about breast cancer (Ashing-Giwa & Ganz, 1997). Work with rural African American communities in North Carolina has found that older women remember the long-standing social and historical conditions of inequality, such as a segregated health care system (Earp et al., 1997; Eng & Smith, 1995). These memories make it especially difficult for rural African American breast cancer survivors to express their quality of life (QOL) concerns, which may be distinct from those of white women.

QOL is recognized as a subjective perception of well-being that is multidimensional and time and context dependent ("The World Health Organization Quality of Life Assessment . . . ," 1995). It has been asserted that perceptions of QOL are influenced by cultural and ethnic factors such as social norms, values, beliefs, and shared experiences (Hassey Dow, Ferrell, Leigh, Ly, & Gulasekaram, 1996). Although the number of African American women who survive long term with breast cancer has increased (Clegg, Li, Hankey, Chu, & Edwards, 2002), few studies have been conducted with this population (Northouse et al., 1999), with most cancer QOL studies recruiting entirely or predominantly white participants. Consequently, insufficient knowledge exists about the influence of ethnicity and culture on QOL (Leedham & Ganz, 1999). At this early stage of understanding African American breast cancer survivors' QOL concerns, the challenge was to clarify the functional significance of race and ethnicity that may differentiate the social and cultural contexts that lead to living in silence with breast cancer.

The Need. The Inspirational Images Project was an offshoot of the North Carolina Breast Cancer Screening Program (NC-BCSP). Since 1991, NC-BCSP has been working with African American communities in rural eastern North Carolina to establish a network of lay health advisers to address several barriers to breast cancer screening (Earp et al., 1997). In response to the need for support for women who have survived breast cancer, NC-BCSP and the

University of North Carolina's Lineberger Comprehensive Cancer Center also sponsored a program that we will call the We-Count Program (pseudonyms are also used for the individuals who partnered and participated in this project), which involved a self-help group for African American breast cancer survivors and their families. We-Count was originally developed and facilitated by NC-BCSP community outreach specialist Helen Rock, who brought to the monthly meetings her own experiences as a breast cancer survivor.

The project described in this chapter builds on relationships developed by means of the academic researchers' work with NC-BCSP and We-Count, through which rapport and trust were established with several breast cancer survivors. As the researchers learned more about survivors and their lives, it became apparent that these women obtained their survivorship support and information almost exclusively through We-Count, because they did not feel comfortable using other resources available in their communities. This was verified by Helen Rock, who often described the onus she felt as the primary resource for numerous African American breast cancer survivors in her community. The goal in forging a partnership between the academic researchers and We-Count was to design and conduct a CBPR study that would enable breast cancer survivors to explore and voice their survivorship concerns so that appropriate interventions could be developed to address them.

Research Method and Project Protocol: A Photovoice Pilot Study. The challenge was to use a research approach that would enable these women to communicate the social and cultural meaning of living in silence with breast cancer. The academic researchers, who were familiar with Caroline Wang's work, broached the idea of photovoice with Helen Rock. She agreed to participate in a pilot study to assess the feasibility of using it with African American survivors in her community. Helen Rock recruited Marian Sweet, another survivor who often cofacilitated We-Count meetings, to participate as well. Helen Rock and Marian Sweet represented variation in age, treatment regimen, time since diagnosis, and experience of recurrence, and so contributed different survivorship perspectives. As the women to whom other women turned for support and information, they also provided insight into how other survivors would react to the photovoice method and made suggestions, based on their own participation, for improving the study protocol.

The pilot study deployed a mini-photovoice project that included an introductory meeting and three sequences of photo-assignments and audiotaped photo-discussion sessions. The photo-assignments included taking at least six pictures of the "people, places and things that make your life enjoyable" and "the small, yet significant things you have encountered as a breast cancer survivor and what you did to cope." The pilot study also included content analysis of taped discussions and a findings feedback session.

During each photo-discussion session, Helen Rock and Marian Sweet shared and talked about the images they had taken. In addition, the first author of this chapter used a structured process guide she had developed specifically for this pilot study to elicit feedback about whether the photovoice method was sensitive to participants' issues; feasible, interesting, and enjoyable; and able to generate findings that accurately reflected participants' survivorship experiences. Some of the process questions asked were: How did you feel using the camera? How did you go about asking people if you could take their picture? How enjoyable was it for you to complete your photo-assignment? What suggestions do you have for improving the project?

During the findings feedback session, the first author reported back the themes that had emerged from content analysis of the photo-discussions (for example, an evolving body image and strategies used to "get back to normal"). Helen Rock and Marian Sweet verified that the findings accurately captured their survivorship experiences, and expressed amazement at how effective the photos had been as triggers for their discussions. For example, during one photo-discussion session, Helen Rock shared a photograph of the clothes iron she used to lift like a weight after her mastectomy. Her motivation was to gain strength and flexibility in her arm so that she could reach up to write on a blackboard and resume teaching.

For Marian Sweet, seeing the picture of Helen Rock's iron encouraged her to share how she shot basketballs to rehabilitate her arm, a topic she had not considered important enough to share with others. Their photographs generated critical discussion about the need for health care providers and insurers to offer postmastectomy physical therapy. For several of the themes, Helen Rock and Marian Sweet discussed how powerful their photographs and discussions would be in helping policymakers and health care providers to understand, discuss, and address survivorship issues.

Both Helen Rock and Marian Sweet expressed their willingness to collaborate in designing and executing a larger photovoice project to benefit survivors and enhance the scope of We-Count. The photovoice process was tailored according to their feedback and guidance on issues ranging from the decision to use disposable cameras to the location and scheduling of photo-discussion sessions. Upon reviewing the cancer and survivorship literature, the researchers found that several of the themes that emerged during the pilot fell under the rubric QOL, which became the focus of the larger project.

Funding Period and Funders. The academic researchers applied to several funding sources. Although they initially received several rejections due to methodological concerns about photovoice and qualitative research, they eventually obtained over $50,000 from multiple funding sources that were open to using innovative and qualitative methods. A $30,000 two-year award from

Komen provided the majority of the funding. Other funding included one- to two-year fellowships and awards from UNC-CH.

Research Methods for Achieving Objectives. The Inspirational Images Project's specific aims were to

1. Engage the breast cancer survivors in exploring how their QOL is perceived and addressed within their own social context

2. Develop a conceptual framework of QOL and the impact of social and cultural factors

3. Engage local policymakers and decision makers in reviewing findings with survivors in order to identify opportunities and initiate steps toward developing culturally appropriate interventions

To achieve these aims, the project followed the qualitative research design of exploratory inquiry. It used the photovoice method to achieve the first and third aims. To achieve the second aim, it used the data collection and analysis techniques of grounded theory.

Grounded theory is theory that is generated from, or "grounded in," data that have been systematically collected through social research (Glaser & Strauss, 1967). In contrast to the process in deductive theory, which is based on a priori assumptions, in grounded theory, hypotheses and the building blocks of theory (concepts, themes, categories, and conceptual linkages) are generated, inductively, from the data and developed throughout the research process. Grounded theory employs theoretical sampling and constant comparison processes (Strauss & Corbin, 1998). Theoretical sampling entails an interplay between data collection and data analyses. As concepts and themes emerge during the analysis of collected data, they are used to inform and guide subsequent data collection. In the constant comparison process, incidents, actions, and events embedded in the data are compared within and across data sources (transcripts, speakers, literature) so that common concepts can be grouped into categories and so that conceptual linkages among categories can be explored and revised through further theoretical sampling. When no new information is generated, *data saturation,* which is the desired endpoint of grounded theory, has been achieved. The final model represents relationships among important concepts that emerged from and are supported by the data (Glaser & Strauss, 1967; Strauss & Corbin, 1998).

The photovoice and grounded theory data collection and analyses were thereby guided by research questions posed to uncover rural African American breast cancer survivors' perceptions of their QOL needs; the physical, psychological, social, spiritual, and cultural factors that mediate these perceptions; the strategies survivors develop to address their QOL needs; the ways that mediating factors influence survivors' strategies; the ways that survivors' strategies, in turn, influence mediating factors; and the points in the survivorship process where opportunities lie for developing intervention(s) to address QOL needs.

Setting. Helen Rock recruited survivors from three rural counties located in the eastern coastal region of North Carolina. At the time of the project, all three counties ranked among the most economically deprived in North Carolina (North Carolina Rural Economic Development Center, 2002), had populations of less than 30,000, and were 45 to 62 percent African American (U.S. Census Bureau, 2000). Although each county had its own hospital, cancer patients and survivors often made journeys of thirty-five to one hundred miles to larger towns for university medical center care and support services and for stores that carried cancer-related products (such as wigs, turbans, and prosthetics) for African Americans (*Breast Cancer Resource Directory of North Carolina*, 2001).

Partners and Their Roles. This project was targeted at a grassroots level, and breast cancer survivors were key partners. As coinvestigators, they shared decision-making power in the research process. The funding from the Komen Foundation enabled the project to hire two indigenous, well-known, and trusted women as paid, part-time community research advisers (CRAs). The original intention was to hire Helen Rock and Marian Sweet, but on September 21, 2000, Marian Sweet died, after experiencing another cancer recurrence. This led the Inspirational Images Project to ask Helen Rock and another woman whom she recommended to serve as CRAs. As individuals who lived and worked in the project setting, the CRAs provided insights on local social and cultural norms that guided and shaped the research process (Goodman et al., 1998; Israel et al., 1998). Specifically, they participated in planning meetings, helped facilitate project-related activities, reviewed all project-related materials, and assisted survivors with the logistics of photovoice (providing transportation to meetings, picking up film for processing, answering questions, and so forth).

In addition to participating in the photovoice pilot study, We-Count members offered support and advising throughout the project, which enhanced its credibility among survivors and within their communities. We-Count also used its community connections to assist the project in securing a comfortable and convenient meeting space and provided access to survivors who would partner on the project and be rich sources of information.

Survivors contributed their expertise as women who had experienced cancer in their rural communities. They helped to guide the data collection and analysis through their participation in the photovoice process. Survivors clarified and interpreted preliminary themes that emerged from analysis of their photo-discussions and assessed the trustworthiness of the final findings and conceptual framework. They also took the lead in disseminating results and forging relationships with influential people through a public forum and showing of their photographs, and they have collaborated in diffusing findings through other means, such as presentations at conferences and publications (López, Eng, Randall-David, & Robinson, 2005).

Academic partners contributed skills and experience as public health investigators and practitioners to design a research protocol that would yield credible and trustworthy findings. They also applied for funding, developed project-related materials, gained human subjects institutional review board approval on these materials, facilitated meetings, analyzed data, coauthored manuscripts and presentations, and worked with the CRAs to oversee the project's day-to-day activities.

Selection and Recruitment of Participants. Helen Rock identified eligible participants from a database she maintained of the women who contacted her for breast health–related assistance, some of whom were members of We-Count. From this pool of survivors, the project used a purposive sampling strategy to recruit women who met the following criteria: they had completed their initial treatment, they were willing to take photographs about their survivorship, they were open to sharing the photos with a small group of survivors, and they were able to commit to attending several meetings spanning several months. We also attempted to recruit women who varied on characteristics that could influence the survivorship experience (such as education, age, time since diagnosis, insurance coverage, and type of treatment).

Helen Rock contacted potential participants and used information from the project fact sheet and informed consent form (see Appendix M) to help describe the project, discuss what participation would entail, and answer questions. Each survivor who showed interest in participating received an invitation to attend an informational training session. With permission, one of the academic partners called each invitee to introduce herself and answer questions. To reduce barriers to participation, the project offered participants transportation and reimbursement for travel expenses.

Implementing the Photovoice Project Using a CBPR Process

There were a number of steps involved in implementing this photovoice project using a CBPR process. These steps were training, data collection and photo-discussions, theoretical sampling, data management and grounded theory analysis, and data feedback and interpretation.

Training Photovoice Participants. Eighteen women were invited to attend either of two training sessions to learn more about the project. This initial encounter promoted rapport and trust among the academic partners, CRAs, and potential participants, that is, community partners. Thirteen women attended, of whom twelve signed an informed consent form and received a disposable camera (another woman, unable to attend either training session, later signed a consent form and joined the project). During the training, the academic researchers and the survivors reviewed the project goals, the photovoice process, and the concept of participatory research in which the survivors would take a role as active partners. The group also discussed the power dynamics and ethical issues associated with using a camera, the importance of assessing personal safety when approaching strangers whom one wished to photograph, and the concept of reciprocating and expressing appreciation by offering copies of photos to photo subjects (Wang, 1999). The women then received their disposable cameras, basic instructions on how to use them, and tips for successful photographs (for example, when in doubt, use your flash). All the participants tried out their cameras by taking pictures of each other, and role-played using the acknowledgment form (see Appendix N) that they would be using to get written permission *prior* to taking a person's photograph (Wang & Redwood-Jones, 2001).

During the training the women developed photo-assignments in order to identify specific aspects of their survivorship they wanted to explore, and to promote reflection on everyday experiences to which they might have become unreflectively accustomed (Koch, 1970). The women decided that their first photo-assignment would be to *take at least six pictures that represent information I wish I would have had as a survivor.*

Prior to ending the training session, the academic partners reminded the women that the CRAs would be contacting them to set a date and time to pick up their cameras for processing. The group then scheduled the first photo-discussion session. During the time between the training and the photo-discussion session, academic partners, CRAs, and survivors were often in mail and phone contact to ensure that participants were comfortable with the photovoice process.

Collecting Data: Photo-Discussion Sessions. The women completed each photo-assignment within one month, and after each assignment the group reconvened for a three-hour photo-discussion session. All sessions were audio-taped, with permission. The sessions typically began by reviewing the project objectives and meeting agenda. One of the academic partners then presented the themes that had emerged from analysis of previous sessions so that survivors could discuss and clarify preliminary findings. This was followed by a "show and tell" during which each participant presented her photographs and explained how they related to the photo-assignment. For example, for the photo-assignment *"people, places and things that have brought me comfort, strength and hope as a survivor,"* one participant explained her motivation for taking a particular photograph this way: "This is a picture of my church and the reason

I took a picture of my church was because the foundation of my faith came from my church."

The group then chose one or two photographs to discuss in depth, guided by SHOWED, a six-step inductive questioning technique (Wallerstein & Bernstein, 1988). The SHOWED questions were

1. What do you *See* in this photograph?
2. What is *Happening* in the photograph?
3. How does this relate to *Our* lives?
4. *Why* do these issues exist?
5. How can we become *Empowered* by our new social understanding?
6. What can we *Do* to address these issues?

This line of questioning helped move the discussion about the photographs from concrete and personal levels to a social analysis of the root causes of issues and finally to the identification of action steps for creating change (Wallerstein & Bernstein, 1988; Wang & Burris, 1997).

Sampling on Theoretical Grounds: Using Preliminary Findings to Guide Future Data Collection. At the completion of each photo-discussion session the women summarized the themes heard. Through the method of theoretical sampling (Glaser & Strauss, 1967), these new themes, as well as themes that emerged during analysis of earlier session transcripts, helped to direct the avenues of inquiry that the women chose to explore during subsequent photo-assignment and photo-discussion sequences. In addition, the women asked themselves, "Given what we have learned so far, what should we explore next? What should be our next photo-assignment?" The answers to these questions helped the women develop their next photo-assignment.

After five photo-assignment and photo-discussion sequences (which occurred over a seven-month period because on two occasions participants opted to continue discussing the same assignment for two sessions), the partners began to hear the same information being repeated. At this point everyone agreed that no new information was being generated and that data saturation had been achieved (Glaser & Strauss, 1967; Strauss & Corbin, 1998).

Conducting Data Management and Grounded Theory Analysis. Data management and analyses were conducted primarily by the first author, with assistance from the CRAs. During photo-discussion sessions, the CRAs numbered and labeled the photographs as they were presented and discussed so that they would correspond with the taped discussion. Immediately after each session the first author listened to the audiotape to review the session and insert notes and reflections (about body language and expressed emotions, for example)

(Sandelowski, 1995). She then had the tapes professionally transcribed, verbatim, and the transcripts became the raw data for grounded theory analysis (Sandelowski, 1995) using the text analysis software Atlas.ti, Version 4.2.

Grounded theory analyses involved reading through the transcripts multiple times and then breaking down the data analytically by specific events, incidents, and actions and giving these elements conceptual labels. For example, a woman's recounting of praying to be cured was labeled "prayed for a cure." Data were then coded within and across the different transcripts and speakers, using the constant comparison method so that related concepts could be grouped into categories. For example, concepts such as "prayed for a cure" and "turning cancer over to God" were grouped into the category "relying on spiritual faith." Theory began to emerge as conceptual relationships among the categories became evident. For example, analysis revealed that the category "relying on spiritual faith" emerged as the strategy used most often by the women to address their QOL concerns. Analysis was complete when most of the categories could be unified around what were found to be central analytical ideas represented in the data (Strauss & Corbin, 1998).

Performing Data Feedback and Interpretation. Although the women did not choose to be involved in reading and coding the transcripts, a review of preliminary findings at each photo-discussion session provided survivors the opportunity to discuss, interpret, and clarify emerging concepts, themes, and conceptual linkages. For example, the group reported that some survivors receive the message from men that having lost their breast, they had "lost their womanhood." Although survivors verified that this theme did indeed emerge from the data provided during their discussions, they clarified that it was not only men but also women who had made survivors feel ashamed about having undergone a mastectomy.

When analyses incorporating data from each of the photo-discussion sessions were completed, a series of wrap-up findings meetings was held during which the women reviewed the final themes and conceptual model. These meetings continued until the women felt the findings credibly depicted what they wanted others to understand about their survivorship experiences (Kvale, 1995; Morse, 1994).

Developing a QOL Framework Grounded in Survivors' Experiences and Perspectives

From the analysis of the photo-discussions, the survivors and the academic partners developed a quality of life framework (Figure 15.1) that brings to light how QOL is intricately tied to the socially ascribed status of being African American, a woman, and a cancer survivor. Through sharing their experiences, survivors illustrated how the three social forces of racism, the stigma of cancer, and the

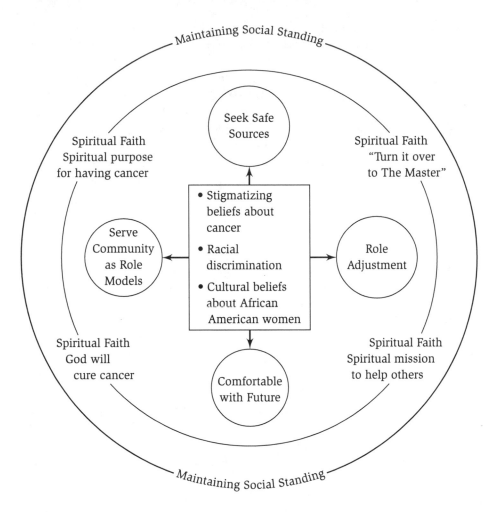

Figure 15.1 Conceptual Framework of Rural African American Breast Cancer Survivors' Quality of Life.

cultural expectations of African American women (depicted in the center of the figure) drive four QOL concerns: seeking safe sources of support, adjusting to the role of "cancer survivor," feeling comfortable about one's future, and serving as a role model to others (depicted in the four central ovals). The framework also reveals two specific individual-level strategies survivors devise to achieve maximum QOL: relying on their spiritual faith (the inner ring of the framework) and maintaining social standing (the outer ring). (For an in-depth discussion of project results and the QOL framework, see López, 2002; López et al., 2005.)

Addressing health issues from an assets-based and ecological perspective is an established principle of the CBPR approach (Green, Richard, & Potvin, 1996; Israel et al., 1998; Stokols, 1996). The QOL framework shows how interventions might build on the personal strategies survivors already employ to maximize QOL. It also illustrates how such interventions may address survivors' concerns by targeting the social forces that operate as policies and practices of local organizations and institutions and as governing norms of these rural communities.

Sharing Findings with Local Policymakers and Decision Makers: Planning and Conducting a Forum

Sharing what is learned through research is an important but often ignored principle of all types of investigation (Flaskerud, 1999; Israel et al., 1998). Congruent with the CBPR principle of disseminating findings to and by all partners (Israel et al., 1998), a specific goal of photovoice is to enable participants to reach local policymakers and decision makers through public forums and showings of their photographs, with the aim of stimulating social action and change (Wang, 1999; Wang & Burris, 1994). Near the completion of the Inspirational Images Project the survivors took the lead in planning and hosting a forum for influential people in their communities who they recognized as advocates of breast cancer survivors.

The forum goals, as set forth by the women, were to

- Share information about the Inspirational Images Project and what was learned about the needs of breast cancer survivors
- Forge relationships among survivors and influential advocates
- Encourage interest in taking action steps toward addressing survivors' needs
- Initiate steps toward taking action by forming task forces
- Establish local sustainability of the project

Identifying and Inviting Forum Participants: Influential Advocates. The project did not recruit *influential advocates* until late in the process because the group wanted the selection to be based on the influence individuals possessed with regard to the specific survivorship issues that emerged during the photo-discussions. As a result, the guests were selected from an extensive list compiled throughout the project and consisting of individuals whom the women had identified as being supportive during their survivorship experience.

From this list of over sixty names the survivors invited forty-three influential advocates. In addition to mailing two invitations to each advocate, the survivors and the academic partners developed an *adopt-an-advocate* process in which academic partners, CRAs, and survivors took responsibility for personally contacting specific advocates. Twenty-seven influential advocates representing diverse professions and interests attended the forum; they were local elected officials, health care providers, clergy, legal service providers, cancer-support agency representatives, and academics.

Presenting Photographs and Engaging in Action-Oriented Discussion. The forum agenda featured photo displays, presentations about the project and what was learned, small-group work, issue prioritization, and future action planning steps. Upon arrival, forum attendees walked around the venue to see photo displays that featured 8-by-10-inch enlargements of the photographs taken and chosen by the women, along with explanatory statements quoted from the women's discussions. The display also exhibited documentary photographs taken during the photo-discussions and forum planning meetings. Several survivors then presented information about the Inspirational Images Project, including the rationale for conducting the project, the data collection and analysis methods, and the findings. Because the conceptual framework was not yet finalized, the survivors and academic partners decided to present a list of ten themes (illustrated with quotations) that survivors felt relayed important information about their survivorship experiences. For example, one of the themes exemplified the significance that both medical and spiritual intervention have in cancer treatment and survival: "The survivor's comfort with her health care provider is strained when her provider does not respect her belief in prayer, and her belief that providers are created to do the Lord's work."

To progress beyond merely presenting findings to the influential advocates to engaging them in discussion about QOL needs and strategies in order to address these issues, the forum participants divided into five small groups. Each group was led by a team of two survivors and focused on one of the ten themes presented earlier. The small-group objectives were to introduce a scenario (based on experiences shared by women during the photo-discussions), use it to trigger discussion employing the SHOWED questioning technique, and then propose three strategies to address the theme discussed.

Prioritizing Needs and Initiating Plans for Taking Social Action. When the participants reconvened, members of each small group summarized the group's scenario and presented its three strategies. All of the strategies were written on sheets of newsprint, posted on a wall, and then grouped into categories. To prioritize future efforts, all attendees came up to the wall to place stickers next to the three strategies they felt were most important to undertake to improve QOL for survivors. The strategies "educating clergy" and "educating male partners" clearly received the most votes.

Several survivors and influential advocates then volunteered to participate on task forces to develop each of these strategies. Members from each task force took a few minutes to schedule where and when they would meet to begin their work. In addition, all the influential advocates and survivors provided their "best meeting times" on blank calendars, so that the partners could schedule another meeting in two to three months. During this future meeting each task force would present its strategic plans and solicit recommendations and support from the larger group.

Prior to ending the forum, all the participants celebrated the Inspirational Images Project with a shared meal and brief speeches from survivors and influential advocates. To sustain the efforts and the new relationships forged among survivors and influential advocates, one of the CRAs accepted responsibility for coordinating future project activities. Although the academic and funding partners would no longer be involved on a daily basis, the academic partners were committed to providing continued support and guidance. Remaining project funds were budgeted to purchase equipment and supplies that would facilitate project management (for example, a computer, a printer, and Internet access).

Carrying Out Other Means of Disseminating Results. Traditionally, dissemination of research findings has been conducted through presentations at scientific conferences and articles in peer-reviewed journals (Flaskerud, 1999). Although not an established goal of photovoice, in the context of a CBPR approach it is incumbent upon investigators to help provide opportunities for research participants to contribute to the further dissemination of results through additional local and scientific arenas (Israel et al., 1998). Survivors, CRAs, and academic researchers in this project have coauthored an academic article (López et al., 2005) and have copresented papers and posters at local and national meetings and conferences. (See Chapter Thirteen for a discussion of the development and implementation of dissemination procedures within a CBPR project.)

CHALLENGES

This project benefited from those who have described elsewhere the challenges they have encountered while using photovoice (for example, time and resource costs, ethical and safety considerations) and the strategies they recommend to address these challenges (Wang, 1999, 2003; Wang & Burris, 1994, 1997; Wang, Cash, et al., 2000; Wang & Redwood-Jones, 2001). In this section we share two specific challenges encountered while using photovoice within a CBPR approach, for which the principles of full participation and equitable decision-making power were paramount.

Achieving equitable decision-making power among all partners throughout the research process. At the beginning several women seemed to cede power and control to the academic partners, while they assumed the role of passive research subjects. For example, although survivors developed their own photo-assignments, several were under the impression that the academic partners had rigid ideas about specific photographs they should be taking. Because researchers did their best to convey otherwise and avoided making explicit suggestions about photographs, the CBPR approach was at first a source of confusion and distress to participants who wanted to make a good impression. This issue was epitomized during a photo-discussion show-and-tell when one woman explained that she had taken a photograph of another survivor because she was "told" to do so.

Determining the optimal time for identifying and recruiting influential advocates so they could be involved and committed to improving survivorship QOL. Although Wang strongly suggested identifying influential advocates early in the photovoice process (Wang, 1999, 2003; Wang, Burris, et al., 1996), the partners in this project recruited advocates near the end of the project. Given the exploratory and inductive nature of the work, it was felt that advocates should be identified during the photo-discussions so that their influence would be relevant to the specific themes that emerged. For example, if advocates had been identified at the outset of the project, one obvious choice would have been to recruit a representative from the local cancer support agency. Yet nobody from this agency was identified by survivors as an advocate. In fact, survivors indicated that they rarely used the agency's resources because they perceived that it catered solely to white women.

Despite the rationale for recruiting advocates later in the project, there were drawbacks to this approach. The partnership did not benefit from the advocates' involvement as partners, co-learners, supporters, or advisers throughout the project, nor was it able to develop lasting and committed relationships with them. For example, a recognized limitation of photovoice is that it does not shift to participants the power to decide policy (Wang, 1999; Wang, Burris, et al., 1996). During the forum, the survivors and the academic partners strove to set the stage for survivors and influential advocates to collaborate in developing and implementing culturally sensitive interventions, but since the formation of the two task forces, it has been challenging to maintain commitment and involvement from advocates who have competing priorities.

IMPLICATIONS FOR PRACTICE

In this section we offer several recommendations for investigators who are interested in conducting a photovoice project using a community-based participatory research approach.

Actively solicit local expertise and support to develop and conduct a photovoice project. From the very beginning of the planning process (conducting the pilot study with Helen Rock and Marian Sweet) and throughout the photovoice process (drawing from insights of CRAs and survivors) to its completion (supporting CRAs to oversee future endeavors), the project benefited from local knowledge, contacts, and insights. As a result the academic partners were able to conduct a project that was appropriate for working with African American survivors in these rural communities.

Devote time during the first few sessions to reviewing the concept of partnership and discussing the distinct expertise and experiences that each partner can contribute in the pursuit of new knowledge. Although it took a while for the community partners in this project to feel comfortable sharing control with academic partners, once they regarded themselves as coinvestigators, they accepted responsibility for taking pictures that directed photo-discussion topics, ensuring the trustworthiness of the findings, identifying influential advocates, planning and conducting the forum, and initiating steps for taking action.

Make every effort to ensure a safe and open environment during photo-discussions. Both academic partners' observations and feedback from the survivors suggest that participants felt free to voice divergent opinions and comfortable with sharing sensitive information about their survivorship experiences. Although we believe that the partnership's ability to establish mutual trust and rapport was, in part, facilitated by a decade of positive relationships forged among academic researchers and African American communities (through NC-BCSP and We-Count), we also realize how fragile even these trusting relationships can be. We suggest establishing agreed-upon group norms to abide by throughout a photovoice project (for example, agree to disagree respectfully and keep what is said during meetings confidential), integrating ample opportunities for group interaction and bonding (for example, icebreakers, refreshment periods, and recognition of cultural events and birthdays), and acknowledging up front the social, cultural, and economic factors that have historically resulted in difficulties achieving and maintaining authentic partnerships (Levy, Baldyga, & Jurkowski, 2003). For example, during the photo-discussion sessions, the survivors and the academic partners tried to openly discuss racial tensions due to the academic partners' not being African American. This facilitated survivors' feeling comfortable with broaching sensitive subjects pertaining to their perceptions of racial discrimination by white people.

Devote time during each photo-discussion session to reporting back preliminary findings from prior sessions. This will provide opportunities throughout the project for all participants to be involved in data analysis and interpretation.

Recruit advocates near the beginning of the research process (Wang, 1999), and strive to engage all partners in carefully selecting these individuals. We also recommend recruiting additional advocates throughout the process as they are identified as influential in regard to salient issues that emerge during photo-discussions.

Involve all partners in planning how the project will be continued in the long term. We suggest that sustainability might be increased through engaging all partners in identifying the program development and capacity-building skills that may need enhancing, and through involving them in deciding how relevant training might be integrated into the project process.

CONCLUSION

Our experience using photovoice demonstrates the utility of this method in investigating the socially sensitive topic of cancer survivorship with African American breast cancer survivors from rural eastern North Carolina. Although the survivors in the project were recruited to represent diversity on a range of sociodemographic characteristics, the photo-discussions facilitated what one survivor described as "fellowship and togetherness." As a more equitable partnership evolved, this trusting bond was extended to all project partners, including academic researchers.

It has been asserted that partners in a participatory research endeavor should benefit from the new knowledge and skills they gain during the research process (Green et al., 1997). We believe that sharing control over the research process and the knowledge gained during the project resulted in survivors' demonstrating increased critical awareness of how broad social and structural factors affect their and other women's lives, and recognizing their need and ability to move beyond simply coping to taking action to influence their personal and social environment (Wallerstein & Bernstein, 1988; Wang, Cash, et al., 2000).

The photovoice method provided the means for survivors to reach and forge relationships with influential people to whom they might not normally have access. The reactions from influential advocates who attended the forum and their willingness to initiate collaborations with survivors, suggest that the women's photographs, and what the women had to say about these photos, powerfully relayed the needs of rural African breast cancer survivors. Although it has been a challenge to sustain the task forces beyond the funding period, several survivors and a few committed influential advocates are using the Inspirational Images Project as a foundation to develop new ways to continue to collaborate, such as through working with churches and civic organizations.

Even as CBPR is increasingly recognized and accepted as a viable means for conducting research, skepticism remains as to the scientific quality of collaborative research (Israel et al., 1998). The same can be said for photovoice, which has been questioned regarding the validity, reliability, and objectivity of its findings (Wang et al., 1998). We contend that in the case discussed here, the quality of the research process, the data, and the findings were enhanced by the use of photovoice within a CBPR approach because the new knowledge gained is grounded in the priorities, expertise, and perspectives of survivors themselves (Israel et al., 1998; Wang et al., 1998). We stress the importance of involving participants in interpreting and assessing the trustworthiness of data and findings. Only by reporting results back to participants so that they can confirm and clarify themes that emerge from their photo-discussions is it possible to establish the credibility of these results (Lincoln & Guba, 1985; Rappaport, 1992).

By sharing this process, we hope that those interested in conducting similar CBPR projects will better appreciate the challenges and benefits of implementing photovoice. We are confident that with local insight, planning, and creativity, photovoice offers a means to realize the underlying principles of successful CBPR partnerships and endeavors. Our experience is but one example of how photovoice can facilitate equitable collaboration and provide a mechanism through which new knowledge can be shared with others to promote taking action for social change.

References

Ashing-Giwa, K., & Ganz, P. A. (1997). Understanding the breast cancer experience of African-American women. *Journal of Psychosocial Oncology, 15*(2), 19–35.

Breast Cancer Resource Directory of North Carolina. (2001). Breast Cancer Coalition of North Carolina and Carolina Breast Cancer Study.

Clegg, L. X., Li, F. P., Hankey, B. F., Chu, K., & Edwards, B. K. (2002). Cancer survival among US whites and minorities: A SEER (Surveillance, Epidemiology, and End Results) program population-based study. *Archives of Internal Medicine, 162,* 1985–1993.

Earp, J. A., Viadro, C. I., Vincus, A. A., Altpeter, M., Flax, V., Mayne, L., et al. (1997). Lay health advisors: A strategy for getting the word out about breast cancer. *Health Education & Behavior, 24*(4), 432–451.

Eng, E., & Smith, J. (1995). Natural helping functions of lay health advisors in breast cancer education. *Breast Cancer Research and Treatment, 35*(1), 23–29.

Ewald, W. (1996). *I dreamed I had a girl in my pocket.* Durham, NC: DoubleTake Books and Center for Documentary Studies.

Flaskerud, J. H. (1999). Disseminating the results of participant-focused research. *Journal of Transcultural Nursing, 10*(4), 340–349.

Freire, P. (1970). *Pedagogy of the oppressed.* New York: Seabury Press.

Glaser, B., & Strauss, A. (1967). *The discovery of grounded theory: Strategies for qualitative research.* Hawthorne, NY: Aldine de Gruyter.

Goodman, R. M., Speers, M. A., McLeroy, K., Fawcett, S., Kegler, M., Parker, E., Smith, S. R., Sterling, T. D., Wallerstein, N. (1998). Identifying and defining the dimensions of community capacity to provide a basis for measurement. *Health Education & Behavior, 25*(3), 258–278.

Green, L. W., George, M. A., Daniel, M., Frankish, C. J., Herbert, C. P., Bowie, W. R., et al. (1997). Background on participatory research. In D. Murphy, M. Scammell, & R. Sclove (Eds.), *Doing community-based research: A reader.* Amherst, MA: Loka Institute.

Green, L. W., Richard, L., & Potvin, L. (1996). Ecological foundations of health promotion. *American Journal of Health Promotion, 10*(4), 270–281.

Hassey Dow, K., Ferrell, B. R., Leigh, S., Ly, J., & Gulasekaram, P. (1996). An evaluation of the quality of life among long-term survivors of breast cancer. *Breast Cancer Research and Treatment, 39*(3), 261–273.

Israel, B., Schulz, A., Parker, E., & Becker, A. (1998). Review of community-based research: Assessing partnership approaches to improve public health. *Annual Review of Public Health, 19,* 173–202.

Koch, K. (1970). *Wishes, lies, and dreams: Teaching children to write poetry.* New York: HarperCollins.

Kvale, S. (1995). The social construction of validity. In *Qualitative inquiry* (Vol. 1, pp. 19–40). Thousand Oaks, CA: Sage.

Leedham, B., & Ganz, P. A. (1999). Psychosocial concerns and quality of life in breast cancer survivors. *Cancer Investigation, 17*(5), 342–348.

Levy, S. R., Baldyga, W., & Jurkowski, J. M. (2003). Developing community health promotion interventions: Selecting partners and fostering collaboration. *Health Promotion Practice, 4*(3), 314–322.

Lincoln, Y., & Guba, E. (1985). *Naturalistic inquiry.* Thousand Oaks, CA: Sage.

López, E.D.S. (2002). *Quality of life needs among rural African American breast cancer survivors from eastern North Carolina: Blending the methods of photovoice and grounded theory.* Unpublished dissertation, University of North Carolina.

López, E.D.S., Eng, E., Randall-David, E., & Robinson, N. (2005). Quality of life concerns of African American Breast Cancer Survivors within rural North Carolina: Blending the techniques of photovoice and grounded theory. *Qualitative Health Research, 15*(1), 99–115.

McIntyre, A. (2003). Through the eyes of women: Photovoice and participatory research as tools for reimagining place. *Gender, Place and Culture, 1,* 47–66.

Morse, J. (1994). Designing funded qualitative research. In N. Denzin & Y. Lincoln (Eds.), *Handbook of qualitative research* (pp. 220–235). Thousand Oaks, CA: Sage.

North Carolina Rural Economic Development Center. *Distressed counties.* (2002). Retrieved October 4, 2002, from http://www.ncruralcenter.org/databank/distressed.htm

Northouse, L. L., Caffey, M., Deichelbohrer, L., Schmidt, L., Guziatek-Trojniak, L., West, S., et al. (1999). The quality of life of African American women with breast cancer. *Research in Nursing and Health, 22*(6), 449–460.

Rappaport, J. (1992). Research methods and the empowerment social agenda. In P. Tolan, C. Keys, F. Chertok, & L. Jason (Eds.), *Researching community psychology: Issues of theory and methods* (pp. 51–63). Washington, DC: American Psychological Association.

Reinharz, S. (1992). *Feminist methods in social research.* New York: Oxford University Press.

Sandelowski, M. (1995). Focus on qualitative methods: Sample size in qualitative research. *Research in Nursing and Health, 18,* 179–183.

Solomon, J. (1995). Introduction. In J. Spence & J. Solomon (Eds.), *What can a woman do with a camera?* London: Scarlet Press.

Stokols, D. (1996). Translating social ecological theory into guidelines for community health promotion. *American Journal of Health Promotion, 10*(4), 282–298.

Strauss, A., & Corbin, J. (1998). *Basics of qualitative research: Techniques and procedures for developing grounded theory* (2nd ed.). Thousand Oaks, CA: Sage.

Streng, J. M., Rhodes, S. D., Ayala, G. X., Eng, E., Arceo, R., & Phipps, S. (2004). Realidad Latina: Latino adolescents, their school, and a university use photovoice to examine and address the influence of immigration. *Journal for Interprofessional Care, 18*(4), 403–415.

U.S. Census Bureau. (2000). *State and county quick facts.* Retrieved February 24, 2002, from http://quickfacts.census.gov/gfd/states/37117/html, http://quickfacts.census.gov/gfd/states/37187.html, and http://quickfacts.census.gov/gfd/states/37015.html.

Wallerstein, N., & Bernstein, E. (1988). Empowerment education: Freire's ideas adapted to health education. *Health Education Quarterly, 15*(4), 379–394.

Wang, C. C. (1999). Photovoice: A participatory action research strategy applied to women's health. *Journal of Women's Health, 8*(2), 185–192.

Wang, C. C. (2003). Using photovoice as a participatory assessment and issue selection tool: A case study with the homeless in Ann Arbor. In M. Minkler & N. Wallerstein (Eds.), *Community-based participatory research for health* (pp. 179–196). San Francisco: Jossey-Bass.

Wang, C. C., & Burris, M. A. (1994). Empowerment through photo novella: Portraits of participation. *Health Education Quarterly, 21*(2), 171–186.

Wang, C. C., & Burris, M. A. (1997). Photovoice: Concept, methodology, and use for participatory needs assessment. *Health Education & Behavior, 24*(3), 369–387.

Wang, C. C., Burris, M. A., & Xiang, Y. P. (1996). Chinese village women as visual anthropologists: A participatory approach to reaching policymakers. *Social Science & Medicine, 42*(10), 1391–1400.

Wang, C. C., Cash, J. L., & Powers, L. S. (2000). Who knows the streets as well as the homeless? Promoting personal and community action through photovoice. *Health Promotion Practice, 1*(1), 81–89.

Wang, C. C., Morrel-Samuels, S., Hutchinson, P., Bell, L., & Pestronk, R. M. (2004). Flint Photovoice: Community-building among youths, adults, and policymakers. *American Journal of Public Health, 94*(6), 911–913.

Wang, C. C., & Redwood-Jones, Y. A. (2001). Photovoice ethics: Perspectives from Flint Photovoice. *Health Education & Behavior, 28*(5), 560–572.

Wang, C. C., Wu, K. Y., Zhan, W. T., & Carovano, K. (1998). Photovoice as a participatory health promotion strategy. *Health Promotion International, 13*(1), 75–86.

Wang, C. C., Yuan, Y. L., & Feng, M. L. (1996). Photovoice as a tool for participatory evaluation: The community's view of process and impact. *Journal of Contemporary Health, 4,* 47–49.

Weiler, K. (1994). Freire and a feminist pedagogy of difference. In P. McLaren & C. Lankshear (Eds.), *Politics of liberation: Paths from Freire* (pp. 12–40). New York: Routledge.

The World Health Organization Quality of Life Assessment (WHOQOL): Position paper from the World Health Organization. (1995). *Social Science & Medicine, 41*(10), 1403–1409.

CHAPTER SIXTEEN

Policy Analysis and Advocacy

An Approach to Community-Based Participatory Research

Nicholas Freudenberg, Marc A. Rogers,
Cassandra Ritas, and Sister Mary Nerney

Many community health problems are caused or exacerbated by policies that make it difficult for individuals, neighborhoods, or organizations to protect well-being (Themba & Minkler, 2003). Increasingly, effective public health advocates must be able to identify, describe, and change health-damaging policies. In this chapter we describe participatory policy research, an approach to community-based participatory research designed to analyze the impact of policies on public health and to use these analyses to catalyze action to change harmful policies. To illustrate the methods used in participatory policy research, we present our experiences working to change policies related to community reintegration of individuals returning from a municipal jail system to urban low-income communities in New York City.

Acknowledgments: The research described in this chapter was supported by grants from the Open Society Institute to Hunter College and from the Centers for Disease Control and Prevention to the Harlem Urban Research Center. All opinions expressed are those of the authors and do not necessarily represent the positions of their institutions or funders. We gratefully acknowledge the suggestions and contributions from the Community Action Board of the Urban Research Center, the Policy Work Group, and the assistance of Salwa Nassar, Nina Aledort, Juliana van Olphen, Eric Canales, Sandro Galea, David Vlahov, and Ann-Gel Palermo.

METHODS FOR PARTICIPATORY POLICY RESEARCH

Policy refers to an organization's planned activity to achieve a goal (Themba & Minkler, 2003). Policies may be public (for example, local, state, or federal government policies) or private (for example, corporate or voluntary association policies); they may be short or long term; and they may come in the form of a single action (for example, a proclamation or law) or multiple actions across agencies (for example, devolution of federal responsibilities to states). Although policies are intentional, a decision not to act or to ignore a problem is also a policy, even if not explicitly articulated. Public health professionals have long been involved in *policy analysis,* an assessment of the health impact of various approaches to solving a problem, and *policy advocacy,* efforts to change policies that harm health (Acosta, 2003; Brownson, Newschaffer, & Ali-Abarghoui, 1997; Christoffel, 2000).

Participatory policy research (PPR) differs from more traditional approaches to policy analysis and advocacy in several ways. First, it actively seeks the involvement of all relevant stakeholders, especially those traditionally excluded from the policy process (Themba & Minkler, 2003). Second, because it starts with community perceptions of the problem, PPR frames policy questions more broadly, often cutting across sectors (for example, health, education, and criminal justice) and levels of government, that is, local, state, and federal (Themba, 1999). Third, like other forms of participatory research, PPR is rooted in the context in which it unfolds, requiring an analysis of the broader historical, social, cultural, and political dimensions of the problem and setting (Greenwood & Levin, 1998). Finally, PPR embraces both analysis and action; it does not stop once analysis is complete (Israel et al., 2003; Ritas, 2003). Each of these defining characteristics emerges from the broader field of community-based participatory research and each shapes the specific methods used to implement PPR.

Involvement of Relevant Stakeholders

The starting point of participatory policy research is to involve all relevant stakeholders in the definition and analysis of the problem and then in action to resolve it. Because those with less power are often excluded from the political process, PPR places a high value on including them in the research and action process. The methods used to elicit and engage different constituencies are similar to those used in other types of research—for example, surveys, public opinion polls, focus groups, in-depth interviews, observation, and community forums—all methods we used in the case described here. Each of these methods has unique advantages and disadvantages (DiClemente & Blumental, 2004), and many researchers describe the benefits of combining several methods to gain a deeper understanding of various viewpoints (Fine & Weis, 1998; Klinenberg, 2002). Key questions that these methods seek to answer are

- What is each group's perception of the problem or issue in the community?
- What is the range of policies that affect this problem or issue?
- What are the perceived costs and benefits of current policy approaches?
- What are the unintended consequences of current policy approaches?
- What changes in policy make sense to the community, and how might these changes affect life in the community?

As in other forms of participatory research, the team of investigators that poses research questions, designs instruments, collects and interprets data, and presents findings to the public should include representatives of the involved groups (Israel et al, 2003; Whyte, 1991). To balance historical inequities in power, the ground rules for making decisions about the research need to give equal voice to team members who have comparatively less formal education, social status, or political power (Chávez, Duran, Baker, Avila, & Wallerstein, 2003).

Broad Frame of Policy Problem

Policy research is indicated when community residents, advocates, policymakers, or researchers identify a problem that is perceived to have significant policy determinants (Themba & Minkler, 2003). Because each particular policy is embedded within many others, researchers need to select where to focus their attention. Several methods can help researchers in carrying out these critical analyses. They include reviews of relevant professional, mass media, government, and advocacy literatures; interviews with government policymakers, administrators, and advocates; and surveys of various constituencies. Each of these was used in the case described here. Several recent analyses of specific public health policies illustrate the varying use of these methods (Dievler & Pappas, 1999; Klinenberg, 2002).

Importance of Context

Not only is each policy linked to a web of other policies, each policy initiative unfolds in a context characterized by a unique history, culture, and politics (Greenwood & Levin, 1998). Policy researchers, especially those investigating the impact of policies on communities, need to understand the relevant dimensions of this context. Participatory policy research has the advantage of involving multiple stakeholders, making it easier to elicit and document contextual factors (Themba & Minkler, 2003). Methods that can be used for this purpose include interviews with long-time community residents, leaders, and activists and reviews of media reports and local history documents. (See Chapter Four for an explanation of the use of in-depth interviews with community residents that is relevant to assessing contextual factors.)

Analysis and Action

Traditionally, research and policy advocacy are seen as separate activities. CBPR principles question this distinction between research and action, and PPR especially insists on the unity of this dialectic (Acosta, 2003). The fundamental rationale for PPR is to understand fully the policy context in order to make improvements. Thus even before beginning to collect data, the research team must ask such questions as these:

- What kinds of information will move various constituencies to action?
- What change strategies have been demonstrated to be effective in this context or on this issue in the past?
- What are the implications of these previous experiences for the research that is needed on this issue?

Research methods that can assist researchers in moving between action and analysis are reviews of formal and informal evaluation studies of previous change efforts; the development of rapid assessment feedback loops between policy implementation and future advocacy; and as in earlier stages, the use of quantitative methods (for example, public opinion polls and surveys) and qualitative methods (for example, in-depth interviews and focus groups) to assess the impact of various change strategies on the policy process.

APPLICATION OF METHODS TO THE PROJECT

In this section we discuss applying methods in a project of reintegrating men and women who have been serving jail sentences into the community. We present an overview of community reentry from jail and discuss the evolution of the participatory research team, the research methods used, and the accomplishments to date.

Overview of Community Reentry from Jail in New York City

Every year almost 100,000 inmates are released from jail or prison to return to New York City communities. Many have been incarcerated for alleged crimes related to homelessness, drug addiction, mental illness, or violent behavior, and few have the education, work experience, or job skills needed to succeed in this nation's economy. Yet most return to their families and neighborhoods, usually within a few weeks or months of arrest, without having received help for these problems (Belenko, 2000; Mumola, 1999; Nelson & Trone, 2000). After having spent nearly $3 billion a year to incarcerate these individuals, the city and state release most inmates with a Metrocard for two subway trips in their pockets and no specific plan for finding help with housing, drug treatment, employment, or health care. Within a year almost half have been incarcerated again (City of New York, Office of Mayor, 1999; Belluck, 1996; Hunter College Center on AIDS . . . , 2002, 2003; Nelson et al., 1999).

New York City (NYC) is not alone in facing problems related to reentry from jail or prison (Beck & Mumuola, 1999). Each year more than 10 million (Kerle, 1998) Americans return home from jail, and about 600,000 return from state and federal prisons. (*Jails* house people after arrest and before trial and those sentenced to less than a year; *prisons* confine people sentenced to more than a year.) Recently, several research reports have documented the social, health, financial, and moral costs of these consequences of U.S. policies of mass incarceration (Butterfield, 2002; Hammett, Roberts, & Kennedy, 2001; National Commission on Correctional Health Care, 2002; Rand Corporation, 2001; Travis, Solomon, & Waul, 2001).

People entering jail or prison bring an extraordinary concentration of health and social problems with them. Surveys show that 80 percent have a drug or alcohol problem, and 15 percent have a diagnosis of serious mental illness (Arrestee Drug Abuse Monitoring Program, 2000; Barr, 1999; Hunter College Center . . . , 2003; City of New York, Office of the Mayor, 2002). Many are victims or perpetrators of family violence, and nationally their rates of both HIV and Hepatitis C infections are about nine times higher than in the general population (Hammett, Harmon, & Rhodes, 2002).

Today, 30 percent of NYC inmates report they have been homeless at some point in the three months prior to their arrest. More than 90 percent are high school dropouts. The cycling of people in and out of jail represents a significant threat to the well-being of many low-income urban communities. Although the causes and consequences of mass incarceration operate at the individual, community, and policy levels, our work in this area and our understanding of the relevant research literature (Freudenberg, 2001b) led us to believe that the policy determinants of unsuccessful reentry were fundamental to the problem. Thus we believed that any reversal of the problem required not only new services for individuals but also changes in public policies regarding incarceration, social services, health care, mental health, substance abuse treatment, and employment (Barr, 1999; Conklin, Lincoln, & Flanagan, 1998).

Evolution of a Participatory Research Team

The work described here has been a collaborative effort among community and advocacy organizations and the Center for Urban Epidemiologic Studies (CUES) at the New York Academy of Medicine; the Harlem Urban Research Center, supported by the U.S. Centers for Disease Control and Prevention and located within CUES; and a community action board that was established within this research center. The mission of the Harlem Urban Research Center (URC) was to make it easier for individuals to find help for a drug problem than to find drugs in Central and East Harlem (Galea et al., 2001). The URC research team used CBPR as well as traditional epidemiological research methods to understand the determinants of substance use at multiple levels (Galea et al., 2001; van Olphen, Freudenberg, Galea, Ritas, & Palermo, 2003; van Olphen & Freudenberg, 2004).

Other participants in the present project included public health researchers at Hunter College and community service providers and advocates in Central and East Harlem (Freudenberg, 2001a; Galea et al., 2001). Later a citywide network, the Community Reintegration Network, developed from this policy change project. (See Table 16.1 for a description of the key partners involved.)

In 2000, several service providers, community residents, researchers, and advocates based in Central and East Harlem in New York City, two of the nation's poorest neighborhoods (McCord & Freeman, 1990), formed the Policy Work Group (PWG). Most of the founders were members of the Community Action Board of the Harlem URC. The PWG goals were to document and then advocate changing the policies that made it difficult for people returning to Harlem from jail to become healthy, productive members of their community.

Over time, the effort to change city policy on jail reentry expanded to include more advocacy and service organizations. In 2002, more than fifty individuals and organizations from around New York City, including service providers, advocates, former inmates and their families, and researchers joined to create the Community Reintegration Network (CRN) to advocate for citywide changes in reentry policy. The CRN was established as the Policy Work Group recognized the importance of working on a citywide as well as a local level. Finally, a third group, the Strategic Retreat on Reentry Policy, was convened in 2002 by two city commissioners who wanted advice on how to change city policy. Several members of the PWG and the CRN were also participants in this process. Thus the efforts described here include both *community-wide* and *citywide* PPR, demonstrating that the boundaries of participatory research sometimes extend outside a specific geographical community.

Methods Used to Understand and Change Reentry Policies

In this section we describe selected methods carried out by the partners listed in Table 16.1 for the purpose of understanding and then changing city policies related to reentry from jail. Table 16.2 summarizes the methods and activities used, and selected activities are described in more detail in the text.

Table 16.1. Key Partners in the Project

Organization	Objectives	Level of Intervention	Types of Members
Harlem Urban Research Center (URC)	Identify and reduce threats to health in Harlem; focus on substance abuse and infectious disease	Community	Researchers
URC Community Action Board (CAB)	Act with URC to improve health in Harlem; advise URC on community priorities and needs; serve as URC liaison to community	Community	Service providers, local leaders, researchers
CAB Policy Work Group (PWG)	Identify policy obstacles to improving health of Harlem residents with substance use problems; act to reduce obstacles	Community	Advocates, service providers, local leaders, researchers
New York City Community Reintegration Network (CRN)	Provide forum for service providers working with people returning from jail; advocate policies to facilitate reentry from jail or prison	New York City	Advocates, service providers, researchers, media
Strategic Retreat on Reentry Policy	Identify and strengthen city policies and practices that can contribute to successful reentry from jail or prison	New York City Government	City commissioners, citywide service providers, advocacy groups

Table 16.2. Methods Used to Understand and Change Jail Reentry Policies

Method	Brief Description	Research Questions
Review of public data on reentry issues	Collection and analysis of government records and data on people in and leaving jail	What are the demographic and other characteristics of people leaving jails? What problems do they face? What services are available for what populations?
Review of relevant legislation and agency regulations	Assessment of relevant public policies that affect reentry	What policies facilitate reentry of people leaving jail?
Survey of service providers	Interviews with sample of 79 Harlem service providers to assess their perceptions of policy obstacles and facilitators to successful entry into drug treatment	What policies affect drug users' ability to get help for their problems? Which policies affect drug users most? Which policies affect the most drug users?
Focus group with people released from jail	Focus groups with 36 individuals recently released from jail or prison to identify postrelease problems	What are the perceptions of people returning from incarceration about what helps and what hinders successful community reentry?
Literature reviews: professional literature, mass media, advocacy reports	Summary and analysis of various types of literature describing problems and successes of reentry from jail	What barriers and facilitators to successful reentry have journalists, public officials, and advocates identified? What successful interventions have been described? To what extent does coverage of other criminal justice issues contribute to or detract from a focus on reentry?
Community forums	Public meetings to discuss the issue of community reentry from jail	What policy changes might activate sectors of the population? How do the experiences of service providers, advocates, and people returning from prison inform the policy debate? What effect does connecting diverse stakeholders have on policymaking?

Public opinion polls	Household and street surveys of community-based populations to understand perceptions of people returning from jail and prison and what they think are the biggest problems facing those reentering	What policies might the general public support in order to promote successful reentry?
Meeting with legislators and staff	Meetings with local city council representatives and chairs of relevant council committees to discuss reentry	What policy changes on jail reentry might city council members be willing to support? What other policy initiatives might affect jail reentry?
Meeting with executive branch officials	Meetings with city agency officials to discuss reentry issues and policies and to assess support for change	What policy changes on jail reentry might these officials be willing to implement? What other policy initiatives might affect jail reentry?
Cost study of incarceration	Assessment by city budget office of full costs of incarceration in New York City	What are the annual costs of incarceration? What are the components of these costs? How has the cost changed over time?
City council hearings	Public hearing on the issue of discharge planning and reentry	What is the level of political support for changes in policy?
Policy reports	Various policy reports advocating changes in city policies that affect jail reentry	What arguments and evidence will persuade various stakeholders to take action to bring about policy change?

Review of Public Data on Reentry Issues. To quantify the dimensions of the problem and to supplement the information collected within the community, PWG members collected data from city agencies such as the Departments of Correction, Health, and Human Resources Administration and the Agency for Children's Services, among others. Simply determining what data were available was often a daunting task, and the service providers, Legal Aid lawyers, and former inmates who were members of the PWG were often more knowledgeable than university researchers in developing strategies for finding the information buried in bureaucratic archives. For the first few years, the difficulty in finding relevant data was complicated by a mayoral administration intent on withholding data from the public. In these situations, getting access to data that had been released in response to prior lawsuits (for example, a class action lawsuit that ultimately forced the city to provide discharge planning services to mentally ill inmates) was sometimes helpful. In other cases, data were simply unavailable because administrators wanted to withhold data that could be used to advocate for policy change or because agencies were failing to track data that might cause political problems.

Review of Relevant Legislation and Agency Regulations. As previously noted, a web of legislation and regulations affected the reentry prospects of people returning from jail. Learning which categories of policy and which levels of government were relevant sometimes proved challenging. For example, it took two years to learn that the New York City Housing Authority's public housing policy of evicting individuals who have been incarcerated was more stringent than the federal legislation required. This discovery, the result of a collaborative legal research effort among service providers, public defender organizations, and administrators of other city agencies, led to an unsuccessful attempt to persuade the NYC Housing Authority to reconsider its eviction policy. As with obtaining public data, having multiple partners at different levels often made it easier to find someone who had a more complete understanding of a particular policy issue.

Survey of Service Providers. To identify policy obstacles that impeded or facilitated clients' attempts to overcome substance use and related problems, we interviewed seventy-nine Harlem-based service providers (van Olphen & Freudenberg, 2004). The URC Community Action Board helped to identify relevant policies to include in the survey, reviewed early drafts of the survey, and recruited respondents from its own and neighboring agencies. The respondents were asked to rate thirty specific policies (in such areas as drug treatment, public assistance, child protective services, housing, Medicaid and managed care, mental health, police, corrections, and probation and parole) as harmful or helpful to their clients, and to assess how the policies acted as barriers to getting services and reducing drug use. Eleven policies in the areas of drug treatment, corrections, and Medicaid were rated as harmful to their clients by more than 50 percent of the respondents. The high percentage of service providers who indicated that several policies affecting reentry were problematic contributed to the PWG's decision to focus on reentry policies as an obstacle to reducing drug use in the community. (See Chapter Five for a discussion of using a survey to identify issues and factors associated with health status.)

Focus Groups with People Returning from Jail or Prison. In order to explore the challenges in successful community reintegration, the PWG researchers conducted six focus groups. The participants were thirty-six men and women who had been recently released from jail or prison. They were asked to describe their experiences with discharge planning and their access to services, employment, and housing prior to and immediately following release from jail. The findings suggested that many people leaving jail are not prepared for release, and once they are released they face a myriad of obstacles to becoming healthy, productive members of their communities. In addition, participants made specific suggestions for improving these services. PWG researchers prepared a brief summary of the findings of the focus groups for PWG and CAB members. Later, these focus group findings helped to guide PWG members' testimony at City Council hearings and informed the recommendations in subsequent policy reports. (The use of focus groups in CBPR efforts is further examined in Chapters Four and Seven.)

Literature Reviews. In order to avoid reinventing the wheel, PWG researchers conducted reviews of various kinds of literature, including mass media coverage of correctional issues in New York City; scientific reports on the health and social needs of people leaving jail and evaluation studies or descriptions of innovative approaches to improving the outcomes of reentry from jail; and policy reports by governmental agencies and advocacy organizations.

Where resources permitted, the PWG researchers prepared brief summaries of these reviews for the group and other interested parties. In several cases discussion of drafts of these summaries and consideration of community perspectives at PWG meetings led to changes in the conclusions. For example, a discussion of barriers to substance abuse treatment after release from jail showed not only that a shortage of appropriate treatment slots existed but that treatment program regulations also served as a deterrent for those returning from jail.

Community Forums. After completing its initial research, the PWG moved into a more interactive phase of PPR, in which PWG members sought to build a community network for change, disseminate the results of their research, and with community partners and residents, develop policy recommendations to bring to city officials. This phase was kicked off with a community forum, held at the URC's home, the New York Academy of Medicine in East Harlem. CAB and PWG members actively recruited participants to attend the forum. The 150 service providers, researchers, people returning from jail and prison, and legal advocates who attended later became the core of the Community Reintegration Network, the citywide alliance that addressed reentry issues. The forum provided information and asked small groups of participants to identify obstacles to reentry and to suggest specific actions for a policy agenda. The recommendations developed in this forum formed the basis of the policy prescriptions later presented to elected and appointed officials. The network was developed by creating a listserv for forum attendees and later was nurtured by convening a planning committee that met monthly to address such issues as housing, job training, and health care.

Public Opinion Poll. In 2002, we persuaded a group conducting a survey to add questions on community reentry to existing telephone polls of random samples of New York City residents in selected low-income neighborhoods. This group was willing to add questions to its surveys both because it had been involved in other URC activities and supported URC goals and because the incremental cost of adding four or five additional questions was relatively low.

The poll was conducted in early 2002 from the New York Academy of Medicine. It surveyed 1,003 random households by telephone in four neighborhoods, including Central and East Harlem. Results showed that almost 40 percent of respondents personally knew someone who had been in jail or prison in the last year, almost a third personally knew someone who had returned from jail or prison in the last year, 12 percent had a household member who had served time, and 8 percent of the respondents themselves had served time behind bars at some time in their lives, confirming that a substantial portion of low-income community residents in New York City had direct and recent experience with correctional facilities and people returning from them. In addition, the poll demonstrated strong support for policies that increase job training and other services for people coming out of jail. More punitive policies had lower levels of support. These data suggested the potential for community support for policy changes in regard to reintegration services and also indicated the importance of public dialogue on these issues.

Meetings with Legislators and Staff. Policy change takes place within both the legislative and executive branches of government. However, because the two branches interact with each other, advocates need to know what policy changes each branch is willing to support. In the case at hand, we wanted to know which policy changes the City Council members were willing to support, council views on mayoral policy initiatives on jail reentry issues, and council willingness to take leadership on these issues. We began by meeting with the City Council members who represented the communities in which the PWG was working. To each meeting, PWG members, both researchers and service providers, brought a discussion agenda, a list of PWG's community members and their letters of support for our efforts, a one-page overview of NYC reentry issues, and a longer analysis of jail reentry issues. City council members gave us advice on whom to meet with in the mayoral agencies, background on related political and policy issues, and suggestions for legislative strategy.

Subsequently, we met with the chairs of three City Council committees: criminal justice, health, and mental health and substance abuse. At the suggestion of one of the Council members with whom we had met previously, we decided to advocate at each meeting for a jointly sponsored, three-committee public hearing on reentry. In particular, the chair of the Criminal Justice Services Committee, which oversees the Department of Correction (DOC), embraced this idea and took the lead; she had already been organizing a hearing on jail discharge planning, and this fit well into her plans. The other committee chairs also supported the idea of a hearing.

Meetings with Executive Branch Officials. Within the executive branch, several members of the PWG met first with the mayor's criminal justice coordinator to discuss our goals and agenda. The most productive meeting was with the commissioner of correction. At this meeting, we discussed previous attempts to improve inmate services such as discharge planning and postrelease follow-up care. We described new research findings that supported the effectiveness of reentry services and suggested that the available evidence showed that services that help people leaving jail to improve their lives and reduce recidivism save the city money. We presented the commissioner with budget savings scenarios developed via discussions with a previous commissioner of correction.

The commissioner was already interested in working for change on jail reentry and was easy to engage in dialogue. But like other officials, he had budget constraints high on his list of concerns. He agreed to host a professionally moderated retreat (the Strategic Retreat on Reentry Policy in Table 16.1) to which he would invite key city agency heads and service providers who could discuss the many pieces of the picture together. The Strategic Retreat process lasted seven months, during which time participants gathered and analyzed data and made suggestions for policy change.

In several instances the research of the community-based PWG informed this process. For example, the findings from the focus groups with former inmates illustrated some of the problems those leaving jail encountered. At the same time, some community service providers in the PWG doubted whether there was a commitment to real change in the Department of Correction and felt excluded from the retreat process, fearing that recommendations from the retreat would favor the larger, citywide service providers at the expense of the smaller, more grassroots agencies.

Cost Study of Jail Services. For elected officials one of the most compelling arguments for reconsidering current jail policies was the high cost of incarceration. As NYC fell into a fiscal crisis in late 2000, policymakers were searching for new ways to save money. PWG researchers' review of existing evidence on the cost of incarceration showed conflicting data, with many costs unaccounted for, so PWG requested the New York City Independent Budget Office (IBO), a public agency independent of NYC's Mayor and City Council, to prepare a report on this issue. The IBO found that the full annual cost for one incarceration, including inmate health care costs, benefits for correctional officers, and debt service on jail capital costs, reached $92,500 in 2002 (City of New York, Independent Budget Office, 2002). More than a year later, the *New York Times* reported on the findings of this IBO study that the PWG had requested (von Zielbauer, 2004), provoking further political discussion of reentry policy.

In another case a community service provider active in the PWG calculated that its own alternatives to incarceration program had saved the city $670,355 and the state $2,269,850 by keeping twelve women out of jail and prison and their children out of foster care for six months. By showing that the agency had saved the city and state far more than the government money allocated to the program, agency staff were able to make a strong case for continued funding and expansion of funding for similar programs.

City Council Hearing. In planning for a City Council hearing, our primary goal was to make recommendations for change that were viable and supported by many stakeholders. The Community Reentry Network (CRN), which included members of the PWG, joined with other organizations to accomplish this goal by convening a planning meeting so that participants could agree on recommendations to be made to the city. More than thirty-six service providers and advocacy organizations and several formerly incarcerated individuals attended this meeting, significantly expanding membership in the CRN.

The CRN planning committee developed twelve recommendations to present to the council to improve reentry policies and practices. This list was circulated to all CRN members by e-mail and modified based on the responses. The CRN also prepared a list of questions for the city agency representatives who were testifying at the hearing and submitted it to the planning committee chair. The network's mobilization effort led to a high turnout and a substantial media presence at the hearing. This media coverage, which was also generated by the public officials themselves, further legitimated jail reentry as a valid political issue in the city.

Policy Reports. At various points the research team produced and distributed policy reports on its work. The first, "Coming Back to Harlem from Jail or Prison: One-Way or Round Trip," described the dimensions of the reentry issue in Harlem and suggested actions various groups can take to address the problem (see Appendix O). Its goal was to encourage various constituencies in the community to learn about and then act to reduce the individual and policy obstacles facing people returning to Harlem from jail or prison. The report was distributed at community meetings, sent to local elected officials, and eventually posted on the CRN's Web site. Later, a second report, entitled "Coming Home from Jail: An Action Plan to Improve NYC Reentry Policies & Programs," was produced by the CRN and Hunter College. Aimed at citywide policymakers and advocates, it described the social and financial costs and consequences of current reentry policies in New York City and suggested various actions to reduce the problem. This too was distributed at meetings and posted on the CRN Web site.

Accomplishments to Date

A full assessment of the impact of the research and advocacy efforts described here is premature. After four years, the project partners have accomplished many goals but still face daunting challenges. First, we have created organizational capacity that has led to action to address the issue of jail reentry at both the community and city levels. This work was part of a broader effort that included many others, but the research, community mobilization, and education carried out by the PWG and the CRN were vital to bringing new attention to this issue. Second, the research conducted and the findings disseminated have helped several constituencies, including community residents, service providers, advocacy groups, and elected officials, to better understand the issue of jail reentry, to suggest feasible solutions, and to advocate for change in the political arena.

Finally, our efforts and those of others have contributed to modest but potentially significant changes in reentry policies and programs: a new job program for people leaving jail, new contracts for service providers to provide discharge planning and follow-up services, and new release procedures (Committee on Fire and Criminal Justice Services, 2004; von Zielbauer, 2003). Many other policy changes are under consideration.

At the same time, however, we have yet to achieve many of the prerequisites for the development of a humane, just, and affordable system for people returning home from jail. We have not yet been able to mobilize substantial portions of community residents to advocate for change in this area; convince officials that a transformation of the system, rather than incremental change, is needed; or develop specific alternative proposals that are both politically feasible and promise significant change. In the years ahead, our participatory policy research and advocacy efforts will turn to these unmet challenges.

LIMITATIONS AND CHALLENGES

We faced a number of limitations and challenges in conducting this PPR effort, which we describe in this section.

There are perils in wearing two hats. Wearing the hats of both researchers and advocates may result in identity confusion for PPR teams and especially for the constituencies with whom they interact. Researchers are expected to be disinterested and "objective." Their credibility is based on their technical expertise, their institutional affiliations, and their independence from interested stakeholders. Advocates' standing is based on their intimate knowledge of the issues and affected populations, their commitment to social justice, their ability to mobilize people for action, and their prior successes in achieving policy change.

A substantial literature exists on the conflicting and overlapping philosophical and theoretical dimensions of these two roles (Aronowitz, 1992; Fine, 1992; Gamson, 1999), but it was the practical issues that impressed us. Municipal policymakers interact regularly with both researchers and activists but judge the two by different criteria. In some cases the very legitimacy of our research team members undermined their credibility as advocates, and vice versa. Although there are advantages for a policy change effort in having a public face that includes both researchers and advocates, there are disadvantages as well.

Each research method has limitations. The research team used a variety of methods, but each had limitations that compromised its ability to influence policy. In most cases these limitations were dictated by constraints of time and money. As a result, although the team accumulated a diverse and multi-faceted chain of evidence to document the impact of current policies, each link of the chain had weaknesses that subjected these findings to challenge. In retrospect, it is possible that putting all the project resources into a single rigorous research effort might have had a greater impact on policy than the multimethod approach we actually employed. Although each of the work components met research standards, their modest scope required us to use a "weight of the evidence" approach that combined findings from several small-scale studies. The alternative would have been a definitive study that demonstrated that a particular solution led to better results, saved taxpayer money, and was politically feasible. Not only were the resources lacking for such an approach but the project partners have yet to identify such a magic bullet solution. Instead, as the policy process unfolded, the research team responded to questions as they emerged. This approach also has value and may be more realistic for a community-based effort that is unable to obtain the substantial up-front resources needed for the experimental approaches that traditional researchers value most highly.

Research or evidence has limited impact on policy. The Policy Work Group and Community Reintegration Network spent considerable time and resources to gather the best available evidence to document problems and suggest directions for policy change. The project partners knew, however, that evidence is only one of many influences on policy. Many elected officials believed that raising the issue of people returning from jail could never win them political support, and no countervailing data on public opinion could convince them otherwise. Similarly, the Mayor's Office became actively involved in modifying the jail release process only when substantial public and private dollars became available for redeveloping the section of the city to which most inmates were released. The prospect of economic development was far more persuasive than years of effort on the part of advocates to document the social consequences of the inhumane release process.

Pressure may exist to frame narrowly. As researchers and advocates, both the PWG and the CRN faced strong pressure from both within and without to frame the problem and the solutions more narrowly. The demand to focus our concern was reasonable: researchers can productively study only one phenomenon at a time, policy advocates have to select priorities if they are to be effective, and limited resources also dictate priorities. At the same time, everything we learned about jail reentry suggested that it was a multilevel, multidetermined problem that required multiple systems and levels of organization to resolve. Our decisions to pursue the investigations in several service sectors (for example, housing, drug treatment, and job training) and populations (men, women, adolescents, and drug users) and to elicit the views of multiple stakeholders made the work take longer. It made it more difficult to articulate simple sound-bite solutions and to respond to policymakers' requests for a specific, "realistic" action agenda.

Defining accountability for different participants may be problematic. The literature on community-based participatory research often assumes that the research team comes from and is accountable to a specific community. In such situations, even though it may be difficult to define mutually satisfactory relationships within the partnership, the stakeholders are known and the scope of action has known boundaries. In practice, however, and especially in policy campaigns, the work often spills into other levels of social organization. This spillover raises such complex questions as: How do researchers balance their accountability to communities and to wider advocacy coalitions? and, What happens when the research or advocacy imperatives at these two levels differ? In our work, we did not choose to create a single organization that crossed these levels or to define formal procedures for making decisions about research or action across levels. In effect, researchers and a few advocates served as the bridge between the two.

LESSONS LEARNED AND IMPLICATIONS FOR PRACTICE

Our experience suggests the following lessons and implications for the use of participatory policy research.

Use multiple methods. The research team used a variety of methods to study the issue of jail reentry, and we believe its portfolio of studies had many advantages. They increased our understanding of the issues, provided different types of evidence to use with different constituencies, allowed us to conduct brief investigations with limited resources, and effectively tapped the various capacities of team members. Having a mix of quantitative and qualitative studies may be especially important not only for methodological reasons but also because different stakeholders value types of evidence differently: for example, agency officials are more likely to be moved by quantitative than qualitative data whereas some elected officials are more moved by the personal narratives that emerge from qualitative data. In planning a policy research project, teams should carefully consider in advance what types of data are needed to influence each relevant constituency.

Look at the costs of policy options. Researchers and advocates with a commitment to social justice sometimes find it distasteful to highlight the costs of policy options, fearing that fiscal arguments will trump health or justice concerns. In our project, the ability to present data on the costs of current ineffective policies added significantly to our ability to engage with policymakers. Even when the cost benefits of more just and humane policies are not as clear as in criminal justice, in the current political climate advocates will always face questions on cost. Understanding these issues and "owning" relevant data increases advocates' effectiveness.

Consider the research team's public face. In every setting, people interacting with participatory policy researchers want to know who "we" are. In our experience, there is no single answer to this question, and PWG and CRN members learned the importance of bringing a representative group to each meeting with elected officials. Researchers or community members alone cannot convey the power or relevance of PPR partnerships, but together they can deliver a strong, well-researched message that clearly comes from the communities that politicians represent. For agency officials, in contrast, the stance of dispassionate researchers may sometimes be more persuasive and be free of the "taint" of politics or advocacy. We suggest PPR teams consider the most appropriate faces and voices for each context. In retrospect, we believe more and stronger community representation throughout the information gathering and dissemination process would have better advanced our policy agenda.

Use research processes to build constituencies for change. A unique benefit of PPR is that it can draw different people into the research and advocacy process. By using methods that explicitly seek to engage new participants, PPR can strengthen both research and advocacy. For example, we collected survey data from community forum participants both to assess the support for various policy options among an activated cross-section of the community and to identify those willing to join the campaign.

Time dissemination of research findings to influence policy process. Although advocates know the importance of timing the release of findings to influence policy, researchers sometimes let research imperatives drive their timing. In retrospect, we believe the project partners could have used many important findings better (for example, the Independent Budget Office cost study and the opinion poll findings) had they focused more on how to use results than on the research process itself. Finding the right balance between research and policy outcomes requires an explicit and ongoing discussion of priorities.

Put research findings in the hands of those who can use them. The research team often spent considerable effort in producing well-researched and well-presented summaries of findings. It spent less time putting these reports into the hands of those who could use them, for example, advocates or legislative staffers. With time we developed a variety of mechanisms for getting our reports out, including conducting briefing sessions in the community, hosting a Web site, distributing copies at community meetings, and holding informal meetings with individual advocates.

CONCLUSION

We believe the primary implications of our experiences for participatory policy researchers who want to change public policies that damage health do not reside in specific guidelines on the use of methods. The critical importance of context makes cookbook approaches to PPR inappropriate. Rather, we have learned the importance of immersing oneself in the many dimensions of a social problem, using a variety of methods to learn more about the problem, engaging with constituencies at all levels of the social and political hierarchy, and developing an ongoing dialogue between the research and advocacy arms of the process.

References

Acosta, C. M. (2003). Improving public health through policy advocacy. *Community-Based Public Health Policy and Practice, 8,* 1–8.

Aronowitz, S. (1992). *Science as power: Discourse and ideology in modern science.* Minneapolis: University of Minnesota Press.

Arrestee Drug Abuse Monitoring Program. (2000). *Annual report on drug use among adult and juvenile arrestees, 1999* (NCJ 181326). Washington, DC: National Institute of Justice.

Axelsson, B. O., Saraf, A., & Larsson, L. (1995). Determination of ergosterol in organic dust by gas chromatography-mass spectrometry. *Journal of Chromatography B: Biomedical Applications, 666*(1), 77–84.

Barr, H. (1999). *Prisons and jails: Hospitals of last resort: The need for diversion and discharge planning for incarcerated people with mental illness in New York.* New York: Correctional Association of New York and Urban Justice Center. Retrieved May 20, 2002, from www.soros.org/crime/MIReport.htm

Beck, A. J., & Mumola, C. J. (1999). *Prisoners in 1998.* Washington, DC: U.S. Department of Justice.

Belenko, S. (2000). The challenges of integrating drug treatment into the criminal justice process. *Albany Law Review, 63,* 833–876.

Belluck, P. (1996, November 17). The youngest ex-cons: Facing a difficult road out of crime. *New York Times,* pp. 1, 40.

Brownson, R. C., Newschaffer, C. J., & Ali-Abarghoui, F. (1997). Policy research for disease prevention: Challenges and practical recommendations. *American Journal of Public Health, 87,* 735–739.

Butterfield, F. (2002, February 11). Study finds steady increase at all levels of government in cost of criminal justice. *New York Times,* p. A14.

Chávez, V., Duran, B., Baker, Q. E., Avila, M. M., & Wallerstein, N. (2003). The dance of race and privilege in community-based participatory research. In M. Minkler & N. Wallerstein (Eds.), *Community-based participatory research for health* (pp. 81–97). San Francisco: Jossey-Bass.

Christoffel, K. K. (2000). Public health advocacy: Process and product. *American Journal of Public Health, 90,* 722–726.

City of New York, Independent Budget Office. (2002). *Memo on costs of incarceration in New York City.* Prepared for Hunter College Center on AIDS, Drugs, and Community Health.

City of New York, Office of the Mayor. (1999). *Mayor's management report: Preliminary fiscal year 1999* (Agency Narratives, Vol. 1). New York: Office of the Mayor.

City of New York, Office of the Mayor. (2002). *Mayor's management report: Preliminary fiscal year 2002* (Agency Narratives, Vol. 1). New York: Author.

Committee on Fire and Criminal Justice Services. (2004, May 3). *Oversight hearing: Discharge planning and community reentry for the city's jail population.* New York City Council. Retrieved May 8, 2004, from http://www.council.nyc.ny.us/attachments/60799.htm

Conklin, T. J., Lincoln, T., & Flanagan, T. P. (1998). A public health model to connect correctional health care with communities. *American Journal of Public Health, 88,* 1249–1251.

DiClemente, R. J., & Blumental, D. S. (Eds.). (2004). *Community-based health research: Issues and methods.* New York: Springer.

Dievler, A., & Pappas, G. (1999). Implications of social class and race for urban public health policy making: A case study of HIV/AIDS and TB policy in Washington, DC. *Social Science & Medicine, 48,* 1095–1102.

Fine, M. (1992). *Disruptive voices: The possibilities of feminist research.* Ann Arbor: University of Michigan Press.

Fine, M., & Weis, L. (1998). *The unknown city: The lives of poor and working-class young adults.* Boston: Beacon.

Freudenberg, N. (2001a). Case history of the Center for Urban Epidemiologic Studies in New York City. *Journal of Urban Health, 78,* 510–520.

Freudenberg, N. (2001b). Jails, prisons and the health of urban populations: A review of the impact of the correctional system on community health. *Journal of Urban Health, 78,* 214–235.

Galea, S., Factor, S., Bonner, S., Foley, M., Freudenberg, N., Latka, M., et al. (2001). Collaboration among community members, local health service providers, and researchers in an Urban Research Center in Harlem, New York City. *Public Health Reports, 116,* 530–539.

Gamson, W. A. (1999). Beyond the science-versus-advocacy distinction. *Contemporary Sociology, 28,* 23–26.

Greenwood, D. A., & Levin, M. (1998). *Introduction to action research: Social research for social change.* Thousand Oaks, CA: Sage.

Hammett, T. M., Harmon, M. P., & Rhodes, W. (2002). The burden of infectious disease among inmates and releasees from US correctional facilities, 1997. *American Journal of Public Health, 92,* 1789–1794.

Hammett, T. M., Roberts, C., & Kennedy, S. (2001). Health-related issues in prisoner reentry. *Crime and Delinquency, 47,* 390–409.

Hunter College Center on AIDS, Drugs, and Community Health. (2002). *Coming back to Harlem from jail or prison: One-way or round trip.* New York: Author.

Hunter College Center on AIDS, Drugs, and Community Health. (2003). *Coming home from jail: An action plan to improve NYC policies & programs.* New York: Author.

Israel, B. A., Schulz, A. J., Parker, E. A., Becker, A. B., Allen, A. A., & Guzman, J. R. (2003). Critical issues in developing and following community-based participatory research principles. In M. Minkler & N. Wallerstein (Eds.), *Community-based participatory research for health* (pp. 53–76). San Francisco: Jossey-Bass.

Kerle, K. E. (1998). *American jails: Looking to the future.* Boston: Butterworth-Heineman.

Klinenberg, E. (2002). *Heat wave: A social autopsy of disaster in Chicago.* Chicago: University of Chicago Press.

McCord, C., & Freeman, H. (1990). Excess mortality in Harlem. *New England Journal of Medicine, 322,* 173–178.

Mumola, C. J. (1999). *Substance abuse and treatment: State and federal prisoners, 1997*(Bureau of Justice Statistics Special Report). Retrieved June 29, 2003, from http://www.ojp.usdoj.gov/bjs/abstract/satsfp97.htm

National Commission on Correctional Health Care. (2002). *The health status of soon-to-be-released inmates: A report to Congress.* Chicago: Author.

Nelson, M., Deess, P., & Allen, C. (1999). *The first month out: Post-incarceration experiences in New York City.* New York: Vera Institute of Justice.

Nelson, M., & Trone, J. (2000, October). Why planning for release matters. In *Issues in Brief* (pp. 1–8). New York: Vera Institute of Justice.

Rand Corporation. (2001). *How the war on drugs influences the health and well-being of minority communities.* Santa Monica, CA: Author.

Ritas, C. (2003). *Speaking truth, creating power: A guide to policy work for community-based participatory research practitioners.* Community Campus Partnerships for Health. Retrieved March 22, 2003, from http://www.futurehealth.ucsf.edu/ccph/commbas.html#Tools

Themba, M. N. (1999). *Making policy, making change: How communities are taking law into their own hands.* San Francisco: Jossey-Bass.

Themba, M. N., & Minkler, M. (2003). Influencing policy though community-based participatory research. In M. Minkler & N. Wallerstein (Eds.), *Community-based participatory research for health* (pp. 349–370). San Francisco: Jossey-Bass.

Travis, J., Solomon, A. L., & Waul, M. (2001). *From prison to home: The dimensions and consequences of prisoner reentry.* Washington, DC: Urban Institute.

van Olphen, J., & Freudenberg, N. (2004). Harlem service providers' perceptions of the impact of municipal policies on their clients with substance use problems. *Journal of Urban Health, 81,* 222–231.

van Olphen, J., Freudenberg, N., Galea, S., Ritas, C., & Palermo, A. G. (2003). Advocating policies to promote community reintegration of drug users leaving jail: First steps in a policy change campaign guided by CBPR. In M. Minkler & N. Wallerstein (Eds.), *Community-based participatory research for health* (pp. 371–389). San Francisco: Jossey-Bass.

von Zielbauer, P. (2003, September 20). City creates post-jail plan for inmates. *New York Times,* p. B1.

von Zielbauer, P. (2004, January 16). Rikers houses low-level inmates at high expense. *New York Times,* p. B1.

Whyte, W. (1991). *Participatory action research.* Thousand Oaks, CA: Sage.

CHAPTER SEVENTEEN

Citizens, Science, and Data Judo

Leveraging Secondary Data Analysis to Build a Community-Academic Collaborative for Environmental Justice in Southern California

Rachel Morello-Frosch, Manuel Pastor Jr., James L. Sadd,
Carlos Porras, and Michele Prichard

Over the last decade California has become a hotbed of environmental justice activism. The fuel behind this political momentum has been effective community organizing and advocacy by a variety of organizations seeking fundamental changes in environmental health policy and regulation at the regional and state levels. In this context it has become clear that the recent focus of California policymakers on questions of environmental justice is politically rooted in the state's changing demographic realities. Legislators representing crucial swing-vote communities are attaining positions of political power that have enabled them to push forward new environmental health and justice initiatives. In 1999, the California legislature passed Senate Bill 115, a measure that directs the Governor's Office of Planning and Research to coordinate environmental justice initiatives across state agencies, including the California Environmental Protection Agency. In light of these political gains, state and local agencies have been seeking feedback from environmental justice groups on how to identify issues and solutions to environmental health problems.

Although regulatory agencies have developed systems to ensure that decision making includes some form of community participation (such as access to

Acknowledgments: The authors wish to thank The California Endowment, the California Wellness Foundation, and the Ford Foundation for their support of the work described in this chapter. We also thank the California Environmental Justice Movement for its inspiring work in promoting progressive social change both within the academic community and the policy arena.

information, public comment periods, and public meetings and hearings), these processes tend to be focused on procedural justice and have not necessarily ensured equitable outcomes in regulatory, zoning, and siting decisions. Ensuring that community participation in these policy and regulatory efforts is effective requires extensive preparatory work, including building capacity and addressing language and scientific literacy needs. Moreover, if governmental agencies are to truly enhance effective public participation in the regulatory arena, they need to recall two key lessons from years of environmental justice organizing. First, diverse communities have important insights and localized knowledge about ways in which environmental hazards may be affecting their health and well-being (Morello-Frosch et al., in press). Second, although scientific analysis is critical to informed decision making, this expertise should not be the sole driver of whether and how agencies respond to environmental health and justice problems (Loh & Sugarman-Brozan, 2002). Community organizations, which have traditionally had to muscle their way into the policy-making and regulatory process, should also be welcomed as a resource for broadening the range of voices and should be empowered to improve community environmental health in the most effective way possible. Community-based participatory research (CBPR) can be an effective means to address this issue, and there are multiple methods that community organizations and their academic partners have developed with the aim of enhancing community engagement in environmental justice issues in policymaking and regulation. The use of secondary data sources is one such method and will be the focus of this chapter.

In 1998, the Southern California Environmental Justice Collaborative (SCEJC) was formed to build a regional initiative to promote environmental health and social justice issues in Southern California. This six-year collaborative involves a community-academic partnership that combines research on regional economic development and environmental health, public policy advocacy, and community organizing. The partners in the collaborative are

- Communities for a Better Environment, a California-based environmental justice organization with strong organizing roots in the South Coast area

- A multidisciplinary academic research team

- Liberty Hill Foundation, a Los Angeles–based community foundation specializing in grant making, technical assistance, and capacity building for community-based organizations

The goals of the collaborative are twofold: to improve environmental health in low-income communities of color in Southern California by conducting community-based participatory research on air quality and environmental justice and to build the capacity of community-based environmental justice advocacy organizations through secondary grant making and training.

This chapter demonstrates how the Southern California Environmental Justice Collaborative has applied a CBPR approach in order to conduct research using secondary data sources. We begin by describing each partner involved and how these groups function as a partnership. We then focus on the role environmental health research plays in the collaborative, discussing the rationale for depending on secondary data analysis and the ways in which the partners collectively develop projects, interpret data, and disseminate study results. We also briefly describe how the collaborative has leveraged data to promote policy change and bolster organizing. We briefly explore how the collaborative's research model has sought to transform traditional scientific approaches to studying community environmental health. We conclude with a discussion of some of the challenges of this research method and the lessons learned from the collaborative's work.

THE PARTNERS IN THE SOUTHERN CALIFORNIA ENVIRONMENTAL JUSTICE COLLABORATIVE

Communities for a Better Environment (CBE), founded in 1978, was one of the first organizations in the country to focus primarily on the human costs of industrial pollution and to promote environmental health as an issue strongly connected to social and economic equity. Although the focus of this chapter is on CBE's work in Southern California, the organization has had, until a recent set of budget cutbacks, over twenty-five staff members in both Northern and Southern California, primarily organizers interspersed with attorneys and research staff. As an environmental justice organization with a strong community organizing base, CBE implements what it terms the *triangle strategy* in its work, integrating organizing, science-based advocacy, and legal intervention. The organization is keenly aware of the pitfalls of relying too heavily on litigation or science-based advocacy, yet it has prioritized developing organizational capacity in these areas to supplement its primary emphasis on community organizing. In short, CBE's triangle strategy is rooted in the theory that science-based advocacy and litigation, when applied under grassroots direction and leadership, can be successfully leveraged to promote effective policy change (Communities for a Better Environment, 2004b).

The Liberty Hill Foundation was founded in 1976 as a community foundation that promotes progressive social change in Los Angeles through grantmaking, technical assistance, and capacity-building activities and through promoting progressive philanthropy in the region. As a partner in the collaborative, Liberty Hill has played a critical role in building regional capacity to support environmental justice organizing through two mechanisms. First, Liberty

Hill provides seed funding to small neighborhood organizations working on environmental justice, to support their organizing and mobilization campaigns. Typically, these grants are the first outside funding received by these grassroots, resident-based groups. The money is often used to pay stipends and phone bills, print leaflets, and provide transportation to legislative and regulatory agencies to provide testimony. Funds have also been used to conduct scientific testing of air and water samples. Second, Liberty Hill sponsors and coordinates the Environmental Justice (EJ) Institute, which offers a series of trainings to grantees and other community members representing nearly sixty grassroots organizations. The trainings involve experts from a variety of disciplines (for example, law, public health, computer science, and environmental health science) and trainers in media advocacy, fundraising, and nonprofit management. Topics have included environmental laws, health risk assessments, community-based research, toxics and hazardous materials, public agency accountability, navigating the policy process, and organizational effectiveness. The key to high participation in the EJ Institute has been the provision of transportation, simultaneous translation services, child care, and meals that enable the mostly low-income community members to attend.

The research team encompasses a multidisciplinary group of collaborators from the University of California, Santa Cruz (Center for Justice, Tolerance and Community), Occidental College (Department of Environmental Studies/ Science), and Brown University (Center for Environmental Studies and Department of Community Health in the School of Medicine). The three researchers bring expertise from the fields of environmental health and epidemiology, economics and urban planning, and environmental science. All three came to the collaborative with experience in working with community partners, and many of their academic endeavors have focused on supporting community economic development and improving environmental policymaking and the regulatory process (Boer, Pastor, Sadd, & Snyder, 1997; Morello-Frosch, 2002; Pastor, Dreier, Lopez-Garza, & Grisby, 2000; Sadd, Pastor, Boer, & Snyder, 1999). All three have committed their academic careers to combining rigor, relevance, and reach—that is, to conducting high-quality research that has relevance for policy and that simultaneously sustains training, outreach, and publication efforts that engage diverse constituencies.

Communities for a Better Environment and Liberty Hill initiated the preliminary conversations with the researchers that culminated in the formation of the Southern California Environmental Justice Collaborative. Southern California has a very active environmental health and justice grassroots and nonprofit community working on a range of issues through advocacy, organizing, and education. Throughout the region, disproportionately high rates of a number of negative health impacts are increasingly being linked to poor air quality, toxic chemicals in consumer products, and the pollution generated from traffic, power plants, and other industrial sites that are a part of the urban environment (Kelly, 2003). Residents in heavily affected neighborhoods have organized to challenge such environmental health problems, yet critical aspects of the EJ advocacy network in Southern California needed to be strengthened in several areas. First, environmental justice issues in the Southern California region had not been addressed in a holistic way that promoted an effective regional voice for community environmental health and social justice. Second, there was a paucity of scientific research documenting the regional character of environmental inequality in Southern California. Therefore, a coordinated regional strategy conducted through a community-academic-foundation collaborative could help build regional capacity and leadership by emphasizing community organizing to create public awareness, voice, and political pressure; to conduct legal and policy work to promote change; and to perform scientific research on environmental health and demographics to help environmental justice groups more effectively engage in data judo with regulators and policymakers. *Data judo* is a process through which communities marshal their own scientific resources and expertise to conduct research and leverage the data necessary to support policy and regulatory change.

After a period of planning and some initial experience working together on small research projects, the collaborative partners (that is, the research team and representatives from CBE and the Liberty Hill Foundation) sought and successfully attained three years of funding support from The California Endowment. The total grant was $1.7 million dollars, with 27 percent of the money supporting the organizing work of CBE; 55 percent going toward training, secondary grant making, and organizational capacity building to support EJ organizing and advocacy work throughout the area; and the balance (18 percent) supporting the generation of air pollution and environmental hazard studies on the South Coast region. This grant was subsequently renewed at a lower level for an additional two years. The collaborative was also able to leverage funding from the California Wellness Foundation to support work on children's health and environmental justice.

DEVELOPING APPROACHES TO CBPR
ON ENVIRONMENTAL JUSTICE

The experience of CBPR is well documented (Arcury, Quandt, & McCauley, 2000; Israel, Schulz, Parker, & Becker, 1998; Minkler & Wallerstein, 2003; Shepard, 2000), and recently, CBPR approaches in the area of environmental justice have gained wider recognition and funding support, largely through the many projects funded by the National Institute of Environmental Health Sciences (Loh &

Sugarman-Brozan, 2002; O'Fallon & Dearry, 2002; Shepard, Northridge, Prakash, & Stover, 2002). Despite the inherent challenges in bridging the academic and activist worlds to collect and interpret scientific data, one key asset of a CBPR approach is that the involvement of communities who directly experience exposures and diseases of concern can promote new avenues of research and encourage innovation in analytical techniques. Further, collaboration allows substantive community involvement in several phases of the research process, including formulating research questions, collecting data, and disseminating results to diverse constituencies and the scientific community through peer-reviewed publications, organizing, community presentations, and the media.

The research goals of the collaborative have been twofold: to conduct relevant and rigorous research on air quality that supports advocacy and organizing and to provide the training necessary to help community-based organizations understand the scientific information that drives the regulatory process and policymaking. Although the collaborative's focus on Southern California is partly shaped by its organizing activities and partners, there are additional justifications for its regional emphasis. Southern California has a unique regulatory history in terms of its ongoing struggle to solve some of the worst air pollution problems in the country and yet still promote economic growth. With the majority of its population now comprising people of color, Southern California has also become a bellwether of demographic and socioeconomic change for both the state and the nation. Finally, a regional focus on environmental justice research is consistent with the fact that industrial clusters, as well as land-use planning decisions, are often regionally rooted (Pastor, Dreier, et al., 2000); thus the equity question is how the social and environmental health effects of urban development are distributed within regions and among the demographically diverse communities that host them (Morello-Frosch, Pastor, & Sadd, 2001).

The collaborative has a unique decision-making structure for prioritizing research projects and determining which to undertake. Essentially, any partner can bring a research idea to the table, but the community partner, CBE, is the final arbiter on questions of research project timing, design, and priorities. Once these decisions are made, the research partners gather data and conduct analysis independently. At times the final study results may not validate CBE's advocacy objectives. Nevertheless, the researchers ensure ample opportunities for discussion with community partner representatives as data analysis occurs in order to hear suggestions on new ways to approach complex analytical questions and to solicit feedback on how study results might be interpreted. This decision-making and feedback structure for the research was developed by the collaborative after substantial preliminary discussion between members of CBE, Liberty Hill, and the research team, held during planning meetings at the outset of the work. This structure was formalized in a written document in order to clarify how the collaborative should prioritize requests for conducting research from environmental justice organizations that worked with CBE but that were not directly involved in the collaborative itself. The need to formalize this structure grew out of an action-oriented research project requested by another EJ organization that was not directly involved in the collaborative to assess the environmental justice impacts of the expansion of the Los Angeles airport on the predominantly African American community of Inglewood. This project was resource intensive, and that led the collaborative partners to see the importance of balancing the collaborative's workload, ensuring that it would focus on its initial commitments to fundamental research on environmental justice issues with regional relevance and would avoid overextending its research resources by reactively responding to multiple requests to conduct specialized projects. Therefore the partners met to discuss, develop, and write a document that clearly spelled out the mechanism they would follow to prioritize and carry out research (see Appendix P). This communication and decision-making process derives from the partners' collective desire to ensure the scientific legitimacy of the research while also ensuring that the questions the collaborative pursues ultimately inform policy and organizing strategies on critical environmental justice issues in the South Coast region.

Structurally, the collaborative has set up several processes to promote ongoing communication, continual internal feedback among partners, and evaluation of its work. Partners meet in person at least three times per year for an entire day to carry out their work, discuss issues or challenges that arise in their projects, plan future endeavors, and assess whether and how they are achieving project goals and objectives. These meetings are supplemented with periodic conference calls as necessary. The collaborative also holds annual retreats to plan new work and to strategize on the most effective way to integrate the partners' research and organizing efforts with political opportunities to promote policy and regulatory change that supports environmental justice. Within this context the community partner plays a leading role in prioritizing and setting goals and objectives for the collaborative's organizing, research, and advocacy work.

The Liberty Hill Foundation has assumed the primary role in managing the administrative work of the collaborative, which includes tracking the budget and expenses, coordinating work on reports to funding agencies, and helping to facilitate strategic planning efforts to ensure that project goals and objectives are met. In addition to its grant-making, training, and capacity-building functions, Liberty Hill also supports the media advocacy efforts of the collaborative.

The collaborative also works with an external evaluator, hired at the outset of the work. She attends all collaborative meetings, helps structure ongoing project planning and community feedback mechanisms, and has been conducting an extensive evaluation of the impact the collaborative has had in the policy arena by interviewing policymakers, regulatory officials, funding agencies, and members of Southern California's environmental justice community. In addition to the evaluator's ongoing feedback at collaborative meetings, she provides a final written process and outcome evaluation to collaborative partners and to our funder. (See Chapter Twelve for an examination of the documentation and evaluation of a CBPR partnership using in-depth interviews and closed-ended questionnaires.)

Identification and Selection of Secondary Data

At the outset of this project, the collaborative partners decided to employ secondary data analysis as the core of their research activities. (See Chapter Sixteen for an examination of the use of secondary data analysis and other methods for analyzing the impact of policies on public health.) Although primary data collection is generally viewed as the gold standard in research, it has some major drawbacks. First, CBE was concerned about the fact that primary data collection requires substantial financial resources and organizational capacity to carry out effectively. Second, primary data collection conducted in collaboration with community-based organizations with a clear stake in study outcomes is vulnerable to misguided criticism from the mainstream scientific community or from skeptical policymakers who seek to marginalize CBPR research by arguing that the methods used suffer from systematic bias or lack objectivity (Anderton, 1996; Foreman, 1998). Given some of the high-stakes policy issues CBE was grappling with at the time, the organization and the researchers agreed that the collaborative should address some of the persistent methodological challenges in the field of environmental justice research by using secondary data, specifically, data already collected by environmental regulatory authorities such as the U.S. Environmental Protection Agency (EPA), the California Environmental Protection Agency (Cal/EPA), the California Air Resources Board, and others. In short, drawing from the experience of other mainstream environmental organizations, CBE and the researchers believed that analyzing the data gathered by the state's government and the national government would be a powerful way to draw regulatory attention to environmental justice issues.

Moreover, using secondary data sources allowed the collaborative to take advantage of major advances in air emissions inventories, such as the Toxic Release Inventory and the EPA's National Air Toxics Assessment and Cumulative Exposure Project, which estimates exposure information on outdoor air pollution on a national scale. Because of "right-to-know" laws that make this air pollution data publicly available, the research team was able to generate numerous studies that have built up the body of evidence on the significance of environmental inequality in Southern California. Secondary data analysis has allowed the collaborative both to economize and stretch its scarce resources for research and to strengthen the power and legitimacy of its arguments in the policy arena by demonstrating that its study results are based on data collected by federal and state agencies, which skeptics may view as more legitimate and scientifically objective.

Analysis of Secondary Data

Part of what the collaborative sought to do is document Southern California's environmental health *riskscape*—that is, demographic and geographical distributions of pollution burdens—in ways that are both analytically rigorous and empirically compelling to residents, researchers, and policymakers. The analytical methods used for this research involved computer-based mapping technology, multivariate statistical analysis, environmental health risk assessment, and spatial statistics. The research team developed myriad indicators for assessing potential environmental inequalities, including location of potentially hazardous industrial emission sources (Pastor, Sadd, & Morello-Frosch, 2002), location of treatment storage and disposal facilities (Pastor, Sadd, & Hipp, 2001; Sadd et al., 1999), and estimated health risks associated with outdoor air toxics exposures (Morello-Frosch, Pastor, Porras, & Sadd, 2002; Morello-Frosch, Pastor, & Sadd, 2001; Morello-Frosch, Pastor, & Sadd, 2002; Pastor, Sadd, & Morello-Frosch, 2002, 2004; Morello-Frosch & Jesdale, 2003). The team used traditional regulatory tools of risk assessment to answer scientific and policy questions about the significance of ambient pollutant concentrations for distributions of cancer and respiratory risks among diverse communities (Caldwell, 1998; California Air Pollution Control Officers' Association, 1993; California Environmental Protection Agency, 1997a, 1997b; "Guidelines for Carcinogenic Risk Assessment," 1986; U.S. Environmental Protection Agency, 1986; U.S. Environmental Protection Agency, Office of Research and Development, 1993). This allowed the collaborative to address the question of whether patterns of environmental inequality existed and which communities bear the largest burdens of potential health impacts.

The research team regularly shared and discussed study results with the other collaborative partners. Results were formally reported, and conceptual issues related to the research findings were regularly discussed at the in-person meetings and the conference calls involving the research team, CBE, and Liberty Hill. Researchers worked with CBE policy staff to solicit input on how interpretations of study results should be communicated to diverse audiences such as other community organizations, the media, policymakers, and key environmental regulatory officials. Manuscripts drafted by the researchers were circulated and shared among collaborative partners and PowerPoint presentations were developed by the researchers and posted on the collaborative Web site to ensure that all partners could access and use this information in their work. Often presentations were developed jointly by CBE and the researchers to target specific audiences. Although the researchers disseminated study results at professional academic conferences, both CBE and the researchers played primary roles in disseminating research results to other environmental justice organizations, the media, policymakers, and regulators.

Dissemination of Research Results to Enhance Community Participation in Environmental Policymaking and Regulation

Communication is critical to the Southern California Environmental Justice Collaborative; it needs to reach specific audiences and then help them make a visceral connection to the issues of environmental justice. Whether the collaborative is publishing study results or conducting "toxic tours" of communities affected by toxics, the interdisciplinary work of the research team, coupled with the advocacy experience of CBE and Liberty Hill, gives the collaborative flexibility in framing messages about community environmental health so they are appropriate for such diverse audiences as public health officials, regulators, urban planners, industry, the media, and policymakers.

In order to apply research results toward promoting policy change, the collaborative has developed various dissemination strategies. (See Chapter Thirteen for a discussion of the development of dissemination procedures in a CBPR partnership.) These include publication in the peer-reviewed scientific and policy literature, media outreach, and development of public outreach materials. All decisions regarding dissemination activities are made collectively by the researchers, CBE, and Liberty Hill. The researchers take the lead on activities related to peer-reviewed publications, and CBE and Liberty Hill take the lead in developing media strategies and community-based outreach. Since the beginning of the collaborative, all partners have agreed to give priority to publishing research in the peer-reviewed literature to ensure that results reach an academic audience as well as public health practitioners; this requires targeting publication toward journals in the fields of public health, sociology, urban planning, economics, political science, and public policy.

Media dissemination strategies have entailed interviews and the strategic publication of opinion page editorials in mainstream press outlets. Coverage of the collaborative's research and organizing work has appeared in the *Los Angeles Times, San Jose Mercury News, Sacramento Bee, Wall Street Journal, California Journal,* and smaller local media outlets. This brought statewide attention to the collaborative's research and its implications for organizing and advocacy. CBE plays a central role in shaping media strategies related to dissemination of research results, often working to ensure that press coverage and op-ed pieces are timed to coincide with campaigns to push policy change at either the local or statewide level. For example, media outreach and the placement of an op-ed piece in the *Los Angeles Times* discussing study results showing the disparate impact of ambient air toxics exposures on residents of color were timed to coincide with major activities in CBE's ultimately successful campaign to strengthen local air quality district rules governing facility emissions of carcinogenic compounds (Morello-Frosch, Pastor, & Sadd, 2001; Pastor, Porras, & Morello-Frosch, 2000). Led by CBE, the collaborative partners developed and implemented a similar media strategy to coincide with public hearings sponsored by Cal/EPA regarding its proposed adoption of an environmental justice guidance document for the agency's programs and offices (California Environmental Protection Agency, Advisory Committee on Environmental Justice, 2003).

Collaborative partners collectively decide authorship for both mainstream press and academic publications. Generally, the community partner, CBE, has opted to coauthor the mainstream press articles (Morello-Frosch, Pastor, & Porras, 2001; Pastor, Porras, & Morello-Frosch, 2000) rather than the research publications, although CBE's executive director did coauthor one academic publication on environmental health that appeared in an *Environmental Health Perspectives* supplement on CBPR (Morello-Frosch, Pastor, Porras, & Sadd, 2002).

Collaborative partners have also developed other materials for dissemination, such as PowerPoint presentations, that can be tailored to diverse audiences. The researchers generally take the lead in crafting these presentation materials and regularly solicit feedback from community partners on content and format. Both community partners and researchers use these materials to conduct presentations, and decisions about which partner is strategically best suited to present particular collaborative work are reached collectively. Presentation materials are circulated electronically and posted on a password-protected Web site so they can be viewed, edited, downloaded, and shared among the collaborative partners. Community partners and researchers have also discussed the possible development of *foto novelas* in English and Spanish. These materials would graphically display key study results in a way that lay groups could understand so they could use this information in their own advocacy efforts; CBE has done this with some of its own work, but the collaborative has not yet produced such a publication. The partners also developed a publication, largely addressed to funders, that discusses the collaborative's CBPR and advocacy strategy and what the partners have learned from their efforts (Communities for a Better Environment, 2004a). The aim of this publication is to disseminate a model of working together that extends beyond the field of environmental justice research; the publication also includes brief descriptions of the substantive study results.

Through the Environmental Justice Institute, administered by Liberty Hill, the researchers have also presented the results of the research conducted under the auspices of the collaborative to the broader environmental justice community in a workshop that highlighted environmental justice concerns in the South Coast region. Moreover, the EJ Institute has provided CBE with an excellent venue for disseminating data collection techniques. In community trainings on establishing "bucket brigades," community organizations are taught to build simple, low-cost air sampling devices using plastic buckets. An ultimate data judo tool, this technology has been used to draw regulatory attention to air pollution problems in neighborhoods where fugitive emissions from nearby industries have not been adequately addressed or monitored (Communities for a Better Environment, 2000; Pastor & Rosner, 2002).

Leveraging Research to Promote Policy Change

The Southern California Environmental Justice Collaborative's strategy of linking research, organizing, and advocacy to promote regulatory reforms and policy change has contributed to some impressive victories at the regional and state levels. For example, the collaborative's study results on the demographic distribution of air toxics and cancer risks in Southern California were leveraged by CBE and other environmental justice groups to compel the regional air quality authority in Southern California to adopt more stringent standards to significantly reduce cancer risks associated with air emissions from industrial facilities (Cone, 2000; Morello-Frosch, Pastor, & Sadd, 2001; Pastor, Porras, & Morello-Frosch, 2000). Each collaborative partner played a central role in this policy victory. The researchers conducted data analysis demonstrating the disparate impact of carcinogenic air toxics on communities of color in the region, and Liberty Hill provided the financial and administrative support to back CBE's successful organizing campaign to tighten the standard. Each partner implemented one piece of an effective, collective media strategy: Liberty Hill leveraged its press contacts to ensure that the public hearings and community testimony were well covered by the media, CBE members conducted interviews with several reporters from mainstream and Latino press outlets, and the researchers worked closely with CBE to craft and place an op-ed piece in the *Los Angeles Times* that provided environmental health arguments supporting the proposed emission rule change.

Perhaps most significant has been the way in which the collaborative has effectively supported CBE's coalition work with other environmental justice organizations statewide that occurs through CBE's participation on the Cal/EPA Environmental Justice Advisory Committee. The state legislature has passed laws requiring Cal/EPA to coordinate environmental justice initiatives with federal efforts and across state agencies. The culmination of one such legislative effort has been the development of a procedural framework for implementing environmental justice programs in the state. The vehicle for this process is the Interagency Working Group on Environmental Justice, composed of the heads of Cal/EPA's boards, departments, and offices that are charged with implementing strategies to address environmental justice in their respective programs. The EJ Advisory Committee, comprising key community, business, and regional government stakeholders, was charged with developing recommendations to the Interagency Working Group on the ways environmental justice could be addressed in various programs. CBE played a critical role as an advisory committee member when it used the collaborative's data and study results to make the case to industry and government stakeholders that more stringent guidelines were needed to address environmental health disparities in the state. This resulted in the committee's consensus decision to make recommendations to Cal/EPA that emphasized

1. Developing resources and programs that promote and enhance meaningful public participation in regulatory decision making that affects environmental health, particularly among communities of color who may face particular challenges to participation, such as language barriers

2. Devising new regulatory and scientific approaches to assess the cumulative health impacts of pollution from multiple emission sources on neighborhoods and vulnerable populations like children

3. Integrating the precautionary principle in environmental regulation and enforcement activities in a more systematic way (California Environmental Protection Agency, Advisory Committee on Environmental Justice, 2003)

The last two recommendations are the most controversial. The precautionary principle means that regulators should be more proactive when scientific evidence strongly suggests, but does not yet fully prove, that a production facility or pollutant may be jeopardizing public health, particularly among communities that are already overburdened by toxics and other health challenges. Similarly, the issue of cumulative impact compels regulators to acknowledge that chemical-by-chemical approaches to regulation may not be protective of public health due to the reality that communities are exposed to numerous pollutants in the air they breathe, the water they drink, and the food they eat, and that it is important to assess exposures and health risks holistically when setting standards to protect vulnerable populations such as children. Integrating the precautionary principle with environmental justice concerns opens the way for disparately affected communities to effectively resist siting decisions that may add to existing neighborhood pollution burdens. Industry stakeholders have argued that the precautionary principle is too cumbersome and will impose undue costs on those who can least afford them because it will result in "overregulation" that decreases economic efficiency and threatens jobs.

As members of the EJ Advisory Committee, industry representatives wrongly assumed that environmental justice stakeholders would not have the data to back up their arguments in favor of adding the precautionary principle to the recommendations proposed to Cal/EPA. Therefore, at CBE's urging, one of the collaborative researchers gave compelling testimony on an environmental health analysis that showed why the precautionary principle should be better integrated into policymaking and regulation. CBE ensured that every committee member received a copy of a peer-reviewed article on the collaborative's study, which gave added validity to the data that were presented at the hearings (Morello-Frosch, Pastor, & Sadd, 2002). This testimony, combined with a massive mobilization of environmental justice organizations throughout the state, compelled a consensus recommendation in favor of the precautionary principle. The significance of this policy victory exemplifies the effectiveness of the collaborative's strategy for social change. Collectively, the partners supported CBE's advocacy efforts by leveraging study results through public testimony, engaging in data judo with industry consultants, and mobilizing local environmental justice communities to participate in public hearings. This integrated strategy ensured that the advisory committee's final recommendations to Cal/EPA addressed the environmental justice concerns of diverse constituencies in the state.

Other successes achieved by the collaborative in the South Coast region include leveraging the collaborative's research linking respiratory risks from ambient air toxics to diminished academic performance in schools. These study results were used to persuade the Los Angeles Unified School District to take a more precautionary approach toward identifying and mediating sites for school construction, and were also employed to validate arguments favoring more equitable distribution of state monies for school construction between suburban and urban school districts (Morello-Frosch, Pastor, & Sadd, 2002). Similarly, research demonstrating the disparate environmental health impact of a planned expansion of the Los Angeles Airport on the predominantly African American community of Inglewood helped persuade the airport authority to take equity issues into account in its environmental impact statement (Pastor & Sadd, 2000).

TRANSFORMING TRADITIONAL APPROACHES TO RESEARCHING COMMUNITY ENVIRONMENTAL HEALTH

The strategy adopted by the Southern California Environmental Justice Collaborative for conducting research and interpreting and disseminating study results has sought to transform traditional approaches to research on community environmental health. In emphasizing secondary data analysis, the collaborative has promoted new approaches to community-based participatory research on environmental justice in three primary ways:

1. *Moving upstream.* An analogy often used to illustrate the role preventive health should play concerns villagers who notice helpless people floating downstream and develop increasingly sophisticated ways to rescue them, yet none of the villagers thinks to venture upstream to find out why people are falling into the river in the first place (Steingraber, 1997). Causally linking pollution

with potentially adverse health effects is a tough challenge in the field of environmental health, particularly when populations are chronically exposed to complex chemical mixtures (Institute of Medicine, 1999). Improving epidemiologic methods is one route to addressing this issue. Nevertheless, environmental justice organizations, including CBE, have argued that in the never-ending quest for better data and unequivocal proof of cause and effect, researchers can lose sight of a basic public health principle—namely the importance of disease prevention (Morello-Frosch, Pastor, & Sadd, 2002). Mindful of this principle, the collaborative has supported dual approaches to environmental health research. The first approach seeks to improve epidemiologic methods, such as exposure assessment, to better understand the relationship between pollution exposures and environmentally mediated disease. (See Chapter Eleven for a discussion of the use of exposure assessment in a CBPR project.) The second approach uses environmental risk assessment and secondary data analysis when there is a paucity of human epidemiological data to show cause and effect between pollution exposures and disease. These dual approaches emphasize employing an "upstream" strategy in environmental health research, and thus avoiding the regulatory paralysis that can occur when definitive human data are lacking, and they also provide crucial tools to keep policymaking and regulation moving forward.

2. *Promoting an ecosocial outlook.* By connecting social inequality with environmental degradation and community health, the collaborative's environmental justice research becomes a framework for understanding the impact of discrimination on the environmental health of diverse communities. This framework also raises the challenge of determining whether disparities in exposures to environmental hazards play an important role in health disparities (U.S. Department of Health and Human Services, 2000; Institute of Medicine, 1999). The collaborative's research focus is broad and looks beyond individual or lifestyle factors, such as smoking and diet, and toward the environmental and socioeconomic factors that shape distributions of people and pollution. It is for this reason that the research team draws extensively from the field of social epidemiology to inform its research on environmental health and social justice (Krieger, 2001). This framework enables the team to examine issues such as segregation, inequality, and community empowerment as possible drivers of environmental inequality (Morello-Frosch, 2002; Morello-Frosch & Jesdale, 2003; Morello-Frosch, Pastor, Porras, & Sadd, 2002).

3. *Ensuring active community involvement.* Communities for a Better Environment is the final arbiter when the collaborative prioritizes research projects, looking at project needs for advocacy work and organizing. This ensures that the type of research the collaborative pursues is relevant to the communities and region it is studying. Nevertheless, implementing CBPR strategies to address environmental health issues facing communities of color invites open skepticism

from critics seeking to challenge the premise of environmental justice and the role of communities in the research process (Foreman, 1998). As a result, the research team and CBE have been vigilant about methodological and statistical strategies in their approach to secondary data analysis and interpretation of results; indeed, the collaborative's research faces scrutiny from diverse reviewers, including academic peers, policymakers, and regulators, and ultimately it must pass the test of community wisdom. Despite the challenges, this approach to connecting community and academic partners through action-oriented research enhances the rigor, methodological integrity, and most important, the relevance of the collaborative's work for environmental policymaking.

CHALLENGES AND LIMITATIONS

The collaborative has had to address certain challenges inherent in using secondary data analysis in the context of a CBPR approach to support organizing and policy advocacy. In contrast to other methods used in CBPR efforts, which engage community partners directly in developing study designs and collecting data, a focus on secondary data analysis, by its very nature, limits the depth of community engagement in the research process. Indeed, limitations on the availability of certain secondary data sources can narrow the scope of research questions that a community partner may be able to pursue. Overcoming this limitation requires the collaborative to build in sufficient time for community partners to review and give feedback on data analysis as it evolves and ultimately to actively engage in framing the interpretation of study results. For example, CBE has been interested in examining environmental justice questions related to asthma severity and incidence in the South Coast region, but comprehensive, individual-level data on the communities of interest have not been readily available. However, by working closely with CBE, the research team was able to address that organization's research question indirectly by conducting an ecological study using noncancer risk assessment to estimate respiratory hazards associated with ambient air toxics exposures among Los Angeles school children (Morello-Frosch, Pastor, Porras, & Sadd, 2002; Pastor, Sadd, & Morello-Frosch, 2002, 2004).

Other challenges to the collaborative's CBPR approach include managing the research needs and expectations of other environmental justice organizations that engage with the collaborative through the Environmental Justice Institute trainings. Owing to the proliferation of neighborhood organizations that are addressing local environmental health concerns, the demand for new, localized research projects is increasing, and meeting this need could easily drain the resources of the research team and of the collaborative as a whole. In any situation of scarce resources, the challenge for the collaborative has been to effectively prioritize the partners' deployment of time and money. After much discussion, the partners collectively decided that a CBPR research strategy based on secondary data analysis would be an effective and efficient approach, one that could promote policy change in a way that would not overwhelm the capacities of the academic partners or unduly burden CBE's organizational resources. Moreover, the collaborative developed a decision-making structure in which its community partner, CBE, has had the ultimate say on prioritizing research projects and shaping strategies for the dissemination of study results. Although this structure compels the academic partners to relinquish some degree of control related to setting the research agenda, it does not require them to compromise the scientific integrity of their analysis.

Therefore, although a small portion of the research undertaken by the collaborative has been specifically related to narrow campaigns, all three collaborative partners agreed at the inception of their work that research would focus mainly on establishing a regional picture of environmental inequity. Prioritizing secondary data analysis on regional and statewide environmental justice questions has provided a body of evidence to support specific actions such as tightening air quality rules, promoting the adoption of cumulative exposure strategies by the state, and pushing for cleaner, safer schools.

LESSONS LEARNED AND IMPLICATIONS FOR PRACTICE

The experience of the Southern California Environmental Justice Collaborative offers some lessons that transcend CBPR approaches to promoting policy change and inform the very nature of productive alliances between funders, community-based organizations, and the academy. The first lesson is to build the base to move policy. Often when community-based organizations engage with academic partners in scientific research and succeed in gaining entry as valid stakeholders in the policy arena, there is the danger that they may abandon the work of organizing. Yet the primary reason community groups are invited to the policy table is the political pressure that is rooted in an organized community base. In their strategic planning, the collaborative partners believed that a CBPR approach emphasizing secondary data analysis rather than primary data collection would allow CBE as the community partner to engage effectively in research without pulling organizational and staff resources away from its core organizing functions. The role of Liberty Hill has also ensured that the collaborative remains vigilant about meeting the need to nurture new community voices, organizing the Environmental Justice Institute, finding seed funding for nascent environmental justice organizations, and providing resources to mobilize communities to participate in public action and debate.

The second lesson is to build organic relationships between partners. This collaborative was not convened in response to a request for proposals. The partners had already formed deep relationships through their prior environmental justice work in the South Coast region. This experience is not something that can be easily replicated, but it does suggest the importance of forming academic-community collaboratives proactively and scaling up those partnerships that are authentic and sustainable. The success of the collaborative's model and the strength of the partner relationships have sustained the collaborative's work, both when funding was abundant and when funding temporarily ran dry. The ability of the collaborative to sustain its research, organizing, and advocacy over the last six years is firmly rooted in the partners' collective commitment to the goals of their work and their unique CBPR method of leveraging secondary data analysis to promote policy change. Using secondary data analysis as the core of a CBPR research strategy enabled the academic partners to keep the research portion of the collaborative active during a temporary lull in the funding stream.

The third lesson flows from the second: make long-term investment in change. There is a tendency among many foundations to think in terms of short-term progress, particularly given the pressures to show accountability, demonstrate measurable outcomes, and make a smooth transition to long-term sustainability. These expectations can have the unintended effect of promoting opportunistic partnerships that have difficulty completing projects or ones that focus primarily on grantsmanship. The Southern California Environmental Justice Collaborative has had the benefit of multiyear investments made by several foundations, especially The California Endowment, the Ford Foundation, and the California Wellness Foundation. This has allowed the partners to think beyond short-term campaigns and work to build a regional framework for social change. Ultimately, building community capacity to promote changes in environmental policy and regulation requires a regional approach. Indeed, shutting down a chromium plating facility operating near an elementary school requires a well-organized neighborhood or parent-teacher organization, but advocating for tighter rules on facility siting and emissions to protect *all* schoolchildren regionwide requires empowering organizations across neighborhoods, racial divides, and economic strata as well as ensuring that they have the technical and organizational capacity to effectively engage in the planning and rule-making process. Achieving this goal requires building in flexibility that allows partners to respond nimbly to opportunities and challenges, shifting directions and resources as necessary.

More important, however, is the partners' desire to support the replication of their collaborative model, with its pillars of research, organizing, advocacy, and community capacity building, to other regions. This long-term goal of replication and ensuring its sustainability requires resources. Although start-up monies have been critical for supporting single-issue campaigns and coalitions, developing a framework to achieve sustainable social and political change for environmental justice requires a significant long-term investment. Some large foundations and governmental agencies like the National Institute of Environmental Health Sciences have taken on this long-term challenge by investing in academic-community collaboratives that promote research that is inclusive and participatory (O'Fallon & Dearry, 2002). Yet much of this work is still conducted on the margins, as few governmental agencies and foundations invest significant resources to support long-term work that *integrates* research and advocacy.

CONCLUSION

The achievements of Southern California Environmental Justice Collaborative show that it is time to mainstream the marginal: academic-community collaboratives that emphasize secondary data analysis in their CBPR approach to promoting environmental justice can be powerful agents for policy change without compromising the standards of rigorous scientific research. These partnerships promote not only good science but science that is focused on important problems that affect the lives of real people, and they do so while enhancing community capacity and participation in research and advocacy—all of which can ultimately improve the regulatory and policymaking process. In light of these results, governmental agencies and foundations need to proactively support such work. Increased long-term investment in this work would also encourage more academic researchers to engage with community organizations in pursuit of scientific research that addresses the real-world environmental health challenges faced by communities of color and the poor. Ultimately, promoting the development of new community-academic collaboratives in other regions nationwide will be critical to broadening constituencies and deepening public understanding of the connections between social justice, racial equality, public health, and environmental sustainability.

References

Anderton, D. L. (1996). Methodological issues in the spatiotemporal analysis of environmental equity. *Social Science Quarterly, 77,* 508–515.

Arcury, T., Quandt, S., & McCauley, L. (2000). Farmers and pesticides: Community-based research. *Environmental Health Perspectives, 108,* 787–792.

Boer, T. J., Pastor, M., Sadd, J. L., & Snyder, L. D. (1997). Is there environmental racism? The demographics of hazardous waste in Los Angeles County. *Social Science Quarterly, 78*(4), 793–810.

Caldwell, J. C. (1998). *Interim methodology to give estimates of potency for Cumulative Exposure Project POM inventories.* Washington, DC: U.S. Environmental Protection Agency.

California Air Pollution Control Officers' Association. (1993). *Air toxics "Hot Spots" program: Risk assessment guidelines.* Sacramento, CA: Author.

California Environmental Protection Agency. (1997a). *Technical support document for the determination of noncancer chronic reference exposure levels.* Berkeley, CA: Author.

California Environmental Protection Agency, Air Resources Board. (1997b). *Toxic air contaminant identification list summaries.* Berkeley, CA: Author.

California Environmental Protection Agency, Advisory Committee on Environmental Justice. (2003). *Recommendations of the California Environmental Protection Agency (Cal/EPA) Advisory Committee on Environmental Justice to the Cal/EPA Interagency Working Group on Environmental Justice.* Retrieved May 12, 2004, from http://www.calepa.ca.gov/EnvJustice/Documents/2003/FinalReport.pdf

Communities for a Better Environment. (2000). *The bucket brigade manual.* Retrieved September 2004, from http://www.cbecal.org/publications/index.shtml

Communities for a Better Environment. (2004a). *Building a regional voice for environmental justice.* Retrieved March 30, 2005, from http://www.cbecal.org/publications/newpublication.pdf

Communities for a Better Environment. (2004b). *Environmental health and justice for California's urban communities.* Retrieved May 12, 2004, from http://www.cbecal.org

Cone, M. (2000, March 18). AQMD tightens cancer rule. *Los Angeles Times,* p. 9.

Foreman, C. (1998). *The promise and peril of environmental justice.* Washington, DC: Brookings Institution.

Guidelines for carcinogenic risk assessment, 51 Fed. Reg. 185, 33992–34003 (1986).

Institute of Medicine, Committee on Environmental Justice. (1999). *Toward environmental justice: Research, education, and health policy needs.* Washington, DC: Author.

Israel, B., Schulz, A., Parker, E., & Becker, A. (1998). Review of community-based research: Assessing partnership approaches to improve public health. *Annual Review of Public Health, 19,* 173–202.

Kelly, W. (2003, May). Environmental justice rising. *California Journal,* pp. 6–7.

Krieger, N. (2001). Theories for social epidemiology in the 21st century: An ecosocial perspective. *International Journal of Epidemiology, 30,* 668–677.

Loh, P., & Sugarman-Brozan, J. (2002). Environmental justice organizing for environmental health: Case study on asthma and diesel exhaust in Roxbury, Massachusetts. *Annals of the American Academy of Political and Social Science, 584,* 110–124.

Minkler, M., & Wallerstein, N. (Eds.). (2003). *Community-based participatory research for health.* San Francisco: Jossey-Bass.

Morello-Frosch, R. (2002). The political economy of environmental discrimination. *Environment and Planning C, 20,* 477–496.

Morello-Frosch, R., & Jesdale, B. (2003). *Racial segregation, ambient air toxics exposures, and estimated cancer risks.* Paper presented at a meeting of the American Public Health Association, San Francisco.

Morello-Frosch, R., Pastor, M., & Porras, C. (2001, June 3). Who's minding the air at your child's school? *Los Angeles Times,* p. M3.

Morello-Frosch, R., Pastor, M., Porras, C., & Sadd, J. (2002). Environmental justice and regional inequality in Southern California: Implications for future research. *Environmental Health Perspectives, 110*(Suppl. 2), 149–154.

Morello-Frosch, R., Pastor, M., & Sadd, J. (2001). Environmental justice and southern California's "riskscape": The distribution of air toxics exposures and health risks among diverse communities. *Urban Affairs Review, 36*(4), 551–578.

Morello-Frosch, R., Pastor, M., & Sadd, J. (2002). Integrating environmental justice and the precautionary principle in research and policy-making: The case of ambient air toxics exposures and health risks among school children in Los Angeles. *Annals of the American Academy of Political and Social Science, 584,* 47–68.

Morello-Frosch, R., Zavestoski, S., Brown, P., McCormick, S., Mayer, B., & Gasior, R. (in press). Social movements in health: Responses to and shapers of a changed medical world. In K. Moore and S. Frickel (Eds.), *The new political sociology of science: Institutions, networks, and power.* Madison: University of Wisconsin Press.

O'Fallon, L., & Dearry, A. (2002). Community-based participatory research as a tool to advance environmental health sciences. *Environmental Health Perspectives, 110*(Suppl. 2), 155–159.

Pastor, M., Dreier, P., Lopez-Garza, M., & Grisby, E. (2000). *Regions that work: How cities and suburbs can grow together.* Minneapolis: University of Minnesota Press.

Pastor, M., Porras, C., & Morello-Frosch, R. (2000, March 16). The region's minorities face major health risks from pollution: Justice demands that the AQMD cut emissions. *Los Angeles Times,* p. 9.

Pastor, M., & Rosner, R. (2002). Communities armed with bucket take charge of air quality. In *Sustainable solutions: Building assets for empowerment and sustainable development,* pp. 15–21. New York: Ford Foundation.

Pastor, M., & Sadd, J. (2000). *Environmental justice and the expansion of the Los Angeles International Airport.* Los Angeles: Communities for a Better Environment.

Pastor, M., Sadd, J., & Hipp, J. (2001). Which came first? Toxic facilities, minority move-in, and environmental justice. *Journal of Urban Affairs, 23*(1), 1–21.

Pastor, M., Sadd, J., & Morello-Frosch, R. (2002). Who's minding the kids? Pollution, public schools, and environmental justice in Los Angeles. *Social Science Quarterly, 83*(1), 263–280.

Pastor, M., Sadd, J., & Morello-Frosch, R. (2004). Reading, writing and toxics: Children's health, academic performance, and environmental justice in Los Angeles. *Environment and Planning C, 2,* 271–290.

Sadd, J., Pastor, M., Boer, T., & Snyder, L. (1999). "Every breath you take . . .": The demographics of toxic air releases in Southern California. *Economic Development Quarterly, 13*(2), 107–123.

Shepard, P. (2000). Achieving environmental justice objectives and reducing health disparities through community-based participatory research and interventions. In *Successful models of community-based participatory research,* pp. 8–28. Research Triangle Park, NC: National Institute of Environmental Health Sciences.

Shepard, P., Northridge, M., Prakash, S., & Stover, B. (2002). Preface: Advancing environmental justice through community-based participatory research. *Environmental Health Perspectives, 110*(Suppl. 2), 139–140.

Steingraber, S. (1997). *Living downstream: An ecologist looks at cancer and the environment.* Reading, MA: Perseus Books.

U.S. Department of Health and Human Services. (2000). *Healthy people 2010: Understanding and improving health.* Washington, DC: Author.

U.S. Environmental Protection Agency. (1986). *Guidelines for the health risk assessment of chemical mixtures.* Washington, DC: Author.

U.S. Environmental Protection Agency, Office of Research and Development. (1993). *Provisional guidance for quantitative risk assessment of polycyclic aromatic hydrocarbons.* Washington, DC: Author.

APPENDIXES

Instructions for Conducting a Force Field Analysis

Adam B. Becker, Barbara A. Israel, and Alex J. Allen III

Force field analysis is a group process activity that enables a group to identify and document the forces for and against reaching a specific desired state of affairs or achieving a specific goal. This process is not one in which solutions per se are identified but one in which the facilitating factors for achieving a goal or objective and the barriers to doing so are enumerated as part of a process of identifying and prioritizing potential action steps. Facilitating a thorough force field analysis can take one to two hours to complete and can be carried out over more than one group meeting.

Procedure

1. Introduce the basic process (described in steps 3 to 6). If possible, practice on a sample proposed change or goal. State both the proposed change and the issue or problem situation to which it relates.

2. Draw this diagram on newsprint, chalkboard, or whiteboard:

Issue or problem: _____
_____

Proposed change (ideal state or goal): _____
_____
_____

Forces for ————————————▶ | ◀———————— Forces against
(the proposed change, ideal | (the proposed change, ideal
state, or goal) | state, or goal)

(List of forces) | (List of forces)

For discussion of the use of this force field analysis activity, see Chapters Three and Four.

3. Following a discussion within the group, write the issue or problem statement identified by the group, in clear and precise language, next to the "Issue or problem" heading in the diagram. Write the group's proposed change or the ideal state or goal (that is, how things would be if the problem did not exist) next to the "Proposed change" heading. Explain the diagram, stating that "forces for" are those that would facilitate the proposed change and "forces against" are those that would be barriers to the proposed change. (Such forces might relate to, for example, individuals, organizations, policies, or community history and context, and they need to be forces that actually exist already in the community.) Ask the group to list the forces that go in these two columns. Discussion of the lists should be withheld until all anticipated forces for and against are listed. The facilitator should write down all the forces identified verbatim in the appropriate columns.

4. Ask the group to identify which "forces for" can be strengthened or harnessed and which "forces against" can be decreased. Circle those forces that seem to be the most important for achieving the ideal state or goal and mark with an "X" those that the group thinks need to be researched and discussed in more depth.

5. As needed, identify group members who will research each force marked with an "X," and ask them to bring their findings back to the next group meeting to share with the group.

6. For each important "force for" ask the group to list as many responses or action steps as possible that would increase its effect. For each important "force against" ask the group to list possible responses or action steps that might reduce its effect or eliminate it completely. The group should then select the most appropriate action steps and make plans for implementing them.

References

Johnson, D. W., & Johnson, F. P. (2003). *Joining together: Group theory and group skills* (8th ed.). Boston: Allyn & Bacon.

Lewin, K. (1944). Dynamics of group action. *Educational Leadership, 1,* 195–200.

Community Member Key Informant Interview Guide

Eugenia Eng, Karen Strazza Moore, Scott D. Rhodes, Derek M. Griffith, Leo L. Allison, Kate Shirah, and Elvira M. Mebane

Introduction: Hello, my name is _____ I'm going to be leading our interview today. This is _____, who will be taking notes and helping me during our discussion. We will be here about sixty minutes to talk to you about living in your community and your opinions concerning the strengths of your community and the challenges it faces. Your insights and opinions on these subjects are important, so please say what's on your mind and what you think. There is no right or wrong answer.

General Information about the Community

1. Please describe your role in the community. (Probe: How long have you lived here?)

2. Describe the community.

3. What do people in the community do for a living? (What is their source of income?)

4. How do people from the community get around?

5. What do people do for fun?

6. How are people involved in politics (for example, voting, talking with community leaders, elections)?

7. How do people of different races (ethnicities or backgrounds) interact within the community?

8. How involved are churches in the lives of people in the community (for example, do people attend church, do they participate in church groups)?

See Chapter Four for a discussion of the development and implementation of this key informant interview guide within a CBPR project.

Assets and Needs of the Community

9. What are some of the best things about the community (for example, resources, agencies, social gatherings or support, physical environment)?

10. What do you think are the major issues or needs community members face (for example, in the areas of children, income, the elderly, safety, housing, disability, health, sanitation, pests)?

11. Which needs do you feel are the most important for the community to address?

12. What do you wish could happen for the community in the next five to ten years?

Problem Solving and Decision Making

13. What kinds of community projects have been started during your time here? How would you explain their success or lack of it?

14. If you were going to try to solve a community problem, who would you try to involve to make it a success?

Services and Businesses

15. What services and programs do community members use? (Do those services come here, or do residents go to them?)

16. What services and programs do community members need?

17. Where do people go to buy things like food, clothing, medicine, and household items?

Recommended Individuals to Interview

18. Is there anyone else whom we should speak with about the community (for example, service providers, residents)? Are you willing to get permission for us to contact them?

    • Describe the specific person or organization.

    • Why do you think their opinions and views would be helpful for us to hear?

Recommendations for Community Forum

19. We plan to conduct a forum this spring to share the information we have gathered with the community. Would you be interested in helping us plan this event?

20. Do you have any ideas regarding how to get people to attend (for example, time, place, publicity)?

21. Who else do you think should help us coordinate this forum?

Additional Information

22. Is there anything else you would like to share about the community?

Thank you again for your participation

Selected New and Revised Items Included in the HEP Survey After Input from the Steering Committee or Survey Subcommittee (SC), Focus Group Themes (FG), or Pilot Testing (PT) of Existing Items

Amy J. Schulz, Shannon N. Zenk, Srimathi Kannan, Barbara A. Israel, Mary A. Koch, and Carmen A. Stokes

Category	*New or revised items (revisions in italics)*
Municipal services [ranked from 1 = poor to 4 = excellent]	[SC, FG] How would you rate the quality of • Street maintenance in your neighborhood, for example, filling potholes or replacing burned-out street lights • Snow removal • Fire department • Trash removal
Recreational resources [ranked from 1 = very safe to 4 = not safe at all]	[SC, FG; Added to existing questions about the presence and quality of parks, playgrounds, and recreational facilities:] • Overall, how would you rate the safety of those [parks, playgrounds, and recreational facilities]?
Sense of community [ranked from 1 = strongly disagree to 5 = strongly agree]	• [FG] I would move out of this neighborhood if I could

See Chapter Five for a discussion of the development and administration of this survey questionnaire using a CBPR approach. See Appendix D for a fuller list of survey categories and more detailed sources, including literature.

Category	*New or revised items (revisions in italics)*
Discrimination	[FG; Added as reasons for unfair treatment, to options initially developed by Williams et al. (1997):] • *your English language skills* • *because you live in Detroit* • *because you were not born in the US*
Police stress [ranked from 1 = never to 5 = always]	• [PT] When police respond [to calls from residents] they don't do anything about the problem • [PT] Police are disrespectful to people in the neighborhood
Immigration stress [ranked from 1 = disagree strongly to 5 = agree strongly]	• [FG] I miss family and friends in (place of birth) • [FG] I worry about family and friends in (place of birth) • [FG] It is difficult for me to be in contact with family or friends in (place of birth) • [FG] I am able to contact (by phone, letters, email, fax) family and friends in (place of birth) • [FG] I worry about being questioned about my legal status or citizenship

Selected HEP Measures by Survey Categories, with Sources and Scale Items

Amy J. Schulz, Shannon N. Zenk, Srimathi Kannan,
Barbara A. Israel, Mary A. Koch, and Carmen A. Stokes

Measure	*Identified by*	*Source*
Neighborhood context		
Municipal services	Steering committee, focus groups	Developed for this study.
Recreational resources	Steering committee, focus group, existing literature	Adapted from East Side Village Health Worker Partnership, Schulz et al., 1998, www.sph.umich.edu/urc, and from REACH Detroit Partnership, www.sph.umich.edu/reach
Food resources	Steering committee, focus groups, existing literature	Adapted from the East Side Village Health Worker Partnership survey, www.sph.umich.edu/urc, and from Michigan Behavioral Risk Factor Survey, Frazier, Franks, & Sanderson, 1992; Gentry et al., 1985.
Sense of community	Steering committee, focus groups, existing literature	Adapted from East Side Village Health Worker Partnership, Parker et al., 2001.
Neighborhood participation	Steering committee, focus groups, existing literature	Items adapted from Goodman et al., 1998; some new items written for this study.

See Chapter Five for a discussion of the development and administration of this survey questionnaire using a CBPR approach. See Appendix C for examples of specific survey questions developed or revised based on community input.

Measure	Identified by	Source
Stressors		
Duke Life Events Inventory	Existing literature, focus groups	Blazer, Hughes, & George, 1987; George, Blazer, Hughes, & Fowler, 1989; Hughes, Blazer, & George, 1988.
General perceived stress	Existing literature, focus groups	Cohen & Williamson, 1988.
Work stress	Existing literature, focus groups	Karasek, Gardell, & Lindell, 1987.
Financial vulnerability	Existing literature, focus groups	James, Keenan, Strogatz, Browning, & Garrett, 1992.
Discrimination	Existing literature, focus groups	Adapted from Williams, Yu, Jackson, & Anderson, 1997; new response categories added based on focus groups (see Appendix C).
Safety stress	Existing literature, focus groups	Schulz, Parker, Israel, & Fisher, 2001; Shulz et al., 2004.
Police stress	Existing literature, focus groups, pilot testing	Items adapted from East Side Village Health Worker Partnership; some new items written for this study.
Family stress	Existing literature, focus groups	Adapted from Schulz et al., 2001, 2004; some new items created for this study.
Immigration stress	Focus groups, existing literature	Adapted items and created new items based on focus groups; Marin, Sabogal, Marin, Otero-Sabogal, & Perez-Stable, 1987.
Neighborhood social environment	Focus groups, steering committee, existing literature, pilot testing	Some new items created based on focus groups; adapted some items from Sampson, Raudenbush, & Earls, 1997.
Neighborhood physical environment	Focus groups, steering committee, existing literature, pilot testing	Some new items created based on focus groups; adapted some items from East Side Village Health Worker Partnership.

Measure	Identified by	Source
Health-related behaviors		
Alcohol intake	Existing literature, focus groups	Block, Coyle, Hartman, & Scoppa, 1994.
Tobacco use	Existing literature, focus groups	Adapted from Centers for Disease Control and Prevention 2004a; Frazier et al., 1992; Gentry et al., 1985.
Physical activity	Existing literature, focus groups	Adapted from Centers for Disease Control and Prevention 2004a; Frazier et al., 1992.
Nutrient intake	Existing literature, focus groups	Adapted from Block, 1994, 1986.
Health screening	Existing literature, focus groups, Steering Committee	Centers for Disease Control and Prevention 2004b.
Social integration and social support		
Social support	Focus groups, existing literature	Strogatz et al., 1997; James, Strogatz, Wing, & Ramsey, 1987.
Spiritual support	Focus groups, existing literature	Pargament, Koenig, & Perez, 2000.
Organizational membership	Focus groups, existing literature	Adapted from East Side Village Health Worker Partnership survey.
Psychosocial indicators		
John Henryism Scale for Active Coping	Existing literature	James et al., 1987.
Beck Hopelessness Scale	Existing literature, focus groups	Beck, Weissman, Lester, & Trexler, 1974.
Anger or hostility	Existing literature, focus groups	Spielberger et al., 1985.
Symptoms of depression (Center for Epidemiological Studies—Depression Scale)	Existing literature, focus groups	Radloff, 1977.
Composite International Diagnostic Interview (CIDI)	Existing literature, focus groups	Wittchen, 1994; WHO, 1991.

Measure	Identified by	Source
Health outcome indicators		
Self-report diagnosis (blood pressure, diabetes, and so forth)	Existing literature, focus groups	Adapted from Centers for Disease Control and Prevention, 2004b.
Physical activity limitations	Existing literature	Roscow & Breslau, 1966.
General self-rated health status	Existing literature, focus groups	Idler & Benyamini, 1997.
Blood pressure	Existing literature, focus groups	Guidelines adapted from James et al., 1992.
Overweight or obesity (height, weight, hip, waist)	Existing literature, focus groups	Guidelines adapted from James et al., 1992.

References

Beck, A. T., Weissman, A., Lester, D., & Trexler, L. (1974). The measurement of pessimism: The Hopelessness Scale. *Journal of Consulting and Clinical Psychology, 42*(6), 851–865.

Blazer, D., Hughes, D., & George, L. K. (1987). Stressful life events and the onset of a generalized anxiety syndrome. *American Journal of Psychiatry, 144*(9), 1178–1183.

Block, G., Coyle, L. M., Hartman, A. M., & Scoppa, S. M. (1994). Revision of dietary analysis software for the Health Habits and History Questionnaire. *American Journal of Epidemiology, 139,* 1190–1196.

Block, G., Hartman, A. M., Dresser, C. M., Caroll, M. D., Gannon, J., & Gardner, L. (1986). A data-based approach to dietary questionnaire design and testing. *American Journal of Epidemiology, 124,* 453–469.

Centers for Disease Control and Prevention, Division of Adult and Community Health, & National Center for Chronic Disease Prevention and Health Promotion. (2004a). *Behavioral Risk Factor Surveillance System online prevention data, 1995–2002* (BFRSS). Retrieved 2004 from http://www.cdc.gov/brfss

Centers for Disease Control and Prevention, National Center for Environmental Health, & Division of Laboratory Science. (2004b). *The National Health and Nutrition Examination Surveys (NHANES)*. Retrieved June 8, 2004, from http://www.cdc.gov/nceh/dls/nhanes.htm

Cohen, S., & Williamson, G. (1988). Perceived stress in a probability sample of the United States. In S. Spacapan & S. Oscamp (Eds.), *The social psychology of health.* Thousand Oaks, CA: Sage.

Frazier, E. L., Franks, A. L., & Sanderson, L. M. (1992). Using Behavioral Risk Factor Surveillance data. In National Center for Chronic Disease Prevention and Health Promotion, Office of Surveillance and Analysis (Ed.), *Using chronic disease data: A handbook for public health practitioners.* Atlanta: Centers for Disease Control and Prevention.

Gentry, E. M., Kalsbeek, W. D., Hogelin, G. C., Jones, J. T., Gaines, K. L., Forman, M. R., et al. (1985). The behavioral risk factor surveys: II. Design, methods, and estimates from combined state data. *American Journal of Preventive Medicine, 1*(6), 9–14.

George, L. K., Blazer, D. G., Hughes, D. C., & Fowler, N. (1989). Social support and the outcome of major depression. *British Journal of Psychiatry, 154,* 478–485.

Goodman, R. M., Speers, M. A., McLeroy, K., Fawcett, S., Kegler, M., Parker, E. A., et al. (1998). Identifying and defining the dimensions of community capacity to provide a basis for measurement. *Health Education & Behavior, 25*(3), 258–278.

Hughes, D. C., Blazer, D. G., & George, L. K. (1988). Age differences in life events: A multivariate controlled analysis. *International Journal of Aging and Human Development, 27*(3), 207–220.

Idler, E. L., & Benyamini, Y. (1997). Self-rated health and mortality: A review of twenty-seven community studies. *Journal of Health and Social Behavior, 38*(1), 21–37.

James, S. A., Keenan, N. L., Strogatz, D. S., Browning, S. R., & Garrett, J. M. (1992). Socioeconomic status, John Henryism, and blood pressure in black adults: The Pitt County study. *American Journal of Epidemiology, 135*(1), 59–67.

James, S. A., Strogatz, D. S., Wing, S. B., & Ramsey, D. L. (1987). Socioeconomic status, John Henryism, and hypertension in blacks and whites. *American Journal of Epidemiology, 126*(4), 664–673.

Karasek, R. T., Gardell, B., & Lindell, J. (1987). Work and non-work correlates of illness and behavior in male and female Swedish white collar workers. *Journal of Occupational Behavior, 8,* 187–207.

Marin, G., Sabogal, F., Marin, B., Otero-Sabogal, R., & Perez-Stable, E. J. (1987). Development of a short acculturation scale for Hispanics. *Hispanic Journal of Behavioral Sciences, 9,* 183–205.

Pargament, K. I., Koenig, H. G., & Perez, L. (2000). The many methods of religious coping: Development and initial validation of the RCOPE. *Journal of Clinical Psychology, 56,* 519–543.

Parker, E. A., Lichtenstein, R. L., Schulz, A. J., Israel, B. A., Schork, M. A., Steinman, K. J., et al. (2001). Disentangling measures of individual perceptions of community social dynamics: Results of a community survey. *Health Education & Behavior, 28*(4), 462–486.

Radloff, L. S. (1977). The CES-D: A self-report depression scale for research on the general population. *Applied Psychological Measurement, 1,* 385–401.

Roscow, I., & Breslau, N. (1966). A Guttman Health Scale for the aged. *Journal of Gerontology, 21*(4), 556–559.

Sampson, R., Raudenbush, S., & Earls, F. (1997). Neighborhoods and violent crime: A multilevel study of collective efficacy. *Science, 277,* 918–924.

Schulz, A. J., Israel, B. A., Estrada, L., Zenk, S. N., Viruell-Fuentes, E. A., Villarruel, A., et al. (2004 November). *Engaging community residents in assessing their social and physical environments and their implications for health.* Paper presented at the annual meeting of the American Public Health Association, Washington, DC.

Schulz, A. J., Parker, E. A., Israel, B. A., Becker, A. B., Maciak, B. J., & Hollis, R. (1998). Conducting a participatory community-based survey: Collecting and interpreting data for a community health intervention on Detroit's east side. *Journal of Public Health Management and Practice, 4*(2), 10–24.

Schulz, A. J., Parker, E. A., Israel, B. A., & Fisher, T. (2001). Social context, stressors and disparities in women's health. *Journal of the American Medical Women's Association, 56*(4), 143–149.

Spielberger, C. D., Johnson, E. H., Russell, S. F., Crane, R. J., Jacobs, G. A., & Worden, T. J. (1985). The experience and expression of anger: Construction and validation of an anger expression scale. In M. A. Chesney & R. H. Rosenman (Eds.), *Anger and hostility in cardiovascular and behavioral disorders* (pp. 5–30). Washington, DC: Hemisphere.

Strogatz, D. S., Croft, J. B., James, S. A., Keenan, N. L., Browning, S. R., Garrett, J. M., et al. (1997). Social support, stress, and blood pressure in black adults. *Epidemiology, 8*(5), 482–487.

Williams, D. R., Yu, Y., Jackson, J., & Anderson, N. B. (1997). Racial differences in physical and mental health: Socioeconomic status, stress and discrimination. *Journal of Health Psychology 2*(3), 335–351.

Wittchen, H. U. (1994). Reliability and validity studies of the WHO Composite International Diagnostic Interview (CIDI): A critical review. *Journal of Psychiatric Research, 28,* 57–84.

World Health Organization. (1991). *International Classification of Diseases (ICD-10).* Geneva: WHO.

Healthy Environments Partnership

Neighborhood Observational Checklist

Shannon N. Zenk, Amy J. Schulz, James S. House,
Alison Benjamin, and Srimathi Kannan

SECTION 1: BLOCK AND OBSERVER DESCRIPTIVE QUESTIONS

Please enter your Observer ID number: _____

What mode of transportation are you using?

1. Walking

2. Driving (only when necessary for safety)

Are you working with a partner?

1. Yes

2. No

What is your partner's name? _____

What are the current weather conditions?

1. Sunny, 85+ degrees

2. Sunny, 65–84 degrees

3. Sunny, <65 degrees

4. Partly sunny, 85+ degrees

5. Partly sunny, 65–84 degrees

6. Partly sunny, <65 degrees

7. Cloudy, 85+ degrees

8. Cloudy, 65–84 degrees

For a copy of the operational definitions and additional information on the Neighborhood Observational Checklist, contact Amy J. Schulz, University of Michigan, School of Public Health, 109 S. Observatory, SPH II, M5134, Ann Arbor, MI 48109. See Chapter Eight for a discussion of the development and implementation of the Neighborhood Observational Checklist by the Healthy Environments Partnership.

9. Cloudy, <65 degrees

10. Rainy

Enter the Block ID number: _____

Referring to the diagram on the block description sheet, how many streets adjoin the block?

1. 1

2. 2

3. 3 streets (triangular)

4. 4 streets (rectangular)

5. 5

6. 6

7. 7

8. 8

9. 9

10. 10

SECTION 2: QUESTIONS ABOUT THE BLOCK FACE

Based on street-level frontage, how is the land used on this block face?[a]
(MARK ALL THAT APPLY)

1. Residential (not vacant)

2. Commercial, business, professional (not vacant)

3. Industrial, warehouse, manufacturing (not vacant)

4. Institutional (e.g., school, church, medical care facility) (not vacant)

5. Parking lot

6. Vacant lot or open space

7. Vacant residential house/building

8. Vacant non-residential building

9. Park or playground

10. Waterfront

11. Expressway

What type of residential housing is on the block face?[a]
(MARK ALL THAT APPLY)

1. High-rise public or private apartment or condominium building (6 stories or more)

2. Low-rise public or private apartment or condominium building (less than 6 stories)

3. Detached single family house

4. Two- or four-family flat

5. House converted to apartments

6. Row house, townhouse, or duplex

7. Housing unit attached to commercial storefront

What type of residential housing occupies the *most space* on the block face?[a]
(MARK ONE)

1. High-rise public or private apartment or condominium building (6 stories or more)

2. Low-rise public or private apartment or condominium building (less than 6 stories)

3. Detached single family house

4. Two- or four-family flat

5. House converted to apartments

6. Row house, townhouse, duplex

7. Housing units over commercial storefront

Are any of the vacant lots or open spaces (not fenced in):
(MARK ALL THAT APPLY)

1. In good condition (well kept)?

2. In poor condition (poorly kept)?

3. Equipped with playground equipment?

4. Used for gardens?

5. Set up with chairs or furniture for socializing?

6. None of the above

Do any of these institutions on the block face face this street?[a]
(MARK ALL THAT APPLY)

1. Church or religious center

2. Medical care facility (e.g., hospital, clinic)

3. Community-based organization, social service agency, or community center

4. Public indoor recreational center or facility

5. None of the above

Do any of these businesses on the block face this street?[a]
(MARK ALL THAT APPLY)

1. Bank

2. Check cashing service

3. Secondhand store/pawn shop

4. Drug store/pharmacy (prescription)

5. Gas station with convenience store

6. Fast food/take out place

7. Other eating place/restaurant

8. Bar/cocktail lounge

9. None of the above

Condition of the sidewalk
(MARK ONE)

1. Good

2. Fair

3. Poor

4. Under construction

5. No sidewalk present

Which of the following are present on the block face?[a]
(MARK ALL THAT APPLY)

1. "Undriveable" car

2. Empty beer or liquor bottle/can or alcohol packaging

3. Cigarette or cigar butt or discarded tobacco package

4. None of the above

Is there strewn garbage, litter, broken glass, clothes, or papers on the block face?[a]
(MARK ONE)

1. Heavy

2. Moderate

3. Light

4. None

Are there any piles of garbage or dumped materials on the block face?

1. Yes
2. No

Are there trees along the block face between the sidewalk and the street?[a]
(MARK ONE)

1. On 100% (all) of the block face
2. On 50–99% of the block face
3. On 1–49% of the block face
4. On 0% (none) of the block face

Is there graffiti on the block face (e.g., on buildings, signs, walls, the sidewalk)?[a]

1. Yes
2. No

Is there evidence of graffiti that has been painted over?[a]

1. Yes
2. No

Are there any murals/paintings on the block face?[a]

1. Yes
2. No

Which of the following sayings, symbols, or murals are visible on the block face (excluding on businesses or institutions)?
(MARK ALL THAT APPLY)

1. Mexican or Latino identity or pride
2. African American or African identity or pride
3. Religious
4. None of the above

Is there a bus stop?

1. Yes
2. No

Are any of the following advertisements visible on the block face?[a,b]
(MARK ALL THAT APPLY)

1. Sign advertising tobacco product

2. Sign advertising beer, whiskey, or other alcohol (not labeling for business)

3. Sign advertising fast food (not labeling for business)

4. None of the above

Are any of the following signs visible on the block face?[a,b,d]
(MARK ALL THAT APPLY)

1. Neighborhood watch, business watch, or crime watch sign

2. Security warning sign

3. Beware of dog sign or see/hear large dog in residential property

4. No trespassing, no loitering, private property, keep out sign, no solicitation, or no handbills sign

5. None of the above

Are any of the following signs visible on the block face?
(MARK ALL THAT APPLY)

1. No dumping sign

2. No commercial vehicles sign (e.g., picture of truck with line through it)

3. None of the above

Are any of the following signs visible on the block face?
(MARK ALL THAT APPLY)

1. *Home* with FOR SALE or FOR AUCTION sign

2. *Home* with FOR RENT sign

3. *Business or commercial/industrial building* with FOR SALE sign

4. None of the above

Are any of the following signs visible on the block face?
(MARK ALL THAT APPLY)

1. Sign or banner with neighborhood name

2. Sign with health message

3. Sign for social, community, or cultural/ethnic event

4. None of the above

Commercial/Industrial/Institutional Buildings

Does any business or institution feature an explicit display of colors (e.g., green/red/white), murals, or symbols oriented toward Latinos?

1. Yes
2. No

Does any business or institution have "Mexican," "Latino," "Cuban," or a Spanish name or surname in the name or a name in Spanish?

1. Yes
2. No

Does any business or institution have a sign or advertisement indicating that they sell Latino or Mexican goods or provide services specifically for Latinos?

1. Yes
2. No

Does any business or institution have a sign or advertisement in Spanish (e.g., a "Se Habla Español" sign) on the building or property?

1. Yes
2. No

Does any business feature an explicit display of colors (e.g., red/green/black), murals, or symbols oriented toward African Americans?

1. Yes
2. No

Does any business or institution have "African," "Caribbean," or "African American" in the name?

1. Yes
2. No

Does any business or institution have a sign or advertisement indicating that they sell African or Caribbean goods or provide services specifically for African Americans?

1. Yes
2. No

How would you rate the condition of *most* of the commercial, industrial, or institutional *buildings* on the block face?[a]
(MARK ONE)

1. Excellent

2. Good

3. Fair

4. Poor/badly deteriorated

5. Abandoned, burned out, unusable

In general, how would you rate the condition of *most* of the commercial, industrial, or institutional *grounds* on the block face?[a]
(MARK ONE)

1. Good

2. Fair

3. Poor

4. No commercial, industrial, or institutional grounds

Are any of the following on the commercial, industrial, or institutional properties?[a]
(MARK ALL THAT APPLY)

1. High mesh fencing with barbed wire or spiked tops OR at least 6-foot-high metal or board fencing

2. Low fencing (under 6 feet)

3. Pull-down/pull-over metal security blinds/shutters or iron grates on the *doors* or entrances

4. Security bars/gratings on the *windows*

5. No fencing or security devices on doors or windows

What proportion of commercial, industrial, or institutional properties on the block face has security devices on the doors or windows?[a]
(MARK ONE)

1. 100% (all)

2. 50–99%

3. 1–49%

4. 0% (none)

Residential Housing

How would you rate the condition of the *best* house/residential *building* on the block face?[a]
(MARK ONE)

1. Excellent
2. Good
3. Fair
4. Poor/badly deteriorated
5. Abandoned, burned out, unusable (and vacant)

How would you rate the condition of the *worst* house/residential *building* on the block face?[a]
(MARK ONE)

1. Excellent
2. Good
3. Fair
4. Poor/badly deteriorated
5. Abandoned, burned out, unusable (and vacant)

In general, how would you rate the condition of *most* of the houses/residential *buildings* on the block face?[a]
(MARK ONE)

1. Excellent
2. Good
3. Fair
4. Poor/badly deteriorated
5. Abandoned, burned out, unusable (and vacant)

Are any of the houses/residential buildings currently being renovated?

1. Yes
2. No

How would you rate the condition of the *best* residential *grounds* on the block face?
(MARK ONE)

1. Good
2. Fair

3. Poor

4. There are no resident-kept grounds

How would you rate the condition of the *worst* residential *grounds* on the block face?
(MARK ONE)

1. Good

2. Fair

3. Poor

4. There are no resident-kept grounds

In general, how would you rate the condition of *most* of the residential *grounds* on the block face?
(MARK ONE)

1. Good

2. Fair

3. Poor

4. There are no resident-kept grounds

What proportion of residential properties has decorations in the yard, on the porch, or on the house/building?[a]
(MARK ONE)

1. 100% (all)

2. 50–99%

3. 1–49%

4. 0% (none)

What proportion of residential properties has security bars/gratings on residential doors or windows or has fences at least 5–6 feet high, clearly intended for security purposes?[a]
(MARK ONE)

1. 100% (all)

2. 50–99%

3. 1–49%

4. 0% (none)

Outdoor Public Recreational Spaces or Equipment

What kinds of outdoor *public use* recreational spaces or equipment are on the block face?[a]
(MARK ALL THAT APPLY)

1. Park

2. Playground (e.g., slide, swings)

3. Sports/playing fields or courts

4. Sports equipment (e.g., goal posts, basketball nets, exercise stations)

5. None of the above

In general, how would you rate the condition of the *public use recreational equipment* on the block face?[a,b]
(MARK ONE)

1. Good

2. Fair

3. Poor

4. There is no public use recreational equipment

In general, how would you rate the condition of the *public use recreational spaces or grounds* on the block face?[a]
(MARK ONE)

1. Good

2. Fair

3. Poor

4. There are no public use recreational spaces or grounds

SECTION 3: QUESTIONS ABOUT THE STREET

Volume of traffic[a]
(MARK ONE)

1. Heavy

2. Moderate

3. Light

4. No traffic

Do you see any "semis"?[c]

    1. Yes

    2. No

Condition of the street[a]
(MARK ONE)

    1. Good

    2. Fair

    3. Poor

    4. Under construction

How noisy is the street?[a]
(MARK ONE)

    1. Very quiet

    2. Fairly quiet

    3. Somewhat noisy

    4. Very noisy

Is there a neighborhood block club sign or do more than 50% of the homes on the street have block club lamps?[c]

    1. Yes

    2. No

Do you see any stray or loose dogs?[d]

    1. Yes

    2. No

Are there any people visible outdoors?[a]

    1. Yes

    2. No

Who did you see?[a]
(MARK ALL THAT APPLY)

    1. Adults (ages 18 and up)

    2. Teenagers (ages 13–17)

    3. Preteens (ages 6–12)

    4. Preschool children (ages 5 and under)

How were you regarded by the people?[a]
(MARK ALL THAT APPLY)

1. Paid little or no attention by those around

2. Treated with suspicion

3. Friendly or helpful responses/greetings

4. Polite responses to your (observer's) questions

5. Asked about what you (observer) were doing in area

6. Verbally or physically harassed

What do you see *adults* doing?[a]
(MARK ALL THAT APPLY)

1. Exercising or doing recreational activities

2. Gardening, doing home maintenance/yard work, working on the car

3. Talking with other adults

4. Sitting or standing on a porch or stoop or in a yard

5. Drinking alcohol or carrying alcohol (e.g., 40 oz)

6. Smoking

7. Walking, but not necessarily for exercise

8. Suspected illegal activity (e.g., drug dealing, prostitution)

9. Other

10. No adults present

What do you see *teenagers* doing?[a]
(MARK ALL THAT APPLY)

1. Exercising or doing recreational activities

2. Gardening, doing home maintenance/yard work, working on the car

3. Talking with other teenagers

4. Sitting or standing on a porch or stoop or in a yard

5. Drinking alcohol or carrying alcohol (e.g., 40 oz)

6. Smoking

7. Walking, but not necessarily for exercise

8. Suspected illegal activity (e.g., drug dealing, prostitution)

9. Other

10. No teenagers present

SECTION 4: QUESTIONS ABOUT THE ENTIRE BLOCK

To what extent did you experience any unpleasant noxious smells during your observation of this block?[a]
(MARK ONE)

1. Quite a bit
2. Some
3. Not at all

To what extent did you experience unpleasant or noxious levels of dirt or dust in the air during your observation of this block?[a]
(MARK ONE)

1. Quite a bit
2. Some
3. Not at all

To what extent did you experience any irritation in your mouth, nose, or eyes from the air on the street during your observation of the block?[a]
(MARK ONE)

1. Quite a bit
2. Some
3. Not at all

Did you see any police officers or police cars during your observation of this block?

1. Yes
2. No

Notes

a. Adapted from the Systematic Social Observation instrument (Morenoff, House, & Raudenbush, n.d.).

b. Adapted from the Brief Neighborhood Observational Measure (Caughy, O'Campo, & Patterson, 2001).

c. Adapted from the Community Action Against Asthma Environmental Checklist (Farquhar, 2000).

d. Adapted from the Block Environment Inventory (Perkins, Meeks, & Taylor, 1992).

References

Caughy, M. O., O'Campo, P. J., & Patterson, J. (2001). A brief observational measure for urban neighborhoods. *Health & Place, 7,* 225–236.

Farquhar, S. A. (2000). *Effects of the perceptions and observations of environmental stressors on health and well-being in residents of eastside and southwest Detroit, Michigan.* Unpublished doctoral dissertation, University of Michigan-Ann Arbor.

Morenoff, J., House, J. S., & Raudenbush, S. W. (n.d.). *Systematic social observation by survey interviewers: A methodological evaluation.* Unpublished manuscript.

Perkins, D. D., Meeks, J. W., & Taylor, R. B. (1992). The physical environment of street blocks and resident perceptions of crime and disorder: Implications for theory and measurement. *Journal of Environmental Psychology, 12,* 21–34.

APPENDIX F

Field Notes Guide

Chris McQuiston, Emilio A. Parrado, Julio César Olmos,
and Alejandro M. Bustillo Martinez

Informant code:
Interviewer name:
Date:
Location of interview:
Time of interview:

Observational notes: What you observe about the informant, the place, or the environment in which the interview takes place, anything that is not recorded by the tape recorder.

Examples

- Description of the location where the interview takes place
- Whether there are other people present during the interview
- Observations about the informant:

  Is he or she nervous? shy? calm?

  Does the informant seem to easily understand the questions that you ask?

Methodological notes: Comments on the process of the actual interview.

Examples

- Comments about the interview guide:

  Changes in the order of questions

  Difficulties with certain questions or themes
- Length of the interview
- Interruptions

Theoretical notes: Refer to the objectives of the interview. Here is where you, the interviewer, start to analyze the information that the informant is giving you. You want to start to answer your basic research questions.

See Chapter Ten for a discussion of the use of these guidelines for taking field notes of ethnographic interviews in the context of a CBPR project.

Examples

- How have gender roles changed as a result of the process of migration to the United States and what do those changes mean for men and for women who experience them?

- How has decision making changed since the individual or couple came to the United States?

- What impact does gender role change have on the sexual behavior of the individual or couple?

- What are the different gender roles and their corresponding attributes as described by the informant?

- How does social or familial support influence a couple's relationship?

- What does the informant know or think about HIV and HIV-related risks?

Here you can also write about new themes that come up from the interview, if the informant talks about ideas that are relevant to the study but are not included in the guide. Try to identify recurring themes—subjects or experiences that the informant talks about repeatedly.

Personal notes: How you felt doing the interview.

Examples

- "I felt uncomfortable asking her about her sex life because this informant is a very religious person."

- "I felt like he answered the questions honestly and openly. He was very open with me, but I did notice that he became hesitant and timid when I asked him questions about his migration history."

- "I felt tired today and started to lose my concentration about halfway through the interview. I asked her if we could take a break for a couple of minutes to have a glass of water so that I could wake up."

Detroit Community-Academic Urban Research Center

In-Depth, Semistructured Interview Protocol for Board Evaluation, 1996–2002

Barbara A. Israel, Paula M. Lantz, Robert J. McGranaghan,
Diana L. Kerr, and J. Ricardo Guzman

INTERVIEW QUESTIONS ASKED IN 1996

1. The Urban Research Center (URC) has been in existence for about a year. Last October was when the first introductory meetings for the URC took place. Can you tell me what you had hoped the URC would accomplish during its first year? What were your expectations for the initial year of the URC?

Probe: Would you say you had high or low expectations for the first year?

2. Has the URC met your expectations for the first year? Has it exceeded these expectations?

Probes: If fallen short of expectations, why do you think this happened? Were your expectations too high to begin with? If exceeded expectations, why do you think this happened? Were your expectations too low to begin with?

See Chapter Twelve and Lantz et al., 2001, for an examination of the development and use of this instrument.

3. What have been the URC's major accomplishments thus far? Name two or more.

4. What have been the major barriers/challenges facing the URC thus far? Name two or more.

5. I would like to know what you hope the URC will accomplish during the next year and then beyond. First, what do you want the URC to tackle and accomplish over the next year? Second, what do you want the URC to have accomplished by the end of the first five years, which will be the fall of the year 2000?

6. What sort of challenges/barriers do you foresee for the URC over the next few years? Do you have any recommendations for how the URC can meet these challenges or reduce these barriers?

7. What have you personally learned from your association with the URC? Has it expanded your knowledge at all, or helped you to develop or refine any skills? Has it helped you professionally in any way?

8. Has your organization's affiliation with the URC provided any tangible benefits yet? What does your organization hope to accomplish by its affiliation with the URC?

9. Could you please give me some examples of exchanges of information/assistance/support between your organization and other organizations in URC? Do you think that these exchanges would have happened without the establishment of the URC?

   Probe for examples that don't involve URC staff or University faculty/staff.

10. What sort of gap or need does the URC have the potential to fill? What would be the consequences of not having a Community-Academic Urban Research Center in Detroit?

11. Evaluation question 1: What would you like to learn from an evaluation of the URC? One way to think about that difficult question is to think about what questions you would like us to be able to answer about the URC four years from now.

   Probe: What do you think an evaluation should try to show?

12. Evaluation question 2: There are six goals of the URC (show them). Do you have any other goals for the URC that are not on this list?

   Probe: What are indicators of success for the URC? What are some indicators of problems or lack of success?

ADDITIONAL INTERVIEW QUESTIONS ASKED IN 1999

1. What factors have facilitated the accomplishments of the URC? What structures and processes instituted by the URC have been important in establishing and maintaining collaborative relationships among the different partners?

2. To what extent has the URC created new relationships among the organizations or partners participating?

3. Do you think that community interests have been represented and assured in the research projects that have been developed and implemented by the URC? Please explain why or why not.

4. To what extent and how has the URC helped communities recognize and work with their assets and local resources in its projects?

5. The last few questions refer to the role of the Centers for Disease Control and Prevention (CDC) in the development of the Detroit URC. In general, how have CDC priorities and policies influenced the direction of the URC? In what capacities has the CDC helped the URC foster and develop community-based participatory research? What recommendations would you give to CDC regarding how to improve their Urban Research Centers program?

6. Thinking about other communities who may want to establish their own partnerships for community-based participatory research, what would you say worked well about the process by which the URC developed its partnership? What would you recommend they do differently?

ADDITIONAL INTERVIEW QUESTIONS ASKED IN 2002

1. In what ways is the work of the URC benefiting the community? How could the URC improve its benefits to or value for the community?

2. Has your organization's affiliation with the URC resulted in any costs or problems for your organization? How about for you personally?

3. During the recent past, the URC has attempted to open up lines of communication with policymakers and policy experts at the local, state and federal level. What do you think of the URC's policy activities to date? What do you recommend for future activities in this area?

4. Future funding from the CDC for URC infrastructure and research projects is uncertain. How do you think the loss of CDC funding would affect the URC? How would it affect your organization's participation in URC activities? How should the URC best explore options for future funding?

Reference

Lantz, P., Viruell-Fuentes, E., Israel, B. A., Softley, D., & Guzman, J. R. (2001). Can communities and academia work together on public health research? Evaluation results from a community-based participatory research partnership in Detroit. *Journal of Urban Health, 78*(3), 495–507.

Detroit Community-Academic Urban Research Center

Closed-Ended Survey Questionnaire for Board Evaluation, 1997–2002

Barbara A. Israel, Paula M. Lantz, Robert J. McGranaghan,
Diana L. Kerr, and J. Ricardo Guzman

General Satisfaction	1997	1999	2001	2002
1. I am generally satisfied with the activities and progress of the URC during the past year.	X	X	X	X
2. I have a sense of ownership in what the URC does and accomplishes.	X	X	X	X
3. I am satisfied with the types of proposals that the URC has submitted.	—	X	X	X
4. I am satisfied with the types of projects that the URC has implemented.	—	X	X	X
5. I frequently think of having my organization sever its affiliation with the URC.	X	X	X	X
6. I have adequate knowledge of the URC budget, URC resources, and how resources are allocated.	—	X	X	X
7. Thus far, the URC has distributed available resources in a fair and equitable manner.	X	X	X	X
8. I would like to have more input regarding the allocation of URC resources.	—	X	X	X
9. The Board of the URC has been effective in achieving its goals.	X	X	X	X

See Chapter Twelve, Lantz et al., 2001, and Schulz et al., 2003, for an examination of the development and use of this instrument.

	1997	1999	2001	2002
10. The URC can have a positive effect on the community.	X	X	X	X
11. Participation in the URC has increased my knowledge and understanding of the other organizations represented.	—	X	X	X

Impact	1997	1999	2001	2002
12. I have increased my knowledge of family and community health issues during the past year.	X	X	X	X
13. Participation in the URC has increased my organization's capacity to conduct community-based participatory research.	—	X	X	X
14. My organization uses knowledge generated by the URC.	—	X	X	X
15. I believe that other, non-member health and human service agencies in the Detroit area *know about* the URC and its initiatives.	—	X	X	X
16. I believe that other, non-member health and human service agencies in the Detroit area *use knowledge* generated by the URC.	—	X	X	X
17. The URC has been effective in informing policymakers and key government officials about the URC and its initiatives.	—	X	X	X
18. It is important that policymakers and key government officials are informed about the URC and its initiatives.	—	X	X	X

Trust	1997	1999	2001	2002
19. Relationships among URC Board members go beyond the individuals at the table, to include member organizations.	—	X	X	X
20. I am comfortable requesting assistance from other Board members when I feel that their input could be of value.	—	X	X	X
21. I can talk openly and honestly at the URC Board meetings.	X	X	X	X
22. I am comfortable expressing my point of view at URC Board meetings.	X	X	X	X
23. I am comfortable bringing up new ideas at the URC Board meetings.	X	X	X	X

	1997	1999	2001	2002
24. URC Board members respect each other's points of view even if they might disagree.	X	X	X	X
25. My opinion is listened to and considered by other Board members.	X	X	X	X
26. In the past year, my willingness to speak and express my opinions at Board meetings has: increased, stayed same, decreased, don't know.	X	X	X	X
27. Over the past year, the amount of trust between URC Board members has: increased, stayed same, decreased, don't know.	—	X	X	X
28. In the past year, the URC Board members'capacity to work well together has: increased, stayed same, decreased, don't know.	X	X	X	X
29. How much trust is there between partners now? A lot, moderate amount, not much, don't know.	—	X	X	X
30. In the next year, how much trust do you expect to see between partners? A lot, moderate amount, not much, don't know.	—	X	X	X

URC Board Decisions	1997	1999	2001	2002
31. I am satisfied with the way in which the URC Board makes decisions.	—	—	X	X
32. All Board members have a voice in decisions made by the group.	—	—	X	X
33. It often takes the URC Board too long to reach a decision.	—	—	X	X
34. Decisions about URC resources are made in a fair manner.	—	—	X	X
35. URC Board members work well together to solve problems.	—	—	X	X

Community-Based Participatory Research and Centers for Disease Control and Prevention (CDC)	1997	1999	2001	2002
36. The URC is following its own community-based research principles in its projects.	—	X	X	X
37. Community interests are well represented in URC activities.	—	X	X	X
38. CDC staff in Atlanta play an important role in helping the URC foster and develop community-based participatory research.	—	X	X	X
39. The CDC is supportive of what we are trying to do in our URC.	—	X	X	X

Organization and Structure of Meetings	1997	1999	2001	2002
40. I find URC Board meetings useful.	—	X	X	X
41. The URC Board meetings are well organized.	X	X	X	X
42. We discuss important issues at URC meetings.	—	—	—	X
43. I wish we spent more time at Board meetings hearing about and discussing URC projects.	—	—	X	X
44. The Board meetings are held too frequently.	X	X	X	X
45. We do not accomplish very much at URC Board meetings.	—	—	—	X
46. I believe that we adequately address all of the agenda items at the URC meetings.	X	X	X	X
47. When I want to place something on the meeting agenda, I am comfortable with the process.	X	X	X	X
48. I would like more of a voice in determining agenda items for the URC Board meetings.	X	X	X	X
49. When the URC Board makes decisions, appropriate follow-up action is taken by staff.	X	X	X	X
50. When the URC Board makes decisions, appropriate follow-up action is taken by URC Board members.	—	X	X	X
51. Certain individuals' opinions get weighed more than they should.	X	X	X	X
52. One person or group dominates at URC Board meetings.	X	X	X	X

References

Lantz, P. M., Viruell-Fuentes, E., Israel, B. A., Softley, D., & Guzman, J. R. (2001). Can communities and academia work together on public health research? Evaluation results from a community-based participatory research partnership in Detroit. *Journal of Urban Health, 78*(3), 495–507.

Schulz, A. J., Israel, B. A., & Lantz, P. M. (2003). Instrument for evaluating dimensions of group dynamics within community-based participatory research partnerships. *Evaluation and Program Planning, 26,* 249–262.

Philosophy and Guiding Principles for Dissemination of Findings of the Michigan Center for the Environment and Children's Health (MCECH) Including Authorship of Publications and Presentations, Policies and Procedures, Access to Data, and Related Matters

Edith A. Parker, Thomas G. Robins, Barbara A. Israel,
Wilma Brakefield-Caldwell, Katherine K. Edgren, and Donele J. Wilkins

A Dissemination Committee (DC) is established that includes 12 members: (6 community partners and 6 University of Michigan faculty): Members unable to attend may designate an alternate to attend in their place.

The DC develops policies and procedures for decision making about dissemination as it applies to MCECH activities and findings. Dissemination activities might be in the form of papers, presentations, news releases, newsletters, or through other resources. Presentations might be to academics, to funding agencies or potential funding agencies, or to community members. We are eager to use these opportunities in a spirit of partnership that lessens the gap between academics and non-academics. Our goal is to have a process that ensures high quality and is fair, inclusive, and allows people to grow in their skills, knowledge, and experiences. It is the university's responsibility to ensure that community partners are involved in decision making. We also recognize this will be a challenge, particularly when decisions need to be made quickly. Having a process where we keep everyone informed means we have to do things a bit differently. We are committed to maintaining feelings of mutual respect and trust and are hopeful that the policies and procedures developed will foster that. If

---

See Chapter Thirteen for an examination of the development and application of these dissemination guidelines.

policies are not followed, the person who did not follow the policy must attend the next Steering Committee meeting and make a clear presentation to the group.

Duties, Rights, and Responsibilities of the DC

- Outlining core articles and presentations based on the original grant and potential conferences and journals for submission, and proposing writing teams including designation of first authorship for these core articles and presentations;

- Reviewing and approving proposals for new articles and presentations from interested members of the research for non-core articles and presentations. These proposals shall include a description of the research questions, variables to be used, members of the writing team and first authorship;

- Developing, in consultation with the MCECH Steering Committee, guidelines and procedures to ensure that information about the project and its findings are presented to the media and at public meetings in a consistent and accurate fashion;

- Reviewing any and all requests for use of data and access to data by members of the research team and outside agencies or persons (e.g., for dissertations, presentations, publications, Freedom of Information Act);

- Determining/prioritizing methods of dissemination of findings to the CAAA Steering Committee and Detroit communities; and

- Developing and implementing strategies to enhance the national and international visibility and prominence of CAAA and MCECH by means such as generating lists of anticipated conferences/meetings, presentation topics, and speakers at which CAAA should present.

Policies/Procedures Developed by the Dissemination Committee

Operating Rules of the Dissemination Committee. While every effort will be made to accommodate Dissemination Committee members' schedules including the use of conference calls, faxes, etc., when necessary, the DC may operate by quorum (simple majority) if the full committee cannot be in attendance. To facilitate input from as many members as possible on key decisions, prior notification of issues and votes by proxy will be accepted from members unable to attend a meeting.

Submission of Non-Core Article for Publication or Abstract for Conference Presentation. The final decision as to whether an abstract and/or article should be submitted, and under whose names, should come to the Steering Committee.

This should preferably be done in person, by presentation to the Steering Committee.

Conference Presentations. When trying to decide which representatives of the project should attend a conference, the criteria of fairness and quality will be used. To ensure fairness, we adopt the "Rose Bowl Principle," and if several people are able to make a high-quality presentation, the person who has never presented will be chosen or if everyone under consideration has previously presented, those who have presented more recently will not be eligible to present. To ensure a high-quality presentation, the following items regarding possible presenters will be considered by the Steering Committee:

- Involvement in project-related activities;
- Length of time of involvement with the project;
- Meeting attendance; and
- Supervisor's evaluation (in the case of project staff).

The actual procedure for deciding who will present at a specific conference is as follows: the Steering Committee or its designees will develop a list of the people who are eligible to attend a conference because of their participation in and knowledge of the CAAA project, and based on the desire to ensure fair participation among all members. Then, based on this list, the decision will be discussed and made at an actual Steering Committee meeting. If the decision has to be made in between Steering Committee meetings (due to time constraints), Steering Committee members will be either called or faxed and approval sought in this way.

In its deliberations, the DC will especially strive for sensitivity to the needs of research team members who are more junior in seniority (e.g., Assistant Professors, Research Scientists, doctoral students) with respect to areas such as authorship and meeting presentations. As part of this sensitivity, opportunities will be organized for members of the research team to deliver practice presentations to other research team members before their scheduled conference presentations.

As an important part of this effort, the DC will develop and update a quarterly project fact sheet written in layperson's language to serve as the main source of information for "informal" presentations in the Detroit community and elsewhere.

Authorship Guidelines. Only those actively participating in the academic work of the project will be eligible for authorship. Active participation means substantial intellectual contribution to the publication in question, and may be measured directly by physical hours of input on acquisition, processing and interpreting of data; or indirectly by time and energy spent supervising a junior researcher in the acquisition, processing and interpretation of data; or a combination of both. Those making such contributions will be recognized in the authorship of manuscripts. Non-academic assistance in the form of funding grants, administrative, and secretarial work will not be the basis of authorship but will be expressly acknowledged in presentations and publications.

Criteria for first authorship are expected to include responsibility for coordinating and facilitating the work of the writing team—e.g., scheduling and facilitating meetings, overseeing data analysis, writing all or most of the first draft of a manuscript, handling communication with journals—together with significant other relevant activity on the CAAA project itself.

Taking the lead on presentations will not necessarily result in lead authorship for resulting manuscripts; this will be decided by the Dissemination Committee in consultation with the writing/presentation team.

Use of Data by Non-SC Members. Any person who gains permission to use any portion of the data set and conducts statistical analyses independent of the work of the data manager must provide written documentation (including statistical programs used, creation of new variables, data output, etc.) to the data manager within a few weeks of the activities conducted using the data.

Media Requests. The DC designates the project manager to serve as the contact person for media requests. She will then contact appropriate SC members, depending on the type of request from the media.

Establishing a CAAA Library. A centralized, accessible, numbered filing system for every manuscript and abstract that is published/produced by CAAA will be established.

Community Action Against Asthma

Fact Sheet on "Particulate Matter"

Edith A. Parker, Thomas G. Robins, Barbara A. Israel, Wilma Brakefield-Caldwell, Katherine K. Edgren, and Donele J. Wilkins

CAAA Steering Committee Partners:

Butzel Family Center

Community Health and Social Services (CHASS)

Detroit Hispanic Development Corporation

Detroiters Working for Environmental Justice

Friends of Parkside

Kettering/Butzel Health Initiative

Latino Family Services

What Is Community Action Against Asthma (CAAA)?

Community Action Against Asthma is a community-based participatory research partnership working to improve the health of children with asthma in the East and Southwest sides of Detroit. The purpose of community-based participatory research projects is to enhance the understanding of issues affecting the community and to develop, implement and evaluate plans of action that will address those issues in ways that benefit the community.

Since 1999, CAAA has been researching air quality and working with families in their homes in Southwest and Eastside Detroit. For the household activities, outreach workers called Community Environmental Specialists (CESs) visit homes of families who signed up to be in the household project. During these visits, the CESs work with the families to educate them about asthma triggers (things that may cause an asthma attack), and to develop a plan to reduce the household environmental triggers for asthma. For the air quality research, CAAA is collecting information on the quality of the indoor and outdoor air in Southwest and Eastside Detroit and looking at the relationship between the quality of the air (primarily particulate matter and ozone), lung functioning, and reports of asthma symptoms of the children enrolled in the household project.

See Chapter Thirteen for a discussion of the development and use of this fact sheet by the CBPR partnership.

United
Community
Housing Coalition

Warren/Conner
Development
Coalition

Detroit Health
Department

Henry Ford
Health System

University of
Michigan
School of
Public Health

University of
Michigan
School of
Medicine

What Is Particulate Matter (PM)?

Particulate matter, a form of air pollution, is particles found in the air. Levels of PM in the air are routinely monitored in urban areas because many of these particles are small enough to be inhaled and reach deep into the lungs of people. The two different sizes of PM routinely measured are PM2.5 and PM10. The emission sources of PM2.5 in urban areas are primarily from combustion sources such as smokestacks (power plants, waste incinerators, etc.) and emissions from cars and trucks. The emission sources of PM10 include these combustion sources and, to a lesser extent, emissions from natural sources such as wind-blown dust.

What Are the Effects of PM on Health?

Many scientific studies have found that exposure to PM at levels currently reported in most urban areas can cause significant adverse health effects, including increased rates of hospital admission due to cardiovascular disease (heart attacks, congestive heart failure, cardiac arrhythmia) and respiratory disease (asthma, pneumonia, COPD), as well as premature death (Samet et al., 2000). In studies specific to inner-city children with asthma, scientists have linked exposure to PM to decreases in lung function and increases in asthma symptoms (cough, chest tightness, wheeze) (Mortimer et al., 2002).

Some recent studies have linked both traffic-related pollutants (including PM) and traffic density with increased hospital admissions for asthma and increased asthma symptoms in children (English et al., 1999; Gehring et al., 2002). Other studies in urban areas, without measuring health status, have found large increases in PM and components of PM specific to diesel truck exhaust measured in schools located along and near highways (Janssen et al., 2001). Several scientific studies are currently under way to better assess the effects that diesel-related components of PM may have on the worsening of symptoms of children with asthma, as well as other health end-points mentioned above.

Michigan Department of Agriculture Pesticide & Plant Pest Management

Funded by:

Environmental Protection Agency

National Institute of Environmental Health Sciences

For more information:

Kathy Edgren, Project Manager Community Action Against Asthma Tel.: 734.615.0494 Toll Free: 877.640. 4064 Fax: 734.763.7379 E-mail: kedgren@ umich.etu

Have the Effects of PM on Health Been Measured in Detroit?

Several studies conducted in Detroit have linked outdoor levels of air pollution (including PM) to adverse health effects (Schwartz, 1994). These also include studies linking daily changes in PM10 with premature death (Lippmann et al., 2000), as well as associations between PM, both PM10 and PM2.5, and increases in hospitalization for cardiovascular and respiratory disease, and also links between exposure to PM10 and decreases in lung function and increases in asthma symptoms (cough, chest tightness, wheeze) for Detroit children with asthma (Mortimer et al., 2002).

What Are the Next Steps in the CAAA Data Analysis?

With all of the CAAA PM data collection coming to an end in 2002 (Keeler et al., 2002), CAAA will be spending the next year combining the PM data with data from the measures of lung function and symptom diaries that each CAAA child and family has filled out. This analysis will help CAAA to determine what effects the PM levels in Southwest Detroit and Eastside Detroit are having on children with asthma in these two communities. For more information on the CAAA project, or to get involved, contact Kathy Edgren toll-free at 877–640–4064.

References

Samet et al. (2000). Fine particulate air pollution and mortality in 20 U.S. Cities, 1987–1994. *New England Journal of Medicine, 343*(24), 1742–1749.

Mortimer et al. (2002). The effect of air pollution on inner-city children with asthma. *European Respiratory Journal, 19,* 699–705.

English et al. (1999). Examining associations between childhood asthma and traffic flow using a geographic information system. *Environmental Health Perspectives, 107,* 761–767.

Gehring et al. (2002). Traffic-related air pollution and respiratory health during the first 2 years of life. *European Respiratory Journal, 19,* 690–698.

CAAA is a part of MCECH, the Michigan Center for the Environment and Children's Health, and is funded by grants from the U.S. Environmental Protection Agency and the National Institute of Environmental Health Sciences.

Janssen et al. (2001). Assessment of exposure to traffic related air pollution of children attending schools near motorways. *Atmospheric Environment, 35,* 3875–3884.

Schwartz. (1994). Air pollution and hospital admissions for the elderly in Detroit, Michigan. *American Journal of Respiratory Critical Care Medicine, 150,* 648–655.

Lippmann et al. (2000). Association of particulate matter components with daily mortality and morbidity in urban populations. *Research Report of the Health Effects Institute, 95,* 5–82.

Keeler et al. (2002). Assessment of personal and community-level exposures to particulate matter (PM) among children with asthma in Detroit, Michigan, as part of Community Action Against Asthma (CAAA). *Environmental Health Perspectives, 110*(Suppl. 2), 173–181.

Community Action Against Asthma

Summary of Air Sampling Data in Your Community and Home, 2000–2001

Edith A. Parker, Thomas G. Robins, Barbara A. Israel,
Wilma Brakefield-Caldwell, Katherine K. Edgren, and Donele J. Wilkins

[Participant's Name]

What Is Particulate Matter (PM)?

Particulate matter, a form of air pollution, is particles found in the air. Some particles are small enough to be inhaled into the lungs. The two different sizes of PM that scientists often measure are called PM10 and PM2.5. PM10, particles that are mostly from natural sources such as wind-blown dust, can be inhaled and get into the nose and larger airways. PM2.5 are smaller-sized particles that are commonly from outdoor sources such as smokestacks, cars, and trucks as well as indoor sources such as cigarette smoke. These smaller particles can also get breathed in, and because they are smaller, they can reach deep into the lungs.

What Are the Health Effects of Breathing in PM?

Scientific studies over many years have found that exposure to high levels of PM can cause significant health effects, including aggravation of asthma symptoms, especially in children and the elderly. Upon learning this, the U.S. Environmental Protection Agency (EPA) developed standards for outdoor air quality in order to "protect public health" with "an adequate margin of safety." The EPA standard for a year-long average of PM10 is 50 micrograms per cubic meter of air ($\mu g/m^3$), while the EPA standard for PM2.5 is 15 $\mu g/m^3$ for a year-long average. The "year-long average" means the typical or usual level of PM measured during the year. These EPA air quality

---

See Chapter Thirteen for a discussion of the dissemination of results to participants in a CBPR study.

standards exist for outdoor levels of PM, but no federal standards exist for inside homes.

What Is the Effect of Cigarette Smoke on the Levels of PM in Homes?

As part of the CAAA study, we have noted that levels of PM measured in homes with smokers are higher than the levels of PM measured in the homes without smokers. Many scientific studies have found that exposure to second-hand smoke may worsen the symptoms of children with asthma.

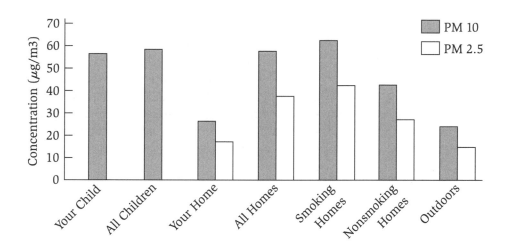

Figure K.1 Average Levels of Particulate Matter in Your Home and Community, 2000–2001.

What Are the levels of PM Measured in Your Community?

As you know, CAAA has made measurements of PM in your eastside Detroit community for over two years. The two-year average level of PM10 measured in your community was 26 μg/m³, well below the EPA standard of 50 μg/m³. On the other hand, the two-year average level of PM2.5 measured in your community was 16 μg/m³, which is slightly higher than the 15 μg/m³ standard set by the EPA (see the data figure on the front page). Though the level of PM2.5 in your community is near the EPA standard, this does not mean that all people with asthma will experience worsening of symptoms. However, some studies have shown health effects in populations "at risk," such as children with asthma, when PM2.5 levels are at or even below the current EPA annual standard of 15 μg/m³. These studies have also shown that certain people are more sensitive than others to the health effects of PM.

What Are the Levels of PM Measured in Your Home and from Your Child's Backpack?

In the figure on the front page, the two-year average level of PM10 measured inside your home was 25 μg/m^3, while the average level of PM2.5 measured inside your home was 16 μg/m^3. These levels are lower than the average levels of PM measured in the homes of other families participating in CAAA. The two-year average level of PM10 measured from your child's backpack was 59 μg/m^3. This level is similar to the average levels of PM10 measured from the backpacks of other children participating in CAAA. While EPA air quality standards exist for outdoor levels of PM, there are no federal standards for PM levels measured inside homes.

What Are the Next Steps in the CAAA Data Analysis?

With all of the PM data collection coming to an end in 2002, we will be spending the next year combining the PM data with data from the AirWatches and diaries that each CAAA child and family has filled out. This analysis will help CAAA to determine what effects the PM levels in your community are having on children with asthma. The key findings from this air sampling study will be made available to you and all other families participating in CAAA. If you have any further questions, please do not hesitate to contact CAAA: 1-877-640-4064 or your CES.

Five Ways to Lower Your Child's Exposure to PM and Other Harmful Pollutants

1. DO NOT smoke in your home or in your car, and DO NOT permit others to do so.

2. DO NOT burn candles or incense in your home.

3. If you have a central furnace, make sure that filters are properly maintained or changed.

4. Remove household dust often from surfaces with a damp cloth. Vacuum carpet, fabric window coverings, and fabric furniture to reduce dust build-up. Be sure area is well ventilated during cleaning or have your child leave the area during cleaning.

5. Limit your child's time spent outdoors on hot sunny days during summer (often called *Ozone Action Days*). These days typically have the highest levels of PM and other harmful pollutants such as ozone.

The Planning Grant

In-Depth Group Interview Protocol: Questions for Community and Coalition Members

Elizabeth A. Baker and Freda L. Motton

Notes

- Have coalition Chair introduce you
- Sign in
- Review guidelines for discussion including consent and ground rules
- Review how information will be used, including (1) data transcription and summary statements and (2) presented back to the coalition to assist the coalition in their planning activities and communicating community strengths and challenges to local and state leadership, and to garner additional resources for communities

Interview Questions

1. How do you refer to the place where you live?

2. What is in this town [however they refer to the area]? Who lives here? How would you describe the people who live in your community? Are there businesses? Services? Schools? How is this area similar to and different from the immediate surrounding areas?

3. When you think about your town [use language they use in referring to the area within which they live], what are some of the strengths or positive things in the community that have helped the community or coalition to create/change/make this a better place?

   - How do the local businesses help?

This protocol was created as part of the Prevention Research Center Special Interest Project—funded by the Centers for Disease Control and Prevention (grant U48/CCU710806), Saint Louis University, and Bootheel Heart Health Coalitions—with input and feedback from other participating centers at the University of Chicago, University of New Mexico, and Tulane University. See Chapter Fourteen for a discussion of the development and application of this in-depth group interview protocol.

- What about
  a. Businesses outside of this town/area?
  b. Schools or educational centers, churches, social agencies, civic groups?
  c. Government offices and officials inside this town?
  d. Government offices and officials outside of this town?

4. What are some of the challenges to creating change?
   - How do the local businesses present challenges?
   - What about
     a. Businesses outside of this town?
     b. Schools or educational centers, churches, social agencies, civic groups?
     c. City hall/government offices and officials?

Inspirational Images Project

Fact Sheet and Informed Consent
Form for Study Participants

Ellen D. S. López, Eugenia Eng, Naomi Robinson,
and Caroline C. Wang

WOULD YOU LIKE TO PARTICIPATE IN THIS RESEARCH PROJECT EXPLORING BREAST CANCER SURVIVORSHIP?

Why am I being asked to participate in this project?

- This project is being done to learn about how African American women in your community who have experienced breast cancer feel about their lives as survivors. The project will give you the opportunity to discuss the challenges you have encountered, what you have done to make your life better, and what more can be done in the future to make sure that you and other women who experience breast cancer have an easier time.

- The purpose of this project is to provide the means for you and a small group of other survivors to voice your needs to local influential people (decision makers and product/service providers).

- The goal of the project is that by sharing your survivorship experiences and concerns with influential people, programs and support services will be developed to better meet your needs and improve the quality of life of African American breast cancer survivors in rural eastern North Carolina.

What will I be asked to do?

- If you choose to participate in the project you and a group of at least ten other survivors will be given disposable cameras so that you can take pictures that "trigger" discussions about your experiences and concerns as breast cancer survivors. At the completion of the project there will be a public forum where you and the other project participants will have

---

See Chapter Fifteen for a discussion of how this form was used to recruit participants into a breast cancer survivorship project.

the opportunity to present your photographs, the information learned from discussing your photographs, and your suggestions on how to address your survivorship needs and concerns to influential people in your community.

How long will this project take? How often will we meet for the project?

- This project should take about 10–14 months to complete and will involve you, the other project participants, and university researchers coming together about once per month. If you choose to participate you will be invited to attend the following sessions:
  - *Project training session* (3 hours): During this session we will all come together to discuss details about the project and what participation involves. If you decide to participate you will be asked to sign the agreement statement on the last page of this form. This will show that you fully understand what being a part of this project entails. You will then receive a disposable camera and tips on how to use it. Then you will have the opportunity to practice using your camera. At the end of the training you and the other project participants will decide on the topic you would like to explore with your cameras. This is called a "photo-assignment." You will also decide on a date and time when you will all come back together to discuss the photographs you have taken.
  - *Photo-discussion sessions* (about 5–7 monthly sessions at 3 hours each): This is where the fun really begins! You, the other project participants and the researcher, will all come together to share and discuss your photos. After several of the photos have been discussed you and the other participants will decide what your next photo-assignment will be.
  - *Findings session* (2 hours): After you and the other participants feel that you have learned enough about your survivorship experiences and concerns we will all come together to discuss the main themes and topics that came from your photos and discussions. As a group, you will then decide how well the themes relay what you want others to understand about your survivorship experiences.
  - *Forum* (4 hours): The forum is the chance for everyone in the project to *celebrate* all that has been accomplished! Most importantly, you will also have the option to present what has been learned during the project to influential people in your community and discuss with them how programs and services can be developed to improve the lives of breast cancer survivors. As a group, everyone will decide *how* to present what has been learned during this project to these influential people. *You do not have to be a part of this presentation if you do not want.*

- *Other public displays of your photos:* You will also have the opportunity to publicly display your photos and the words you used to describe them so that even more people in your community can learn about how women experience breast cancer. If you *do* choose to display your photographs and words, you will decide what photographs to display, how they should be displayed, and where they should be displayed (e.g., public library, town hall). *You do not have to participate in any public displays to be a part of this project.*

Will you be taping our photo-discussion sessions?

- Yes. What you have to say during the photo-discussions is important, therefore the sessions will be audiotaped. If you ever want to have the tape recorder turned off for a while during the discussion sessions just say so, and it will be turned off immediately.

Are there any risks involved with taking part in the project? Will I feel uncomfortable?

- Taking part in the project *should not* put you at risk for physical harm. You *may* feel uncomfortable going out to take pictures, but any concerns you may have will be discussed during project meetings. Also, you may feel uncomfortable discussing your breast cancer. *You will never be required to discuss any issues that make you feel uncomfortable.*

What will I get out of taking part in the project? Will I get paid?

- You will *not* be paid to be in the project. You *will* be offered light refreshments at each discussion session. You will also receive copies of every photograph you take for the study. Further, any film left over in your camera can be used to take pictures of anything or anyone you would like for free.

Do I have to pay for anything to take part in the project?

- You will *not* have to pay for anything to take part in the project. You can use the cameras at no cost to you. You will also be reimbursed for any travel expenses involved with getting to and from the meetings. The only cost for being in the project is the time you allow for taking the photographs and coming to project related meetings.

Will people know that I took part in the project?

- To ensure *confidentiality,* if you wish, you can pick a made-up name to use during the project so that nobody will see your real name associated with the project. Further, what people say during the discussions is confidential, so it will be required that you never tell any specific things that are said by other group members during these discussions.

Do I have to participate? Can I stop being in the project whenever I want?

- No. You *do not* have to participate in this study. Further, you are free to stop being in the project at any time, for any reason.

Has this study been approved by the University of North Carolina at Chapel Hill?

- Yes. This study has been approved by the University of North Carolina at Chapel Hill (UNC-CH) School of Public Health Institutional Review Board on Research Involving Human Subjects.

What if I have any questions about the project or my participation?

- If you ever have any questions about this study, please feel free to contact the [contact person's name, phone number, e-mail address].

Do you have any questions about the project?
☐ Yes (write questions below or ask contact person)
☐ No

If you are interested in participating in this project, <u>please read the following agreement statement very carefully.</u> Then, if you would still like to participate, please sign and date this form and return it to [contact person's name]. You will be given a copy of this form to keep in case you have any questions or concerns at a later date.

Agreement statement:

By signing this consent form, I agree to participate in the project. I also understand and agree that unless otherwise notified in writing, the University of North Carolina at Chapel Hill assumes that permission is granted to use my photograph(s) and text from project-related sessions for *project-related* presentations, publications, exhibits and/or other educational purposes.

Participant Signature _____ Date _____

Staff Signature _____ Date _____

Inspirational Images Project

Consent for Adults Who May Appear in Photographs

Ellen D. S. López, Eugenia Eng, Naomi Robinson, and Caroline C. Wang

MAY I TAKE YOUR PICTURE?

What am I being asked to do?

- You are being asked to give me your permission to take your picture.

Why are you taking these pictures?

- I am part of a group of breast cancer survivors and university researchers that is exploring breast cancer survivorship. We are taking pictures that we can bring back and share with our group. We hope the pictures will help us to discuss topics about survivorship that might normally be difficult to bring up.

How will you use the pictures?

- After I have taken my pictures, I will share them with the group, and we will discuss why I took them, and how they relate to survivorship issues. There is also the possibility that some of the photographs I take will be included in public exhibits or presentations.

Will people know that I had my picture taken for your project?

- Your name will never be revealed during any of the discussions, presentations or exhibits. Still there is the chance that somebody may recognize you.

What will I get out of having my picture taken for your project?

- All pictures will be kept in a secure place by one of the researchers and me. If you wish, I will send you a copy of the picture I take. *If you would like a copy, please write your name and address at the end of this form.*

See Chapter Fifteen for a discussion of how this form was used to obtain permission to take a photograph.

Do I have to allow you to take my picture?

- No. You do not have to allow me to take your picture.

Has this project been approved?

- Yes. This project has been approved by the University of North Carolina at Chapel Hill School of Public Health Institutional Review Board on Research Involving Human Subjects.

Who can I contact if I have any questions about the project?

- If you ever have any questions or concerns please call [*contact person's name, number*].

If you are willing to have your picture taken, please read the following agreement statement very carefully. Then, please sign and date this form and return it to me. I will give you a copy of the form for your records.

Agreement statement:

By signing this consent form, I agree to have my pictures taken. I also understand and agree that unless otherwise notified in writing, the University of North Carolina at Chapel Hill assumes that permission is granted to use my picture(s) for *project-related* discussions, exhibits and presentations.

Your Signature _____   Date _____

Photographer's Signature _____   Date _____

If you would like a copy of your picture(s) please print your name, street number, street name, city and zip code.

_____

_____

_____

_____

Thank you!

Community Reintegration Network

Policy Report—Coming Back to Harlem from Jail or Prison: One-Way or Round-Trip

Nicholas Freudenberg, Marc A. Rogers,
Cassandra Ritas, and Sister Mary Nerney

THE CYCLE OF INCARCERATION IN EAST AND CENTRAL HARLEM

Each year more than 7,500 people—29 every weekday—are released from jail and prison to return to Central or East Harlem. How we receive these returning residents can have a big impact on our families, our neighborhoods, community health, and our feelings of safety. The way the city organizes services for these folks affects both how well they do and the amount of money available for other things like education, housing, and job training.

Currently, New York City jails more than 100,000 people and spends more than one billion dollars annually, only to have the majority of released inmates re-arrested and returned to jail within a year.

A first step towards fixing this problem is to open a dialogue with the many groups involved in the issue. Harlem residents, inmates and their families, community service providers, employers, elected officials, city health and law enforcement agencies, religious leaders, and correctional staff all need to be part of the solution.

In this brochure we present facts about inmates returning to Harlem. We explain why we feel this is an important community issue and we suggest how city government, community organizations, and citizens can act to increase the likelihood that people leaving jail or prison do not return. We are members of the Community Reintegration Network (CRN) a group of Harlem health workers, community residents, policymakers and researchers working to create more effective, humane, and fiscally responsible policies to reintegrate inmates. We ask your help in working to create a community where people who have done their time can become active citizens rather than return to jail.

See Chapter Sixteen for a discussion of how this policy report was used to educate policymakers and community members about jail reentry issues.

FACTS ON PEOPLE RETURNING FROM JAIL AND PRISON

Many Harlem residents are in the criminal justice system.

Each year, more than 11,000 Harlem residents spend time in jail or prison, one in every 8 households. When people go to jail the charges may be drug possession or sales, burglary or assault. But for many the deeper cause is lack of opportunity due to poverty, unemployment, addiction, inadequate education, or mental health problems. The war on drugs locks people up without addressing the causes of addiction and developing solutions. The focus on arrest and imprisonment creates a cycle that is hard to break. Already communities facing many stresses see more and more of their residents losing the most valuable years of their life to jail and prison, a loss they cannot afford.

Treatment can prevent reincarceration.

In the year 2000, 2,719 Harlem residents were arrested more than once, and 1,500 people were arrested three or more times. About half of those released from jail are re-arrested within a year; and 43% of those coming out of prison are back behind bars within three years. Most inmates are released without receiving help for their problems with drugs and few receive education or gain skills that could help them succeed in school or work. About 80% of NYC jail inmates have a drug or alcohol problem at the time of their arrest, yet less than a quarter get help for this in jail. Even fewer get help in the state prisons. Numerous studies show that drug treatment for inmates can reduce drug use and re-arrest while saving money. Also, researchers have shown that some jail-based violence prevention programs can reduce violence significantly, yet only a handful of violent offenders participate in this kind of program. With so little treatment and rehabilitation available, is it surprising that the majority of ex-offenders are re-arrested within a year, repeating the cycle of incarceration, release, and crime?

Many people in jails and prisons have serious under-treated health problems.

Because of our crime policies, jails concentrate people with health and social problems. Jail inmates have HIV infection rates ten times higher than the population as a whole. More people with mental illness are in jail than in mental hospitals and more drug users are behind bars than in treatment programs. Ten years ago, jails actually contributed to the spread of tuberculosis. Most inmates receive inadequate medical care behind bars and few get effective referrals to the post-release health care they need.

Keeping people locked up costs a lot.
The City spends more than $90,000 to keep one person in jail for a year and the state spends about $32,000 to keep a person in prison. Thus, the City spends almost $93 million each year on Harlem's jail inmates and the state $160 million each year on Harlem's prison inmates for a total of more than $250 million a year. The average jail incarceration of 41 days costs the city $10,332. For the cost of one incarceration, the city could pay for 3 Harlem residents to attend City University of New York for a year; for the cost of 10 incarcerations, it could build a new low-income housing unit; and for the cost of 100 incarcerations, it could provide job training vouchers for up to 200 Harlem residents.

Some government policies make life hard when you get out of prison and jail.
While many people are struggling to get their lives together after incarceration, too often government policies end up guaranteeing failure. Convicted felons and their families can be evicted from public housing and end up homeless. After incarceration, people lose Medicaid, making it more difficult for them to take care of illness or treat diseases that can spread. Employers discriminate against ex-cons, making legal work tough to find. NYC jails release inmates at 5 am in the morning, not the time to find drug treatment, medication, health care, a place to sleep, or food. As a result, many inmates return to the people and places that got them in trouble and land in jail again.

IT'S TIME FOR CHANGE: CURRENT POLICIES HURT OUR COMMUNITY, DON'T HELP EX-INMATES GET BACK ON THEIR FEET, AND COST TOO MUCH

Central and East Harlem have numerous strengths: strong families, children with promise, dedicated community service providers, diverse cultures, and a history of struggles against oppression and discrimination. But every resident knows that our communities also face serious challenges. The CRN believes that too often current policies on reentry of people returning from jail and prison create barriers rather than build our community. These policies hurt our community in the following ways:

- **Families fall apart because members coming out of jail and prison don't get enough support.** Many men and women getting out of jail or prison want to work and contribute to their family yet lack the skills needed to succeed in the job market. Others who could have been helped to become better parents, husbands, or wives instead repeat the same destructive patterns. Young men who want to break free of a gang return home with no better options. Children who want to be able to depend on their parents are again disappointed by drug use, neglect or broken promises, creating another generation of anger and mistrust. Even inmates highly motivated to make changes in their lives can slip back into old ways when they return to the situation that got them in trouble to begin with. And when families break up, communities suffer.

- **Failure to plan for reentry harms community health.** By providing inadequate care for infectious diseases inside and after release, our correctional system misses an important opportunity to curb the epidemics that have devastated our neighborhoods in the last two decades. The man who could have learned he was HIV infected, started medication, and acted to protect his partners, returns to infect others. The person with mental illness who could have been connected to community treatment goes back on the streets. The pregnant drug-using woman who might have been helped to find drug treatment, health care and prenatal care goes home with no plan in place. Each of these missed opportunities guarantees pain and heartbreak for the victims, more health problems for the community, and higher costs for all of us.

- **Ignoring community reintegration wastes hundreds of millions of dollars of taxpayer money.** The $250 million a year New York spends to incarcerate Harlem residents is a poor investment since so many return to crime. After release, services for homeless people, emergency room visits and repeated arrests cost millions more. Any company that invested so much in "fixing" a problem that immediately required the same "repair" (incarceration) would rightly be forced out of business. Yet New Yorkers accept this waste because most elected officials fear that addressing the needs of returning inmates may make them look soft on crime. But policies that fail aren't tough, they're wasteful and ineffective and they make our communities less safe, not safer.

- **Our current approach to corrections violates our society's standards of fairness and justice.** The term "corrections" represents a fair approach that has been abandoned. Organizing a correctional system around punishment and revenge diminishes everybody without solving the problem. It "corrects" nothing and helps nobody. Society has always claimed the right to punish people who break the law, but it also has a responsibility to rehabilitate violators. By making it easier for ex-offenders to participate in their communities productively than to return to crime, our city can set a standard for social justice in keeping with American values.

WHAT CAN WE DO TO MAKE THE TICKET ONE-WAY INSTEAD OF ROUND-TRIP?

To reduce the number of people who leave jail or prison with a round-trip ticket to come back will require inmates, families, businesses, neighborhoods, community service providers, faith-based organizations, and city agencies to do something different. Here are some of our ideas. Can you find something you can do? Suggest other ideas?

Inmates

Make a plan before you leave jail or prison.

Join a program while you're in—drug treatment, job training, any way to improve yourself.

Look for people who can help you get your life together.

Churches and Religious Organizations

Adopt a returning inmate and help him find a job or a place to live.

Provide counseling and support groups for returning inmates.

Welcome people who have done their time and want to change their lives, and preach this value to your congregation.

Visit people while they are still incarcerated.

Families of Inmates

Help a family member, friend, or neighbor getting out of jail to find a home, a job, or a place to get help for a drug problem.

Community Service Providers

Establish special services for people coming out of jail.

Send staff to jails or prisons to recruit clients when they return to your area.

Support families with a returning inmate.

Establish services for women and their children to reconnect after incarceration.

City Agencies and Elected Officials

Reduce the policy barriers that keep returning inmates from getting the help they need.

Create meaningful and universal treatment and discharge planning programs in jails and prisons.

Provide support to community groups who can help keep people out of jail.

Support programs that help rather than punish returning inmates who try to get their lives together.

Citizens and Taxpayers

Register to vote, and vote for candidates that care about and support humane reentry policies.

Visit someone you love who's behind bars to help him or her plan for release.

Urge your elected officials to support programs to keep people out of jail. Ask them to justify spending $90,000 a year to keep someone in jail or $32,000 in prison, more on corrections than on higher education.

For more information on the Community Reintegration Network or to join our group, contact: [*name and contact information for Community Action Board staff listed here.*]

Southern California Environmental Justice Collaborative (the Collaborative)

Partnership Agreed upon Mechanism for Deciding on Research Activities

Communities for a Better Environment, Liberty Hill Foundation, and The Research Team

While all the partners want to protect the time allocated for fundamental research, we have agreed that the contours or subjects of action research should be largely determined by Communities for a Better Environment (CBE). While the research team could decline a particular task for various reasons, and research load should emerge, as noted below, from joint conversations, it is our collective sense that CBE has the best notion of the overall organizing agenda and therefore can indicate what action research would be most useful. Of course, trade-offs will need to be acknowledged: more work on a particular research project will lead to less on another. It is probably the responsibility of the research team to raise these trade-offs and it is our collective responsibility to take them seriously and make hard choices.

Criteria for deciding to take on research tasks:

1. Primary responsibility of the researchers would be to CBE.
2. Partners must bring action research ideas to the whole Collaborative.
3. Research must be affiliated with environmental justice (EJ) campaign work in Los Angeles.
4. Research must be relevant to the goals of the Collaborative.
5. Research should be influenced and prioritized by its relevance to projected EJ policy outcomes defined by the Collaborative.
6. At least one conference call and one face-to-face meeting by the whole Collaborative are needed to decide to take on an action research task.

See Chapter Seventeen for a discussion of how this document was developed and used to guide the work of the collaborative.

7. CBE should lead in tying action research tasks to organizing agenda.

8. Trade-offs in the action research arena should be discussed and acknowledged.

9. The research team should continue making progress on the fundamental research front, sharing both results and research designs for discussion and agenda-setting on this front as well.

10. The Collaborative must build in a process to popularize and disseminate research results (multi-lingual fact sheets, posters, maps, newsletters).

11. Research should include an analysis of cumulative exposure.

In this process we must:

1. Create a dialogue to fully integrate, cross-train, and dialogue between CBE and the researchers.

2. Create a plan to share the Web and other technology with activists and community members to improve their ability to access needed information.

3. Coordinate the community-focused research projects and the state policy research and an action plan with CBE.

4. CBE should frequently engage in interval analysis (including Power analysis) to reflect on whether policy goals are being reached.

5. CBE should plan their participation as facilitators for the EJ Institute.

NAME INDEX

SUBJECT INDEX